Trauma Interventions
in War and Peace
Prevention, Practice, and Policy

International and Cultural Psychology Series

Series Editor: **Anthony Marsella**, *University of Hawaii, Honolulu, Hawaii*

A Continuation Order Plan is available for this series. A continuation order will bring delivery of each
new volume immediately upon publication. Volumes are billed only upon actual shipment. For further
information please contact the publisher.

Trauma Interventions in War and Peace
Prevention, Practice, and Policy

Edited by

Bonnie L. Green
Georgetown University Medical Center, Washington, D.C.

Matthew J. Friedman
National Center for PTSD, White River Junction, Vermont and Dartmouth Medical School, Hanover, New Hampshire

Joop T.V.M. de Jong
Transcultural Psychosocial Organisation, Amsterdam, The Netherlands

Susan D. Solomon
National Institutes of Health, Bethesda, Maryland

Terence M. Keane
National Center for PTSD, Boston, Massachusetts and Boston University, Boston, Massachusetts

John A. Fairbank
UCLA–Duke University National Center for Child Traumatic Stress, Durham, North Carolina

Brigid Donelan
United Nations, New York, New York

Ellen Frey-Wouters
International Policy Research Institute, Riverdale, New York

With *Special Consultant* Yael Danieli
Senior Representative to the United Nations, ISTSS

Kluwer Academic / Plenum Publishers
New York, Boston, Dordrecht, London, Moscow

Library of Congress Cataloging-in-Publication Data

Trauma interventions in war and peace: prevention, practice, and policy/edited by Bonnie
L. Green ... [et al.]; with Yael Danieli.
    p.   cm. — (International and cultural psychology)
Includes bibliographical references and index.
ISBN 0-306-47723-8 — ISBN 0-306-47724-6 (pbk.)
    1. Post-traumatic stress disorder.   2. War—Psychological aspects.   3.
Peace—Psychological aspects.   4. Mental health services.   I. Green, Bonnie L.   II.
International and cultural psychology series.

RC552.P67T72 2003
616.85'21—dc21

    2003044646

Prepared in close collaboration with several United Nations agencies and bodies.
The views expressed are those of the authors and do not necessarily reflect
the views of the United Nations.

ISBN HB: 0-306-47723-8
PB: 0-306-47724-6

©2003 Kluwer Academic/Plenum Publishers, New York
233 Spring Street, New York, New York 10013

http://www.wkap.nl/

10 9 8 7 6 5 4 3 2 1

A C.I.P. record for this book is available from the Library of Congress

Permissions for books published in Europe: *permissions@wkap.nl*
Permissions for books published in the United States of America:
permissions@wkap.com

Printed in the United States of America

We dedicate this book to all those who have experienced war, disaster, abuse, and social deprivation, and to those striving to prevent and relieve their suffering.

IN MEMORIAM

In memory of Rosalie Wolf, lead author of the chapter
Abuse of Older People, who died in June 2001,
and who spent the last months of her life
studying and writing about elder abuse.

Contributors

Salma Ali, Executive Director, Bangladesh National Woman Lawyers Association, House #60/A, Road #27, Dhanmondi R/A, Dhaka—1029, *Bangladesh*, bnwla@bdonline.com

Nozomu Asukai, Research Director, Tokyo Institute of Psychiatry, Department of Stress Disorders Research, 2-1-8 Kamikitazawa, Setagaya, Tokyo 156-8585, *Japan*, asukai@prit.go.jp

Florence Baingana, Senior Health Specialist (Mental Health), The World Bank, 1818 H. Street NW, Washington, DC 20433, *USA*, fbaingana@worldbank.org

Nancy Baron, Co-Director, Global Psychiatric and Psycho-Social Initiatives (GPSI), P.O. Box 1360, Sarit Center, 0606 Nairobi, *Kenya*, drnancy@imul.com

Ellen Bassuk, President, National Center on Family Homelessness, 181 Wells Avenue, Newton Center, Massachusetts 02459, *USA*, ellen.bassuk@familyhomelessness.org

Gerry C.J. Bennett, Professor in Health Care of Older People, Barts and The London, Queen Mary's School of Medicine and Dentistry, Academic Office, 1st Floor Alderney Building, Mile End Hospital, Bancroft Road, London E1 4DG, *United Kingdom*, gerry.bennett@thpct.nhs.uk

Adriana Cavalcanti de Aguiar, Coordinator for Educational Development, University Estacio de Sá Medical School, Rua Visconde Silva 321/301, Humaitá, Rio De Janeiro, RJ ·22271–090, *Brazil*, adriana.aguiar@post.harvard.edu

Lia Daichman, Consultant Gerontology and Geriatrics, Associated Professor of Psychology of Ageing, Faculty of Psychology, University of Belgrano, Arenales 1391, 8th Floor "B," (1061), Buenos Aires, *Argentina*, lsdaichman@fibertel.com.ar

Yael Danieli, Director, Group Project for Holocaust Survivors and their Children, 345 E. 80th St., Apt. 31-J, New York, New York, *USA*, YAELD@aol.com

Joop T.V.M de Jong, Professor of Mental Health and Culture and Director, Transcultural Psychosocial Organisation, Keizersgracht 329, 1016 EE Amsterdam, *The Netherlands*, jdejong.tpo@pom.nl

Purnaka L. de Silva, Head, Leadership Programmes in North America, United Nations University, 2 United Nations Plaza, New York, New York 10017, *USA*, pldesilva@hotmail.com

Brigid Donelan, Conflict Resolution Focal Point, SSII, Social Integration Branch, Division for Social Policy and Development, DESA, United Nations, New York, New York 10017, *USA*, donelan@un.org

Mary Ann Dutton, Professor of Psychiatry, Department of Psychiatry, Georgetown University Medical Center, 620 Kober-Cogan Hall, 3800 Reservoir Road, NW, Washington, DC 20057, *USA*, mad27@georgetown.edu

Evelyn Eisenstein, Director, Clinica de Adolescentes, Rua Barao de Lucena 32, Rio de Janiero 22260-020, *Brazil*, ceiias@yahoo.com.br

Brian Engdahl, Counseling Psychologist, Veterans Affairs Medical Center (116B), 1 Veterans Drive, Minneapolis, Minnesota 55417-2300, *USA*, brian.engdahl@med.va.gov

John A. Fairbank, Co-Director, UCLA-Duke University National Center for Child Traumatic Stress, Associate Professor of Medical Psychology, Department of Psychiatry and Behavioral Sciences, Duke University Medical Center, DUMC Box 3454, Durham, North Carolina 27710, *USA* jaf@psych.mc.duke.edu

Ellen Frey-Wouters, Executive Director, International Policy Research Institute, 284 College Road, Riverdale, New York 10471-3051, *USA*, RBInstitute@gc.cuny.edu

Matthew Friedman, Director, National Center for PTSD, VAM and ROC 116D, 215 North Main Street, White River Junction, Vermont 05009, Departments of Psychiatry and Pharmacology, Dartmouth Medical School, *USA*, matthew.friedman@dartmouth.edu

Merle Friedman, South African Institute for Traumatic Stress, P.O. Box 1082, Saxonwold 2132, *South Africa*, merle@icon.co.za

Lisa A. Goodman, Associate Professor, Department of Counseling Psychology, Boston College, School of Education, Campion 310, Chestnut Hill, Massachusetts 02467, *USA*, goodmalc@bc.edu

Bonnie L. Green, Professor of Psychiatry, Department of Psychiatry, Georgetown University Medical Center, 310 Kober-Cogan Hall, 3800 Reservoir Road, NW, Washington, DC 20057, *USA*, bgreen01@georgetown.edu

Virginia Aldige Hiday, Professor, Department of Sociology, North Carolina State University, Raleigh, North Carolina 27695-8107, *USA*, ginny_hiday@ncsu.edu

Stacey Kaltman, Assistant Professor of Psychiatry, Department of Psychiatry, Georgetown University Medical Center, 613 Kober-Cogan Hall, 3800 Reservoir Road, NW, Washington, DC 200057, *USA*, sk279@georgetown.edu

Soeren Buus Jensen, Co-Director, Global Psychiatric and Psycho-Social Initiatives (GPSI), P.O. Box 1360, Sarit Center, 0606 Nairobi, *Kenya*, sbjensen@infocom.co.ug

Terence M. Keane, Chief, Psychology Service, National Center for PTSD and Professor of Psychiatry, Psychology, and Behavioral Neuroscience, Boston University, Veterans Affairs Medical Center 116B, 150 S. Huntington Avenue, Boston, Massachusetts 02130-4826, *USA*, terry.keane@med.va.gov

Dean Kilpatrick, Professor of Psychiatry, Medical University of South Carolina, Department of Psychiatry, 171 Ashley Avenue, Charleston, South Carolina 29424-0002, *USA*, kilpatdg@musc.edu

Kim Mueser, Professor, New Hampshire-Dartmouth Psychiatric Research Center, Main Bldg., 105 Pleasant Street, Concord, New Hampshire 03301, *USA*, kim.t.mueser@dartmouth.edu

R. Srinivasa Murthy, Professor of Psychiatry, National Institute of Mental Health and Neurosciences, P.B. No. 2900, Bangalore 560 029, *India,* murthy@nimhans.kar.nic.in

Gladys K. Mwiti, Counseling Psychologist and Executive Director, Oasis Counseling Center and Training Institute, P.O. Box 76117, Nairobi, *Kenya,* and Clinical Psychology Student, Fuller Graduate School of Psychology, Fuller Theological Seminary, Pasadena, California, glmwiti@fuller.edu

Madhabika B. Nayak, Visiting Scholar and Associate Scientist, Public Health Institute, Alcohol Research Group, 2000 Hearst Avenue, Suite 300, Berkeley, California 94709-7175, *USA,* mnayak@arg.org

Fran Norris, Research Professor, Department of Psychiatry, Dartmouth Medical School, National Center for PTSD, VA Medical Center MS 116D, 215 N. Main Street, White River Junction, Vermont 05009, *USA,* fran.norris@dartmouth.edu

Vikram Patel, Senior Lecturer, London School of Hygiene and Tropical Medicine, Sangath Centre, 841/1 Alto Porvorim, Goa 403521, *India,* vikpat@goatelecom.com

Bukelwa Selema, Medical, Surgical and Psychiatric Nurse, Director of the Zama Centre, P.O. Box 8196, Putfontein 1513, *South Africa,* zama@mweb.co.za

Derrick Silove, Professor and Director, Psychiatry Research and Teaching Unit, School of Psychiatry, University of New South Wales, at Liverpool Hospital, Liverpool, New South Wales, *Australia,* d.silove@unsw.edu.au

Patrick Smith, Research Fellow, Department of Psychology, Institute of Psychiatry, de Crespigny Park, London SE5 8AF, *United Kingdom,* p.smith@iop.kcl.ac.uk

Susan Solomon, Senior Advisor, Office of Behavioral and Social Sciences Research, National Institutes of Health, One Center Drive, Room 256, Bethesda, Maryland 20892, *USA,* ssolomon@nih.gov

Zahava Solomon, Professor, Bob Shapell School of Social Work, Tel Aviv University, Ramat Aviv, 69 978, *Israel,* solomon@ccsg.tav.ac.il

Daya Somasundaram, Professor of Psychiatry, Department of Psychiatry, Faculty of Medicine, University of Jaffna, *Sri Lanka*, dayasoma@panlanka.net

Rune Stuvland, Managing Director, Center for Crisis Psychology Oslo, Kr. Augustsgt. 12, 0164 Oslo, *Norway*, rune.stuvland@krisepsykologi.no

Madeline Tashjian, 16 Karapet Ulnetsu St., Yerevan, 375037, *Armenia*, tashjian@umcor.am

Stuart Turner, Chair, The Traumatic Stress Clinic, 73 Charlotte Street, London W1T 4PL, *United Kingdom*, s.turner@traumaclinic.org.uk

Denise Valenti-Hein, Adjunct Professor of Psychology, University of Wisconsin Oshkosh, Oshkosh, Wisconsin 54901, *USA*, valentih@uwosh.edu

Elena Varavikova, 11 Dobrolyudova Str., Moscow 127254, *Russia*, eva@varavik.msk.ru

Panos Vostanis, Professor of Child and Adolescent Psychiatry, University of Leicester, Westcotes House, Westcotes Drive, Leicester LE3 OQU, *United Kingdom*, Pv11@leicester.ac.uk

Peter Warfe, Director, Preventive Medicine and Rehabilitation Centre, Deakin, ACT, *Australia*, peterwarfe@pmrc.com.au

David Wolfe, Professor, Department of Psychology, University of Western Ontario, London, Ontario N6A 5C2, *Canada*, dawolfe@uwo.ca

Rosalie Wolf, Previously Executive Director, Institute on Aging, Umass Memorial Health Care, 119 Belmont Street, Worcester, Massachusetts 01605, *USA* (Deceased)

Sahika Yuksel, Professor, Istanbul-Psychosocial Trauma Programme, Psychiatry, Faculty of Medicine, University of Istanbul, Topkapi-Istanbul, *Turkey*, sahikayuksel@turk.net

William Yule, Professor of Applied Child Psychology, University of London, Institute of Psychiatry, de Crespigny Park, London SE5 8AF, *United Kingdom*, w.yule@iop.kcl.ac.uk

Foreword

Peace of mind is a most precious resource, without which neither rich nor poor can know happiness. Yet mental health is undervalued and routinely taken for granted. Moreover, we allow war, torture, violence, poverty, disease, discrimination, and domestic abuse to undermine it. The wounds inflicted by these great human ills sicken the individual psyche, tear families apart, and send shock waves through society. Natural disasters, too, can cause sudden and acute trauma. Often, the damage—a chronic and relentless loss of dignity, self-esteem, and hope—is transmitted from one generation to the next: a sad and painful legacy indeed.

Scientists, scholars, and medical and other professionals are seeking continuously to know more about mental health, and to apply their knowledge. All of us, vulnerable human beings that we are, need to work together to ensure that the environment we live in is conducive to peace of mind, and free of the horrors that jeopardize mental well-being.

This publication grew out of the commitment of the United Nations and others to this cause, and is the product of a series of lively meetings that the authors held at UN Headquarters with civil society groups, government officials, and United Nations staff—a dialogue that coincided with the World Health Organization's focus on mental health in 2001. I hope it will be a valuable resource for practitioners, policymakers, and United Nations field and headquarters staff wherever trauma strikes, and wherever peace of mind is threatened.

KOFI A. ANNAN
Secretary-General of the United Nations

Preface

There was a time when few people had heard of posttraumatic stress. As is true with many other emotional and psychological experiences, many people would not have given a name to the consequences of trauma, and some would not have accepted their reality. Yet most people have experienced individual or social traumas in the sudden death of a close relative, for example, or through motor vehicle accidents or unemployment. Many have lived through natural disasters or civil conflicts. Media coverage of these events may have broadened awareness of what it is like to live under threat, as is the case for tens of millions worldwide—for people in Cambodia, the Sudan, Rwanda, Colombia, the Balkans, and Western Asia. The list could go on. No country is free of stress and trauma, whether it is at war or in peace.

The World Summit for Social Development acknowledged the pervasiveness of societal stress, and at its five-year review, in 2000, States called for strengthening the capability of relevant United Nations bodies *"to promote measures for social integration in their post-conflict management strategies and activities, including in their research, analysis, training and operational activities, so as to better address trauma recovery, rehabilitation, reconciliation and reconstruction"* (A/RES/S-24/2).

This book has been driven by a growing recognition throughout the international community of the insidious and potentially long-lasting effects of traumatic stress. It has evolved through the close collaboration of United Nations and professional organizations including, in particular, the International Society for Traumatic Stress Studies (ISTSS) and the Transcultural Psychosocial Organization (TPO). These entities have ensured the involvement of experts from throughout the developing world, including Argentina, Bangladesh, Brazil, South Africa, Sri Lanka, Turkey, and Uganda. They collaborated with several leading research and service centers, many of which have made generous in-kind and financial contributions to the project.

The United Nations provided seed money for the project, and staff from many United Nations agencies and bodies have participated in the conceptual design as well as in peer review of the chapters. Early drafts were presented at a forum during the humanitarian segment of the Economic and Social Council in July 2000, and a *Proposal for Psychosocial Policy and Practice in Social and Humanitarian Crises* was made available during the Commission for Social Development in February 2002 (subsequently re-formulated as *Guidelines*). The Division for Social Policy and Development and the Office for the Coordination of Humanitarian Affairs jointly launched and supported the project. These and several other United Nations agencies or bodies have contributed a "Voice" to the book's different sections, in which they reflect on traumatic stress from their different perspectives and explain some of their own related activities.

The book, in short, evolved through a four-year dialogue among researchers, practitioners, and policy-makers, and I am indeed pleased to thank all those involved, both the individuals and the institutions. Special thanks are due to Ellen Frey-Wouters, who first proposed the project, and to my colleague Martin Barber, who provided crucial institutional and moral support for it from the outset. In short, all participants in this enterprise have given it their best in the hope that the final product—together with the discussions it evoked along the way—will help increase understanding of traumatic stress and lead to better prevention, practice, and policy.

JOHN LANGMORE
Director, Division for Social Policy and Development
Department of Economics and Social Affairs
United Nations
December 2001

Acknowledgments

This book is a joint effort of the United Nations and the International Society for Traumatic Stress Studies (ISTSS), with strong contributions from the Transcultural Psychosocial Organisation and the National Center for PTSD. It has involved the creativity and effort of scores of individuals over its three years of development and fruition. We would like to express our gratitude to all of those individuals and institutions that made this book possible, especially the many authors from around the world who contributed their scholarship, as well as their field and clinical experience, to our offering of best practices in responding to trauma. Ellen Frey-Wouters, ISTSS representative to the UN, conceptualized and initiated the project, with seed money from the United Nations Department of Economic and Social Affairs (DESA). It became a reality through the continuing support of John Langmore, Director, Division for Social Policy and Development, DESA, and Martin Barber, then Director, Policy and Advocacy Development Branch, Office for the Coordination of Humanitarian Affairs (OCHA), to whom we express our most sincere appreciation. Their leadership and support included hosting two meetings at the UN for the editors and authors, as well as their invaluable guidance and encouragement. We would also like to thank Hana Shishtawy and Imma Guerras-Delgado from OCHA for their assistance on substantive and coordination issues at different stages of the project. Other UN personnel who were involved in the evolution of the project were gracious enough to provide the "Voices" that appear throughout the book. We are also deeply grateful to Kofi Annan, Secretary General of the UN, for providing the Foreword to the book.

Several organizations provided support for the project as well. The ISTSS provided organizational, financial, and administrative support. The Transcultural Psychosocial Organisation provided the model underpinning the work, and helped identify important contributors to the book.

The National Center for PTSD in White River Junction, VT provided financial support and much of the coordination for the project. In particular, we
would like to thank Jan Clark and Sandra Mariotti for their coordinating,
scheduling, and manuscript assistance. The Office of Behavioral and Social
Sciences Research of the National Institutes of Health in the US provided
funding for the project, as did the International Policy Research Institute
in Riverdale, New York.

We appreciate the active collaboration and support of Christiane Roll
and Sharon Panulla from Kluwer, who shepherded the book through its
many stages of development and completion. Anthony Marsella, series
editor, was enthusiastic and supportive from the beginning and we greatly
appreciate his ongoing encouragement. Yael Danieli, Special Consultant,
provided valuable feedback at several stages of the project that strengthened the content of the book. Two anonymous reviewers provided helpful
feedback after the first draft. We also thank Sue Bencuya for her excellent
and timely copyediting assistance

Last, but not least, we express our deep gratitude to Stacey Kaltman,
Assistant Professor of Psychiatry at Georgetown University Medical
School, for her work as Assistant Editor to the book. Her contributions
were substantive and extensive, as well as clerical and administrative, and
she provided much of the "glue" that kept the project on target and integrated over the past year.

THE EDITORS

· Contents

I. OVERVIEW

II. ABUSE AND TORTURE

III. WAR AND DISASTERS

IV. UNITED NATIONS PERSONNEL

V. SUMMARY AND CONCLUSION

Part I

Overview

WHO: FROM THE HEALTH PERSPECTIVE

Trauma has serious implications for health and more specifically for mental health. The situations that cause trauma vary enormously—from wars, terrorist attacks, and natural disasters that affect whole communities to torture, abuse, and interpersonal violence that affect a few at a time. However, all of these events result in a wounded psyche, with serious immediate and long-term consequences to mental health. The resultant burden on individuals, families, and communities is enormous. A volume that analyzes the various facets of trauma, and reviews strategies toward the prevention of its occurrence as well as its impact, is a valuable and a very welcome contribution. The editors and authors of this volume deserve full praise for undertaking this massive and difficult but timely task.

From the health perspective, it is most unfortunate that often the very events that traumatize whole communities also destroy or incapacitate the health care system, leading to very little or no health care being available in the face of a much larger need. On the other hand, for individually experienced trauma, the health care system may be intact, but it is often remarkably inaccessible and unresponsive to the trauma victim. This is especially true for mental health care, which is still largely institutional with associated stigma and neglect of human rights. In either case, there is a need to make the health care system more responsive to the needs of trauma victims and more prepared and resilient in emergencies.

World Health Organization (WHO) has been active in the area of mental health care for trauma victims including refugees and those affected by disasters. Dr. Gro Harlem Brundtland, the Director General of WHO, emphasized the need of mental health care for the "50 million refugees and displaced persons worldwide" (Brundtland, 2000). In October 2000, WHO organized the first-ever International Consultation on Mental Health of

1

Refugees and Displaced Populations in Conflict and Post-Conflict Situations. The year 2001 was devoted by WHO to mental health, with the theme for the World Health Day and the World Health Report (WHO, 2001a) being mental health. This emphasis was appropriate in view of the serious deficiency of mental health resources in the world (WHO, 2001b). WHO also organized Round Table discussions on aspects of mental health by the Health Ministers of its Member States in May 2001, during the World Health Assembly. The Ministers highlighted the mental health needs of those affected by traumatic events—among them refugees, internally displaced persons, and women and children facing domestic violence and sexual exploitation. The Ministers called for action to prevent mental disorders and to promote mental health among populations affected by wars, conflicts, and violence (WHO, 2001c). These advocacy efforts have resulted in an enhanced awareness of the mental health needs of populations affected by traumatic events at the highest political level within countries. WHO also provides technical advice and assistance to Member States for improving their mental health services, including emergency assistance. WHO works in close collaboration with other UN agencies, Non-Governmental Organizations, and experts in this field, including many involved in the preparation of this volume.

SHEKHAR SAXENA
Department of Mental Health and Substance Dependence
World Health Organization
Geneva, Switzerland

REFERENCES

Brundtland, G.H. (2000). Mental health of refugees, internally displaced persons and other populations affected by conflict. *Acta Psychiatrica Scandinavica, 102*, 159–161.
World Health Organization (2001a). *The World Health Report 2001: Mental health: New understanding, new hope.* Geneva: Author.
World Health Organization (2001b). *Atlas: Mental health resources in the world 2001.* Geneva: Author. WHO/NMH/MSD/MDP/01.1.
World Health Organization (2001c). *Mental health: A call for action by World Health ministers.* Geneva: Author. WHO/NMH/MSD/WHA/01.1.

Chapter 1

Introduction

Susan D. Solomon

Most people will experience a traumatic event at some time in their lives. The front page of any newspaper attests to the fact that extremely stressful experiences are quite common. Conflicts like those in Kosovo, Bosnia, Rwanda, Afghanistan, and the Sudan, terrorist attacks like those on the US World Trade Center and Pentagon, the Tokyo sarin gas and US anthrax releases, the chemical and nuclear disasters in Bhopal and Chernobyl—all demonstrate the ability of human-caused catastrophes to devastate and disrupt the lives of vast numbers of people.

And the all-too-frequent news accounts of earthquakes, hurricanes, and floods display the power of nature to cause traumatic stress on a massive scale as well. Other types of traumatic experiences, like rape, child abuse, and torture, are so commonplace that they are no longer front-page news, in part because they typically happen to individuals and families one-by-one. Yet these experiences are no less emotionally traumatic for their many victims.

Trauma Interventions in War and Peace: Prevention, Practice, and Policy is intended to guide practice and public policy for individuals and communities exposed to traumatic events. With problem areas on every continent affecting every ethnic and age group, there is a need to identify strategies that can be employed to mitigate the effects of traumatic stressors on these

Note: The opinions or assertions contained herein are the private ones of the author, and are not to be considered as official or reflecting the views of the National Institutes of Health.

populations, as well as on those people who encounter extremely stressful experiences in the performance of a variety of roles central to the mission of the United Nations.

In its 1948 *Universal Declaration of Human Rights*, the UN General Assembly affirmed that all human beings are born free and equal in dignity and rights. They proclaimed that no one should be held in slavery, or subjected to torture or to cruel, inhuman, or degrading treatment or punishment. All were held to be entitled to equal protection of the law, to move about freely, to found a family, to own property, to express their views, and to practice their chosen religion. All were also held to be entitled to the indispensable economic, social, and cultural benefits of their country, including an adequate standard of living, employment, education, and health care. In the years since 1948, governments have adopted many instruments that reinforce these fundamental human rights (see http://www.unhchr.ch; http://www.un.org/rights/HRToday).

Traumatic events can violate all of these basic human rights. Experiences such as torture, domestic violence, rape, elder abuse, and child neglect threaten human dignity, liberty, and security. Events like war, political repression, terrorism, genocide, poverty, and disaster deprive individuals of their homes, their families, their work, their schools, their places of worship, and their access to education and health care. In its Copenhagen Programme of Action, the World Summit for Social Development (March 1995) recognized the need to address these growing threats to mental and physical well-being, as follows:

> Notwithstanding the instances of progress, there are negative developments that include social polarization and fragmentation; widening disparities and inequalities of income and wealth within and among nations; problems arising from uncontrolled urban development and the degradation of the environment; marginalization of people, families, social groups, communities and even entire countries; and strains on individuals, families, communities and institutions as a result of the rapid pace of social change, economic transformation, migration and major dislocations of population, particularly in the areas of armed conflict.
>
> Furthermore, violence, in its many manifestations, including domestic violence, especially against women, children, older persons and people with disabilities, is a growing threat to the security of individuals, families and communities everywhere. Total social breakdown is an all too real contemporary experience. Organized crime, illegal drugs, the illicit arms trade, trafficking in women and children, ethnic and religious conflict, civil war, terrorism, all forms of extremist violence, xenophobia, and politically motivated killing and even genocide present fundamental threats to societies and the global social order. These are compelling and urgent reasons for action by Governments individually and, as appropriate, jointly to foster social

cohesion while recognizing, protecting and valuing diversity' (United Nations, 1995, paragraphs 68 and 69).

As the World Summit for Social Development made clear, most traumatic experiences are not random, unexplained events. Indeed, most are the result of poverty, unemployment, and social disintegration. While some traumatic stressors, like natural disasters, may seem to occur in a random fashion, even these events are more likely to be experienced by, and to be traumatic for, individuals and communities with fewer resources.

And women are always among the most vulnerable, regardless of circumstances. A recent United Nations Population Fund publication (2000) gives some idea of the horrors women and girls still routinely face as a result of their unequal status. This report indicates that each year women undergo an estimated 20 million unsafe abortions, resulting in 78,000 deaths; at least one in three women are beaten, coerced into sex, or abused in some way; one in four women is abused during pregnancy; at least 60 million girls are listed as "missing" as a result of infanticide, neglect, or other factors; and as many as 5,000 women and girls are murdered yearly in so-called "honor" killings by members of their own families. Recognizing this gender disparity, the Fourth World Conference on Women, held shortly after the Social Summit in 1995, called for a gender perspective to be mainstreamed in all United Nations work as the most effective way of ensuring equality between men and women. A gender perspective has also guided the authors of the chapters in this book.

In 2000, the General Assembly's five-year review took a closer look at these issues. It agreed inter alia to address trauma recovery, rehabilitation, reconciliation, and reconstruction among its "further initiatives" pertaining to social integration in post-conflict activities. It noted that greater attention should be given to children, including unaccompanied refugee minors, displaced children, children separated from their families, those acting as soldiers, and those involved in armed conflicts (United Nations, 2000).

Like the UN, the World Health Organization (WHO) has recently highlighted the importance of attending to the psychological consequences of traumatic events. The WHO devoted its entire 2001 report to mental health in order to make "one clear emphatic statement. Mental health—neglected for far too long—is crucial to the well-being of individuals, societies, and countries . . . " While this report does not focus on trauma per se, it notes that factors that determine the prevalence, onset, and course of all mental disorders include poverty, conflict, disasters, and social environment (see Chapter 2; WHO, 2001).

SCOPE AND RELATION TO UN MANDATE

Because traumatic experiences can take so many forms, this book focuses on interventions for a variety of trauma populations, including abused children; victims of crime and violence; abused elderly; traumatized mentally and physically disabled; victims of torture; children in armed conflict; refugees; internally displaced citizens; victims of disaster; former combatants, as well as current members of the military and prisoners of war; and UN peacekeepers, civilian police, and medical and humanitarian personnel. While other important traumatized populations (e.g. victims of genocide, racism, sexism, and political repression) have not been given a separate chapter focus, many of their issues have been integrated into this book. Whether or not they are the subjects of separate book chapters, all of these traumatized populations are exposed to experiences that have the potential to exact a tremendous emotional toll.

This volume represents an initiative that was undertaken by the International Working Group on Trauma on behalf of the International Society for Traumatic Stress Studies, the Transcultural Psychosocial Organisation, the International Policy Research Institute, the National Center for PTSD at the US Department of Veterans' Affairs, and the Office of Behavioral and Social Sciences Research at the US National Institutes of Health, in conjunction with the Division for Social Policy and Development of the Department of Economic and Social Affairs and the Office for the Coordination of Humanitarian Affairs of the UN Secretariat. The initiative's genesis was the World Summit for Social Development, held in Copenhagen in 1995. This meeting represented a landmark shift by governments to support policies that promote a people-centered framework for social development and justice. Among its 10 commitments, the *Copenhagen Declaration* pledged to eradicate poverty in the world and to give special priority to the rights and capabilities of vulnerable and disadvantaged groups. In 1991, the General Assembly had already provided "Principles for the protection of persons with mental illness and the improvement of mental health care" (General Assembly resolution 46/119; see www.unhchr.ch). The *Copenhagen Declaration* extended these principles by making a commitment to promote universal and equitable access to quality physical and mental health care.

COMMON RESPONSES TO TRAUMATIC EXPERIENCES

The *Global Burden of Disease* report gives some indication of the extent to which trauma affects physical health (Murray & Lopez, 1996). The authors developed a measure of disease burden that incorporates both premature death and disability. Using this as a measure of years of healthy life lost, their estimates indicate that traumatic events are in themselves ever-increasing causes of disease burden. In determining changes in rank for the leading sources of disease burden for all age groups worldwide from 1990 to 2020, the authors project that traumatic experiences like traffic accidents will rise in importance from 9th to 3rd place, war will rise from 16th to 8th place, and violence will rise from 28th to 12th place.

Injuries and death are the most obvious manifestations of trauma's impact on physical health. But trauma exposure takes a more hidden toll. Studies of combat veterans, rape victims, refugees, hostages, disaster victims, and women with a history of physical and sexual abuse have found that the physical complaints of trauma victims are many and often serious, over and above any injuries sustained during the traumatic event (Golding, 1994; Kimerling & Calhoun, 1994). For example, recent research on Vietnam war veterans demonstrates a link between exposure to severe stress and the onset of coronary heart disease (Boscarino & Chang, 1999). And traumatized individuals have considerably higher numbers of persistent physical problems, including chronic pain, gastrointestinal disorders, headaches, and seizures, than non-traumatized individuals (Friedman & Schnurr, 1995). Not surprisingly, then, research also indicates that trauma survivors are disproportionate users of the health care system. Studies have found more physician visits and higher hospitalization rates among former prisoners of war, rape victims, survivors of Nazi concentration camps, disaster victims, battered women, combat veterans, and crime victims than among the general population (Friedman & Schnurr, 1995), which may translate into substantial health care costs.

Traumatic experiences can have other devastating consequences on victims' lives, as well as on the lives of those who love them. Over and above its impact on physical health, a traumatic experience can result in marital, occupational, and financial problems for its survivors. The cumulative effects of all of these problems can be lethal: recent studies of refugees, disaster victims, prisoners of war, and other traumatized populations suggest that victims are at excess risk of displaying suicidal behavior for several years after the traumatic event (Ferrada-Noli, Asberg, Ormstad, Lundin & Sundbom, 1998).

Fortunately, most individuals exposed to extreme events and conditions are remarkably resilient. Even after fairly severe traumatic events, a majority will cope effectively if provided with the opportunities and resources to rebuild their lives. However, traumatic experiences can cause serious psychological damage in some survivors. And certain experiences, especially those of human origin, can be so severely traumatic that they may exceed the emotional capacities of even the most hardy.

Exposure to extreme stressors may result in a variety of emotional responses, ranging from low level distress to severe stress reactions that can evolve into chronically disabling conditions like posttraumatic stress disorder (PTSD) (see Chapter 2). According to the recent report estimating the current and future global burden of disease, psychiatric conditions such as depression and alcohol use now account for 5 of the top 10 causes of disability worldwide (Murray & Lopez, 1996). That report notes that while the traditional killers—communicable diseases and malnutrition—are on the wane in developing countries, mental illnesses and injuries are on the rise. And while the addictions receive less attention in this book, these behaviors are intimately involved as well, both as causes and consequences of traumatic events. Problems of violence associated with the production and marketing of drugs are rampant in South, Central, and North America, as well as in Asia and Europe. Moreover, addiction to alcohol or drugs can complicate recovery and lead to additional violence in the home and community. Managing substance abuse is therefore fundamental to addressing the consequences of traumatic exposure.

CAREGIVER AND COMMUNITY EFFECTS

Trauma exposure is a burden not only for victims but also for those who try to assist victims in wartime and peace. Traumatic events may affect the missions of both the United Nations and non-governmental organizations (NGOs), through their negative effects on the mental health of UN and NGO staff. Like the UN, NGOs have an important role in helping victims cope with traumatic events (Danieli, Rodley, & Weisaeth, 1996). Over 44,000 international NGOs, such as the Red Cross, Médecins Sans Frontières, the World Federation for Mental Health, Amnesty International, the Save the Children Fund, and Oxfam, serve as intermediaries between governments and individuals, often providing trauma victims with information and direct services (see http://iberia.vassar.edu/vcl//electronics/etc/gov/un.html). Both UN and NGO personnel may be traumatized by their exposure to the human consequences of interpersonal violence, war, disaster, and deprivation. And they may experience additional stressors, such as frustration, uncertainty, guilt, hostility, or separation from family. The effects of these accumulating stressors may be further exacerbated by inadequate preparation and training or insufficient emotional support. Failure to address these emotional problems may result in a myriad of negative consequences for the individual, including distress, insensitivity, family disruption, and burnout. There may be economic and social consequences for the UN and NGOs as well, in the form of increased turnover, deteriorating performance, inefficiencies, increased costs, and loss of credibility (see Chapter 14). Thus the need for effective interventions for both trauma victims and their caregivers is immense.

As the above discussion indicates, failure to attend to psychological problems following trauma exposure can jeopardize the recovery of individuals caught up in these events. But traumatic experiences also a take a cultural and societal toll, and policy makers must address the psychological consequences for communities as well for individuals. Like individuals, social organizations and cultural groups may become distressed and disintegrate under the pressures of extreme and persistent exposure to traumatic experience. As described in Chapter 3, prolonged and inescapable violence can lead to an erosion of the basic fabric of society. When communities fragment, cultural defense mechanisms such as roles and status are lost. Elders, non-violent men, and women no longer occupy positions of power and influence. Instead, individuals may revert to ethnicity, nationalism, tribalism, and fundamentalism to survive, and the community may be overtaken by an ethic of militarism and conflict. A cycle of increasing violence may erode familiar societal structures and eliminate previously safe relationships. This context can give rise to predatory teenage gangs, scapegoating of minorities, increased violence against women, and intergenerational transmission of mental and physical health problems.

Recent conflicts have been overwhelmingly concentrated in poor countries. Following on poverty and war, these countries have been faced with populations of refugees and internally displaced persons. Between 1990 and 1993, there were an estimated 18 million refugees and, in the same period, twice as many internally displaced persons (De Jong, 1995). It is not surprising then that exposure to trauma is extremely costly, not only to the victims, but also to society as a whole.

A recent estimate of the financial cost—to Americans alone—of only one type of trauma, criminal victimization, is $105 *billion* annually; this includes medical costs, lost earnings, and public program costs related to victim assistance (Miller, Cohen & Wiersma, 1996; Solomon & Davidson, 1997) . War trauma also has a negative impact on employment and earnings: American Vietnam veterans with a diagnosis of PTSD were found to be over ten times more likely to be unemployed than veterans without PTSD. Veterans with PTSD were also earning 22% less per hour than their counterparts without PTSD (Fairbank, Ebert, & Johnson, 1999). Similar adverse workplace outcomes have been described for South African survivors of childhood sexual abuse (Ortlepp & Nkosi, 1993) and Scandinavian victims of spousal abuse (Hensing & Alexanderson, 2000).

Taken together, these findings demonstrate the enormous economic burden that both individuals and societies shoulder as a result of trauma exposure. These findings suggest that the resources involved in responding to traumatic experiences could be better employed by preventing their occurrence through policies and programs that promote social development. Because traumatic stressors usually arise in an environment of social deprivation, it is not only morally and ethically preferable, but also more cost-effective, to promote social and economic development, rather than waiting to respond to traumatic stress after it occurs.

The above discussion illustrates how trauma can adversely affect communities. However, it is also true that communities can affect the level of trauma experienced by their members. Indeed, the community itself may be the agent of traumatic events, as in the case of torture and genocide. Organized political violence affects not only the targeted individual, but also the victim's family and community, since agencies attempting to offer support to victims of political oppression may themselves become targets. And some cultures support actions that others regard as violations of individual human rights: for example, by tacitly condoning genital mutilation, domestic violence, and child abuse. Communities may also violate the economic, social, and cultural rights of their citizens, e.g., through failure to warn of an impending hurricane, failure to provide housing strong enough to withstand an earthquake, mismanagement of resources during famine, or failure to attend to the cultural needs of refugees. The International Covenant on Civil and Political Rights, and the International Covenant on Economic, Social, and Cultural Rights, illustrate the UN's commitment to both the civil and political rights prioritized by Western countries, and the economic, social, and cultural rights prioritized by developing countries. The authors of this book view the preservation of both sets of rights as important goals of preventive interventions.

But it should also be noted that communities can serve as agents of healing as well as harm. Indeed, perhaps the most valuable lesson of this book is the value of collaborating with the leadership of communities in building interventions to address the sequelae of traumatic events, to ensure that the most appropriate and acceptable interventions will be developed.

INTERVENTION STRATEGIES

The goal of this book is to generate more awareness of the knowledge acquired about traumatic stress over the past two decades, and to suggest intervention strategies that can be of use to social organizations and public policy makers. The book recognizes that some of the issues that arise in collective and humanitarian emergencies may differ from those that emerge in social and interpersonal level ones. For example, collective events may be more acute in nature and broad in scope, such as war and disaster (see Chapters 10–14). In contrast, events that are experienced largely at the individual, interpersonal, and family levels, such as rape and child abuse, tend to pose chronic, ongoing problems for a society (see Chapters 5–9). Interpersonal and collective experiences pose different challenges in designing strategies for intervention. In addition, intervention strategies must take into account the variability in resources available in different geographic regions. To address this level of complexity, contributors to this book represent developed, transitional, and developing countries, with authors drawn from Argentina, Australia, Bangladesh, Brazil, Canada, India, Israel, Japan, Kenya, the Netherlands, Norway, Russia, South Africa, Sri Lanka, Turkey, Uganda, United Kingdom, and the United States. The materials are designed to be generic and applicable to a wide range of countries, with different approaches and sensitivities to problems stemming from traumatic experiences. However, cultural differences, as well as the degree of development and sophistication of the health and welfare systems in each nation, will greatly affect the feasibility and appropriateness of implementing different kinds of programs.

While this book places particular emphasis on trauma intervention in developing countries without a strong mental health infrastructure, it is also intended to pertain to vulnerable groups in high-income countries. Even within the wealthiest countries, there are many who live in abject poverty. The economically and socially deprived are always among the most vulnerable to experiencing traumatic events, and to the mental and physical health consequences of these events (see Chapter 3). Unfortunately, they also tend to be those least likely to get help for such problems.

Many of the traumatic stress interventions described in this book are preventative ones (see Chapter 4 for an in-depth discussion). Prevention efforts may be subdivided into three types: primary prevention, secondary prevention, and tertiary prevention (Kaplan & Sadock, 1985). Ultimately primary prevention—i.e., preventing the trauma itself—is the only truly effective intervention for traumatic stress. Prevention of large-scale conditions such as extreme poverty, or catastrophic events such as war and human rights violations, resides mainly with those with national and international decision-making responsibility and authority to implement policies supporting equitable development, de-escalation of hostilities, arms control, and human rights. Such policy can also be effective in preventing trauma at the individual, family, and community levels, for example, by recognizing that actions such as elder abuse, spousal violence, and child sexual assault are criminal behaviors. Policies that promote programs to prevent these kinds of behaviors might include efforts toward early education of parents and children, as well as elimination of inhumane living conditions, which foster and perpetuate violence.

For the most part, this book deals with secondary prevention, which may be defined as any effort to shorten the course of traumatic responses by early identification and rapid intervention (Kaplan & Sadock, 1985). Our major concern is in fostering natural resiliency. For many survivors, removing obstacles to self-help, or providing for basic needs such as food, shelter, education, and health care, may be the only intervention needed. This type of secondary prevention may also involve reparations, provision of a safe and healthy recovery environment, and reunion of family and community members. The underlying goal is to empower victims to participate in their own recovery efforts so as to regain both a sense of control over their lives and an orientation toward the future.

When more direct emotional help is also needed, traumatic stress services should be integrated with other systems providing assistance to victims. Successful secondary prevention requires that help be geographically, economically, and culturally accessible to those who need it (De Jong, 1995). It may involve working with primary heath care providers, who can then train others, to design and establish a traumatic stress program suitable to the local culture. This book will describe model secondary prevention programs along these and other lines that can be implemented at the community, family, and individual levels. However, the magnitude of psychosocial and emotional problems may be vast following large-scale catastrophes such as disasters, war, and forced migration, as well as in prolonged conditions of poverty, powerlessness, and discrimination. Although professionals working in the mental health arena are seldom trained or prepared to work at a broader community or national level, the scale of these emergencies—now occurring in both war and peacetime—may require abandoning dyadic interventions (e.g., one-to-one psychotherapy) for those that can be implemented via community action, using a public health approach (De Jong, 1995).

While the book emphasizes secondary prevention, it also includes tertiary prevention: i.e., efforts to reduce chronicity of emotional problems through active rehabilitation, and the prevention of complications such as health, work, or family problems (Kaplan & Sadock, 1985). Although mental health treatment holds the promise of shortening the duration of impairment, most people with emotional problems resulting from traumatic exposure do not receive it. Because primary health care workers in both developing and developed countries are the ones most likely to treat people exposed to traumatic events, health care workers offer an important point of intervention. They can be trained to ask patients about trauma exposure and to recognize its psychosocial and psychiatric consequences. Many low-income countries lack mental health care referral facilities. A multi-systemic approach may therefore be needed, wherein primary health care workers turn to other sectors such as education, social services, women's affairs, rural development, or religion to implement both secondary and tertiary preventive strategies.

In fact, as tertiary prevention providers, traditional healers may offer several advantages over trained psychiatrists for those with trauma-related psychosocial problems (De Jong, 2001). These advantages include greater availability and accessibility, more time for patients, and a shared worldview that strengthens the therapist-patient relationship. While psychiatrists in low-income countries have to struggle to establish a position of trust and respect, healers such as medicine men, shamans, and cult or religious leaders already occupy positions of ascribed authority within a given community. They are also often able to understand and attribute problems in a way that increases social status, rather than conferring a stigmatizing label of mental illness.

There are also important benefits associated with non-Western treatment facilities. For example, Ilechukwu (1991) suggests that while African governments seldom value psychiatric villages as highly as the Western-style medical hospital when it comes to allocating resources, psychiatric villages offer many advantages: they are cheaper to build, to maintain, and to accommodate patients. They also have a lower admission threshold, and they do a better job of facilitating contact with the patients' normal social environment than the Western-style hospital. Since treatment is more in line with the daily life of patients, they are likely to feel less alienated, especially when one or several family members participate in the therapeutic program. In the chapters that follow, the authors note the cultural advantages of traditional healers and facilities for trauma victims with non-psychotic psychosocial problems.

While this book describes many different forms of intervention, we humbly acknowledge that we do not have the final word on how to intervene in either developing or developed countries. Our goal is to bring together the best existing evidence on how victims of traumatic experiences can be helped, with the awareness that there is much to learn and much more work to be done in this critically important area.

In his foreword to this book, Secretary-General of the UN Kofi A. Annan has noted that we routinely allow events such as war, torture, violence, poverty, disease, discrimination, and domestic abuse to undermine our "peace of mind...a most precious resource, without which neither rich nor poor can know happiness." We share his hope that this book will help promote environments conducive to peace of mind, by providing strategies to intervene with trauma survivors at the point when intervention is most needed.

REFERENCES

Boscarino, J.A., & Chang, J. (1999). Electrocardiogram abnormalities among men with stress-related psychiatric disorders: Implications for coronary heart disease and clinical research. *Annals of Behavioral Medicine, 21*, 227–34.

Danieli, Y., Rodley, N.S., & Weisaeth, L. (Eds.) (1996). *International responses to traumatic stress.* Amityville, NY: Baywood.

De Jong, J.T.V.M. (1995). Prevention of the consequences of man-made or natural disaster at the international, the community, the family and the individual level. In S. E. Hobfoll & M.W. De Vries (Eds.), *Extreme stress and communities: Impact and intervention* (pp. 207–227). Dordrecht, Netherlands: Kluwer Academic Publishers.

De Jong, J.T.V.M. (2001). Remnants of the colonial past: The difference in outcome of mental disorders in high- and low-income countries. In D. Bhugra & R. Littlewood (Eds.), *Colonialism and mental health.* New Delhi: Oxford University Press.

Fairbank, J.A., Ebert, L., & Johnson, G.A. (1999). Socioeconomic consequences of traumatic stress. In P.A. Saigh & J.D. Bremner (Eds.), *Posttraumatic stress disorder: A comprehensive text.* Boston: Allyn and Bacon.

Ferrada-Noli, M., Asberg, M., Ormstad, K., Lundin, T., & Sundbom, E. (1998). Suicidal behavior after severe trauma. Part 1: PTSD diagnoses, psychiatric comorbidity and assessments of suicidal behavior. *Journal of Traumatic Stress, 11*, 103–112.

Friedman, M.J., & Schnurr, P.P. (1995). The relationship between trauma, post-traumatic stress disorder and physical health. In M.J. Friedman, D.S. Charney, & A.Y. Deutch (Eds.), *Neurobiological and clinical consequences of stress: From normal adaptation to post-traumatic stress disorder.* Philadelphia, Pa: Lippincott-Raven Publishers.

Golding, J.M. (1994). Sexual assault history and physical health in randomly selected Los Angeles women. *Health Psychology, 13*, 130–138.

Hensing, G., & Alexanderson, K. (2000). The relation of adult experience of domestic harassment, violence, and sexual abuse to health and sickness absence. *International Journal of Behavioral Medicine, 7*, 1–18.

Ilechukwu, S.T.C. (1991). Psychiatry in Africa: Special problems and unique features. *Transcultural Psychiatric Research Review, 28*, 169–218.

Kaplan, H.I., & Sadock, B.J. (Eds.) (1985). *Comprehensive textbook of psychiatry (4th ed.).* Baltimore, MD: Williams & Wilkins.

Kimerling, R., & Calhoun, K.S. (1994). Somatic symptoms, social support, and treatment seeking among sexual assault victims. *Journal of Consulting and Clinical Psychology, 62*, 333–340.

Miller, T.R., Cohen, M.A., & Wiersma, B. (1996). *Victim costs and consequences: A new look.* Washington, DC: United States Department of Justice, National Institute of Justice.

Murray, C.J.L., & Lopez, A.D. (Eds.) (1996). The global burden of disease: A comprehensive assessment of mortality and disability from diseases, injuries, and risk factors in 1990 and projected to 2020. Cambridge, MA: Harvard School of Public Health on behalf of WHO and the World Bank (distributed by Harvard University Press).

Ortlepp, K., & Nkosi, N.D. (1993). The relationship between spouse abuse and subjective job-related variables in a sample of employed women. *South African Journal of Psychology, 23*, 145–148.

Solomon, S.D., & Davidson, J.R.T. (1997). Trauma: Prevalence, impairment, service use, and cost. *Journal of Clinical Psychiatry, 58 (suppl 9)*, 5–11.

United Nations (1948). *Universal Declaration of Human Rights.* General Assembly resolution 217 A (III).

United Nations (1995). *Copenhagen Declaration and Programme of Action: World Summit for Social Development.* New York, NY: United Nations Department of Public Information.

United Nations (2000). *Report of the Ad Hoc Committee of the Whole, twenty-fourth special session of the General Assembly* (A/S-24/8/Rev/1). Annex, section III, paragraph 75.

United Nations Population Fund (2000). *The State of World Population 2000. Lives together, worlds apart: Men and women in a time of change.* New York, NY: United Nations Publications. http://www.unfpa.org/publications/swp.htm.

World Health Organization (2001). *World Health Report 2001. Mental health: New understanding, new hope.* Geneva: WHO Publications Center.

Chapter 2

Traumatic Stress and Its Consequences

Bonnie L. Green

STRESS AND TRAUMATIC STRESS

Stress is experienced when individuals lose resources that are highly valued, like loved ones, possessions, social connections, and community resources, or have those resources threatened in some way (Hobfoll, 1991). While the experience of any major event can be stressful because it requires change, researchers have focused on those events, or stressors, that are both undesirable and unexpected as being the most difficult to accommodate and resulting in the most negative reactions in terms of scope and severity (e.g., Pearlin, 1982). These types of noxious or threatening events and losses, such as divorce or separation, job disruption, injury and illness, and ruptured relationships, which tax the individual's capacity to cope effectively, are associated with unpleasant or distressing psychological, behavioral, and physiological reactions. While any of these events individually may present a challenge to coping capabilities, their accumulation or repetition is known to have a more powerful and negative impact than any single event (Pearlin, 1982).

Individual stressor events occur in social and economic contexts that need to be taken into account in understanding their impact. In conditions of rapid social change, people may be physically uprooted or experience the weakening and disruption of social ties. They may also have an alien culture imposed on them (or be forced to accommodate to one), eroding established forms of social organization (Pearlin, 1982) and creating conditions conducive to the occurrence of individual negative life events. Those at the lower end of the economic ladder are at particular risk for experiencing chronic or repeated stressors (Turner, Wheaton, & Lloyd, 1995). Adapting to these experiences becomes more difficult over time, probably due to the lack of time needed to recover from one event before another occurs, as well as the lack of material resources with which to cope. For the poor, this unrelenting chronic stress goes on over long periods and is interwoven into the fabric of day-to-day life.

Definitions of traumatic stressors, which are more extreme, **emphasize harm, injury, and encounters with death, either by having one's own life threatened, or by experiencing the death of others.** Van der Kolk (1987) focuses on the sense of safety that is lost after a traumatic encounter, suggesting that trauma involves a loss of faith that there is order and continuity in life. Death and violent loss, with associated feelings of fear, helplessness, and horror, are at the core of experiences defined as traumatic stressors. In the chapters that follow, we make the basic assumption that the events under discussion will be perceived as extremely stressful for most individuals, disrupting their lives in some way. These traumatic events, like disaster, war, crime, torture, rape, and abuse, are those on the continuum of stressors that may be particularly severe, and/or those that disrupt whole communities.

While stressful events challenge an individual's usual modes of coping and often require adjustment and adaptation, more extreme or traumatic stressors may make much larger demands. These more severe stressors often expose individuals to overwhelming levels of perceived danger and fear. They may create such disruption that the usual coping strategies do not work, and adjustment to them may not be possible. When coping capabilities are so overwhelmed, there may be permanent damage. Repeated exposure to very stressful circumstances, or chains of circumstances, may increasingly deplete resources, so that individuals and communities experience a downward spiral of events and consequences that is difficult to reverse.

Within extremely stressful experiences, there are a number of components that may put individuals at even greater risk for negative emotional and physical consequences. These include a specific threat to a person's life, experiencing severe physical harm or injury, or being a victim of harm that is intentionally perpetrated, like rape, torture, or assault. Additional experiences that may be particularly traumatic are exposure to the unnatural or grotesque death of others, including multiple or violent deaths, witnessing or hearing about death or violence done to a loved one or a member of one's social group, or inadvertently causing the death of others (Green, 1993).

COMMUNITIES AT RISK FOR TRAUMATIC STRESSORS

As with more general stressors, poor individuals and communities with few resources are particularly at risk (see Chapter 3). Even events like natural disasters do not strike randomly. For example, statistics from the International Federation of Red Cross and Red Crescent Societies (2002) clarify that while countries of low human development have accounted for only one-fifth of the total number of disasters from 1992–2001, they account for over half of all disaster fatalities. On average, 13 times more people die per disaster in low development countries than in high development countries. Developing countries are also much less likely to have the resources with which to respond to such events. This lack of resources heightens the likelihood that the impact will be prolonged for months or even years after the initial assault, compounding the effects. When the proportion of victims is large relative to community resources for responding, help necessarily must be brought in from the outside, increasing the likelihood of dependency on non-residents. Even within higher-income countries, those more vulnerable to begin with are more likely to experience disastrous events. For example, those with less education and lower incomes are more likely to be in harm's way due to having to live in substandard housing, being in poorer health due to lack of access to health care, or needing to live in more violent areas or to pursue riskier occupations.

In addition to contributing to non-interpersonal traumas like disasters and accidents, poverty contributes to the risk for experiencing interpersonal traumatic events as well. For example, child prostitution usually grows out of the family's need for basic resources such as food and shelter for its other members (see Chapter 5). Poor elders or disabled persons may be more at risk for abuse because families or communities may be unable to provide a safe place for them to live and receive care. For these reasons, it is important, and probably cost-effective as well, to include social development as a method for reducing the occurrence of traumatic stress in the first place, in addition to treating individuals and communities after they have been exposed.

Women and girls are at higher risk for certain types of violent encounters, particularly those involving physical or sexual violence that is perpetrated within families. The UN has recognized this increased risk through several initiatives, including the United Nations *Declaration on the Elimination of Violence against Women*, adopted by the General Assembly in 1993. This document defines violence against women as "any act of gender-based violence that results in, or is likely to result in, physical, sexual or psychological harm or suffering to women, including threats of such acts, coercion or arbitrary deprivation of liberty, whether occurring in public or private life" (Article 1 of General Assembly resolution 48/104 of 20, December 1993). States are required to exercise due diligence to prevent, investigate, and punish acts of violence against women. While women are more likely to experience rape and child abuse, men are more likely to encounter extra-familial physical violence and combat (e.g., Kessler, Sonnega, Bromet, Hughes, & Nelson, 1995).

Much of the research on trauma has focused on specific events or finite periods of exposure (e.g., a tour of duty in the military) in which the event or events come to an end and the person is out of actual danger when the health care system intervenes. However, many persons and communities worldwide have a different experience. They suffer from prolonged traumatic stressors such as war, famine, domestic violence, and abuse, as well as from ongoing stressors such as sexual or political oppression, and they face ongoing dangers that are constant and real, and where the likelihood of escape is remote. The sources of such trauma are multiple and complex: disasters and external enemies; violence from within their own communities, homes, and families; and life-threatening health concerns such as malnutrition and the HIV/AIDS epidemic. These disadvantaged communities may be defined regionally, or may represent subgroups within a larger community that are excluded from the mainstream in some way because of race, ethnicity, religion, language, etc. Globalization may also threaten communities with inequality across and within countries as well, with the persistence of poverty and deprivation, and with the weakening of social cohesion (Desai, 2000).

One of the most damaging aspects of traumatic events such as war and disaster for communities is its potential for disrupting existing support networks, leading to isolation and loneliness. With evacuations, failures of communication, and relocation, ties with friends and family are affected, as well as ties with one's home and geographic community; and these disruptions of social networks occur at a time when the need for such networks and support is at its highest (Solomon, 1986). In situations of individual interpersonal trauma such as domestic abuse, the lack of a strong social network may contribute to the opportunity for individuals or families being isolated and victimized. Conversely, strong community and social supports are likely to reduce trauma to individuals, by serving a monitoring function, where community members are aware of the abuse and can intervene, as well as by putting pressure on leaders to develop or enforce laws or prohibitions on abusive behavior. Danieli (1998b) also notes that because culture influences the way traumatic stressors are experienced and responded to, the continuity of culture can play a protective role in facilitating healing. The destruction of culture through war, colonialism, political oppression, and other mechanisms impairs or prevents the healing process in communities and individuals exposed to external traumatic stressors. Indeed, the suppression, loss, or destruction of culture, in and of itself, may be the source of the trauma (Danieli, 1998b).

On the other hand, while communities may provide support and comfort in many circumstances, they may also be sources of additional stress or trauma, or they may interfere with coping and healing. Culture as a source of trauma or stress arises when it imposes rigid norms or standards on subgroups or individuals who deviate in some way from the culture of those in power, as seen recently in Afghanistan. Individuals who have experienced a trauma that is associated with shame in the community (e.g., rape) may find themselves outside of the social protection of the culture; indeed, they may experience devaluation or aggression from those enforcing the culture. The same may be true for those who have values, lifestyles, or customs that are outside the usual or traditional practices.

EMOTIONAL REACTIONS TO TRAUMATIC STRESSORS

Just as more common stressors have behavioral, emotional, and physiological effects on individuals that can lead to emotional distress or physical illness, experiencing traumatic events may have profound effects on the body, and on mental and emotional well-being. While people are remarkably resilient in many ways, and are able to adapt to a wide range of events and circumstances, some of the events described in this book may overload the body and mind's capacity to adapt. While many escape serious problems, coping with extreme stress can take a high toll, requiring more extraordinary strategies and resources than coping with routine stressors, and placing much greater demands on individuals and communities. At the extreme, fear, and subsequent failures at coping and adaptation, can have profound and possibly irreversible effects. Traumatic exposure may cause direct injury to the body, or it may exert its influence on mental health through impaired cognitive, emotional, and behavioral functioning. Severe emotional distress can cause chemical and biological alterations in the brain and in the body's biology and physiology (Friedman, Charney, & Deutch, 1995), which, in turn, may affect general physical health.

The emotional impact of traumatic stressors may also be passed on psychosocially to later generations through families, as, for example, when family members recount events that occurred in the adult generation, behave in certain ways toward their offspring due to their own traumatic experiences, develop certain emotional styles that influence their children, or transmit conscious or unconscious values, fantasies, and beliefs

(Danieli, 1998a). However, children of survivors of traumatic events do not necessarily have more formal psychiatric disorders than others in the community (Levav, 1998; De Jong, 2001a). Intergenerational transmission may also occur through cultural mechanisms, as the young are introduced to oral histories, religious rituals, and traditions that are affected by the group's exposure to a particular traumatic event or series of events (Danieli, 1998a).

Posttraumatic reactions are manifested in a variety of ways, and these differ from one individual to the next. Almost everyone is affected in some way by exposure to very serious and life-threatening events, but only a subset of these will develop ongoing emotional and physical health problems. An even smaller group will actually develop mental disorders. Common reactions to traumatic events in the immediate aftermath include fear, surprise, sadness, shock, anger, helplessness, confusion, and numbness. These often abate in the weeks and months following an event. Table 2.1 (from Young, Ford, Ruzek, Friedman, & Gusman, 1998, p. 110) contains a list of reactions (repeated in Chapter 14) that are commonly seen after stressful and traumatic events have been experienced. They include symptoms in the domains of biological, cognitive, emotional, and psychosocial reactions.

Common symptoms that may last weeks or months, or even longer, following traumatic exposure include being plagued by recurrent and disturbing images and recollections of the trauma that come involuntarily, and that may interrupt normal thought processes. Traumatized individuals

Table 2.1. Common Stress Reactions

Emotional	Biological
Shock	Fatigue
Anger	Insomnia
Disbelief	Hyperarousal
Terror	Somatic complaints
Guilt	Impaired immune response
Grief	Headaches
Irritability	Gastrointestinal problems
Helplessness	Decreased appetite
Despair	Decreased libido
Dissociation	Startle response
Loss of pleasure from regular activities	
Cognitive	*Psychosocial*
Impaired concentration	Alienation
Confusion	Social withdrawal
Distortion	Increased stress with relationships
Intrusive thoughts	Substance abuse
Decreased self-esteem	Vocational/occupational impairment

may dream about the trauma, or even feel that it is happening to them again. They may be particularly sensitive to reminders of the event, like weather conditions, geographic locations, date or time of the year, people who look like perpetrators, or particular sounds or smells associated with the event, including viewing the devastation or aftermath of an event they lived through (e.g., being in a war or disaster zone). They are likely to avoid these reminders if they can, and they may become numb or unresponsive emotionally, unable to enjoy or maintain relationships with loved ones. Individuals may be psychologically and physically aroused following a traumatic event, and thus have trouble sleeping and concentrating, be irritable, be constantly on guard for something else to happen, and react too easily, or overreact, to sudden noises or movements. If a sufficient number of these symptoms occur together in the same person for a sufficient period of time, a diagnosis of posttraumatic stress disorder (PTSD), an anxiety disorder, may be given. This diagnosis is described in the international classification systems (ICD-10, World Health Organization, 1992; DSM-IV, American Psychiatric Association [APA], 1994). Experiencing traumatic events has also been associated with a range of other mental health problems such as depression, other types of anxiety, and substance abuse (Green, 1994). Moreover, exposure to traumatic events and trauma-related disorders may be associated with considerable functional impairment and disability, and with physical health symptoms (e.g., Schnurr & Green, in press; also see below). However, as noted, most people who are exposed to traumatic events do not develop full-blown psychiatric disorders.

Repeated traumatization, especially that which is deliberately perpetrated and involves situations of "captivity" (such as torture, child abuse, or domestic violence), may lead to additional symptoms and complaints. These include chronic somatic symptoms, difficulty regulating and controlling emotions, impaired personal relationships, and prolonged symptoms of dissociation (an alteration in how one experiences the external world or oneself, such as feeling that time is moving very slowly, feeling like a robot, forgetting parts of the experience, or feeling detached from one's body) (e.g., Herman, 1992).

A recent study of the general population of the United States (Kessler et al., 1995) indicated that about half had been exposed to some type of traumatic event in their lifetime, and that 8% of individuals between the ages of 15 and 55 have developed PTSD at some point. In a large epidemiologic study of refugees, internally displaced persons, and post-conflict survivors from Algeria, Cambodia, Ethiopia, and Gaza, using the same instrument, De Jong and colleagues (2001) found rates of PTSD ranging from 16%–38%, or double to quadruple those in the US. However, rates of exposure to severe interpersonal violence were higher in those survivors as well. Exposure to violence, type of violence, and demographic factors varied across samples, as did specific risk factors for disorder. Conflict-related events after the age of 12 were significantly related to PTSD in all four samples. Other studies focusing on specific samples of trauma survivors around the world, such as those surviving terrorist attacks, civil wars, rape, abuse, and torture, also report these higher (that is, compared to the general population) rates of PTSD, sometimes reaching 25–60% of survivors in given trauma-exposed populations (e.g., De Girolamo & McFarlane, 1996; Green, 1994; Kessler et al., 1995). More details about prevalence of the different types of traumatic events, and rates of PTSD and other disorders associated with specific types of events, are described in the following chapters of this book.

RISK FACTORS FOR REACTIONS TO TRAUMA

Individuals at greatest risk for chronic emotional problems following traumatic events include those with poorer social support, those who are divorced or widowed, those with comparatively lower education and income, with other current family stressors, with more previous exposure to traumatic stressors, and more previous mental health problems, in addition to those whose trauma was more severe (e.g., Brewin, Andrews, & Valentine, 2000; Kessler et al., 1999). While most individuals exposed to traumatic events do not develop PTSD or other psychiatric disorders, risk factors for developing PTSD have been documented in the historical, family, genetic, biological, and psychosocial domains. Higher rates of psychiatric disorder are associated with low economic status in developed and developing countries alike (e.g., Araya, Rojas, Fritsch, Acuna, & Lewis, 2001; Holzer et al., 1986; WHO International Consortium in Psychiatric Epidemiology, 2000). This may be explained, at least in part, by the higher levels of day-to-day stressors experienced by these individuals, a factor linked to the development and persistence of mental disorders (see Chapter 3). On the other hand, comparing psychiatric epidemiology studies in low and high-income countries, De Jong (2001b) found few differences in rates of disorder. This suggests that the risk factors just discussed may operate primarily within settings or cultures, or that those differences in exposure from one country to the next cancel out income differences.

Many studies have also indicated that women have higher rates of PTSD, rates that are about twice those found in men (e.g., Kessler et al., 1995). It has been suggested that this may be due to the fact that mental disorders are associated with being poor, and the poor tend to be women and children. Moreover, women tend to be more highly exposed to violence and oppression, and to events, like rape, that are associated with high rates of PTSD (Kessler et al., 1999). However, controlling for type of exposure did not eliminate gender differences. An additional, and not mutually exclusive, explanation lies in the distribution of mental disorders between men and women. In most studies, women are found to have higher rates of mood disorders (i.e., depression) and anxiety disorders than men, while men are more likely to be substance abusers (e.g., Kessler et al., 1994; WHO International Consortium in Psychiatric Epidemiology, 2000). Thus, PTSD, because it is an anxiety disorder, would be expected to be more prevalent in women. However, this relationship with gender does not always hold. For example, De Jong et al. (2001) found expected gender differences in PTSD rates (i.e., women with more PTSD) in Cambodia and Algeria; however, they found no gender differences in Ethiopia, and, in Gaza, men had more PTSD. These findings are more supportive of the notion of differential exposure. Those authors indicated that the men from Ethiopia and Gaza were more likely to have been involved in conflict situations than the women, and had experienced more torture and trauma during their flights from their countries of origin. Thus, the issue is a complicated one, in all likelihood with multiple and overlapping explanations.

It is important to reiterate that the nature of the exposure plays a critical role, especially when the trauma is severe and repeated. Ongoing, chronic exposure, especially to trauma that is perpetrated interpersonally, rather than being an impersonal act of nature, confers the highest risk for ongoing negative consequences (Green, 1994, Green et al., 2000).

PHYSICAL HEALTH CONSEQUENCES

In addition to direct physical harm and emotional distress, experiencing traumatic stressors is also associated with a wide range of adverse physical health outcomes. Research has linked exposure to traumatic events with the experience or perception of poor health, as well as with poorer daily functioning and physical limitations, chronic medical conditions, and physician diagnoses (Green & Kimerling, in press).

For example, in a follow-up study of Norwegian concentration camp survivors, Eitenger (1973) found that Holocaust survivors, on average, were sicker, were more often sick, and aged and died earlier than refugees who had not been in the camps. In populations with access to regular medical care, history of trauma has been shown to predict more use of physician services and higher health care costs. Studies in the United States have linked exposure to childhood trauma such as sexual and physical abuse with health outcomes in very large samples (e.g., Felitti et al., 1998). History of traumatic childhood experiences was associated with poorer health in general, with greater functional disability, and with more physical distress. Patients with trauma histories received more diagnoses for medical and psychiatric disorders, including obesity, cancer, heart disease, and other chronic illnesses, and reported more suicide attempts. Further, childhood trauma histories were associated with more smoking and substance abuse, as well as other risky behaviors with health consequences, such as early pregnancy, number of sexual partners over one's lifetime, and sexually transmitted diseases.

Gender-based violence and fear of abuse has also been linked to gynecological disorders, unsafe abortion, pregnancy complications, miscarriage, low birth weight, and pelvic inflammatory disease; and women in abusive situations may be at risk for unwanted pregnancy and sexually transmitted diseases, including HIV/AIDS (Heise, Ellsberg, & Gottemoeller, 2000).

Findings of increased negative health outcomes are similar to those in war veterans, whose combat experiences are associated with physical health complaints and conditions, and with physician-diagnosed medical disorders as well (Green & Kimerling, in press). Several studies have examined complex models of the relationship between trauma and physical health, and have indicated that psychiatric disorders commonly associated with exposure to severe trauma, like depression and PTSD, are important links (Schnurr & Green, in press; Schnurr & Jankowski, 1999). Some of the negative behaviors that may follow trauma, like increased smoking or alcohol use, have adverse health consequences as well, and may be an additional pathway between experiencing a trauma and developing health problems or chronic health conditions. Some of the same mechanisms are likely to be operating in low-income countries as well, particularly if the exposed populations have poorer health to begin with, and less access to regular health care.

CULTURAL ISSUES

We make the assumption in this volume that traumatic stressors, like having one's life threatened, losing family members violently, and being injured, would be disturbing to almost everyone—that these types of experiences are universally distressing. On the other hand, specific types of events may be differentially traumatic across cultures, and the way in which specific losses and stressors are perceived and processed may vary depending on the culture of the individual and the community. For example, a recent study of Tibetan refugees in India showed that the experiences rated as most traumatic were those associated with religion (e.g., destruction of religious signs), rather than the life-threatening experiences named above, although those were rated as very traumatic as well (Terheggen, Stroebe, & Kleber, 2001). In Buddhist and African cultures with a belief in reincarnation, the loss of a family member may have a different impact. The loss of an older loved person with children and some accumulated wealth can be acceptable in African animist cultures, since the person will travel to the reign of the ancestors and occupy an intermediary position between the living and the dead. On the other hand, the death of a child in the same culture is a disaster. Similarly, political conviction may be an important factor in grief or mourning as has been described in Gaza or among Albanian Kosovar families, where a deceased family member may be regarded as a martyr. Such conviction may alleviate the loss, yet it may also complicate the mourning process. Even exposure to the grotesque (Green, 1993) can be mediated by religious convictions such as the role of karma in Buddhism in Asia or divine persecution during the Holocaust (De Jong, 2002). There are also cultural variations in how distress is expressed (see below). Further, the culturally shared values and beliefs of community members may affect how the events impact the community as a whole, as well as its capacity to respond. For example, De Vries (1995) gives an example of the expansion of a traditional medical system to accommodate and respond to a new threat. Raids from another tribe, the Masai, were causing distress among the Digo of the East African coast. Sometimes this distress was expressed in ad hoc trance dances. Eventually, the traditional healers gave this specific distress a name, and incorporated it within the traditional healing rituals, formalizing the dances, which were then used to relieve the distress.

It is notable that most of the work systematically documenting responses to traumatic events has been conducted in Western and industrialized societies, where values tend toward autonomy and individualization. Therefore, descriptions of outcomes following traumatic events in the literature are culturally bound. In the developing world, interdependency of community and family are often more highly valued. People from traditional cultures are more likely to perceive themselves as part of a larger whole; and they may view illness and trauma to be externally caused and ongoing, and thus linked to the larger society (De Vries, 1995). These differing worldviews are important to incorporate into planned interventions in order for them to be accepted and useful. It is possible that community level responses to traumatic events (like rituals and public ceremonies) would be relatively more effective and appropriate for traditional societies or cultures, while individual interventions (like psychotherapy) may be better suited, or more accepted, for psychosocial problems in industrialized nations , although each presumably has its place in each setting. Spirituality or religion may play a larger role in non-Western cultures as well (De Vries, 1995; Terheggen et al., 2001), and may provide an important avenue for intervention.

Cultures may place differing emphasis on particular symptoms, assign unique meanings to the stressor experience and its intensity, or to the expression of distress, and shape the general tone of emotional life to which a person should aspire, making it difficult to distinguish among moods, reactions, symptoms, and disorders (Kirmayer, 1996; Manson, 1997; Van Ommeren et al., 1999). Research has documented many of these cultural variations, including the ways in which causes of symptoms are perceived, the nature of the illness, onset patterns, symptom expression, extent of disability, course, and outcome (Marsella & Yamada, 2000). These cultural variations have implications for cross-cultural research in the areas of use of Western diagnostic instruments, inclusion of local idioms of distress, culturally appropriate translation, and standardized use of exclusionary and skip rules of diagnostic instruments (De Jong, 2002) With regard to responses to traumatic events, somatic and dissociative symptoms in particular may have quite different meanings depending on their cultural context. Kirmayer (1996) has identified several ways in which Western systems of classification are problematic with regard to somatically expressed distress. First, separating physical symptoms from emotional distress reflects distinctions that are not made in all cultures. Second, in many cultures, physical or somatic symptoms and attributions are commonly used as "idioms of distress," or folk categories, to convey a wide range of personal and social concerns that may or may not have anything to do with individual distress or mental disorder. Third, the nature and scope of physical symptoms, theoretically and in illness models, varies considerably across cultures (Kirmayer, 1996). The range of physical symptoms associated with mental distress is much wider than is commonly recognized in Western models. However, the effects of traumatic exposure on physical health just discussed suggest that the separation of the physical from the emotional is probably artificial even in Western cultures.

Dissociative symptoms, as well, take very different forms in different cultures. While they are often described as indicating more severe distress or pathology in Western cultures, they are commonly part of religious and healing cults that offer oppressed groups (often women) an avenue for protest and a measure of power or leverage within relationships, or these may be sanctioned as coping strategies in times of stress (Kirmayer, 1996). Cultural factors also may influence the propensity to dissociate as a response to stress. In societies where individuals receive practice in dissociation in religious or artistic performances, or where it is appropriate or expected to experience trance, these experiences are less likely to be indicators of disorder than in societies where such experiences are not encouraged (Kirmayer, 1996). In situations of massive stress in developing countries, large numbers of people may show symptoms of dissociation, varying from individual possession as an "idiom of distress" to classical fugue states and epidemics of mass psychogenic illness. In these countries one often still sees the classical dissociative phenomena described by Janet or Freud (De Jong, 2002).

Cultural practices may also be the conveyer of traumatic experiences for certain of its members. Indeed, culturally sanctioned practices (e.g., female genital mutilation, as it is called outside of countries in which it is practiced, dowry death, or oppression of women through intimidation and physical violence) may be directly perceived as traumatic stressors by some of those who experience them. In some cases, outsiders, including those who are preparing to intervene following a catastrophe, or to aid those undergoing these practices, may see them as violations of human rights. Anthropologists and others struggle with how to reconcile clashes between "cultural relativity" and universal understandings of human rights. Attempting to avoid ethnocentrism, those intervening in other, dissimilar, cultures may appropriately acknowledge and embrace cultural differences, as we have just suggested. Yet when cultural practices result in differential treatment of certain subgroups within a society (women, the poor, minorities, indigenous groups), outsiders may reasonably raise questions about who benefits from these traditions (Nagengast, 1997). Nagengast suggests that while the *concept* of human rights applies to everyone, the actual content is more ambiguous, with historical, economic, and political considerations. She concludes that, for the time being, it is better to "promote dialogue such that universal values capable of insuring the integrity of all humans emerge" (p. 363).

Like Nagengast, we do not pretend to have good answers in situations where human rights and cultural sensitivities seem to clash, and dialogue about these difficult issues must be continued. These are extremely difficult and sensitive areas, requiring even higher degrees of thoughtfulness and planning than culturally specific interventions in general. For all of the reasons just discussed, the cultural context of the traumatic exposure, and reactions to it, need to be a starting point for the exploration and integration of any intervention that hopes to succeed.

While the effects of individual and community trauma may be profound, appropriate and timely interventions may prevent some of the worst effects or may shorten their impact. Some of the immediate impacts of traumatic exposure may be unavoidable; however, many of the long-term impacts can be prevented. It is these prevention and early intervention strategies that are addressed in the present volume, first, in a general context (See Chapter 4), and then, as associated with each different type of trauma.

REFERENCES

American Psychiatric Association (1994). *Diagnostic and statistical manual of mental disorders* (4th ed.). Washington, DC: Author.

Araya, R., Rojas, G., Fritsch, R., Acuna, J., & Lewis, G. (2001). Santiago Mental Disorders Survey: Prevalence and risk factors. *British Journal of Psychiatry, 178*, 228–233.

Brewin, C.R., Andrews, B., & Valentine, J.D. (2000). Meta-analysis of risk factors for post-traumatic stress disorder in trauma-exposed adults. *Journal of Consulting and Clinical Psychology, 68*, 748–766.

Danieli, Y. (1998a). Introduction. In Y. Danieli (Ed.), *International handbook of multigenerational legacies of trauma*. New York: Plenum.

Danieli, Y. (1998b). Conclusions and future directions. In Y. Danieli (Ed.), *International handbook of multigenerational legacies of trauma*. New York: Plenum.

De Girolamo, G., & McFarlane, A. (1996). The epidemiology of PTSD: A comprehensive review of the international literature. In A.J. Marsella, M.J. Friedman, E.T. Gerrity, & R.M. Scurfield (Eds.). *Ethnocultural aspects of posttraumatic stress disorder: Issues, research, and clinical applications* (pp. 33–85). Washington, D.C.: American Psychological Association.

De Jong, J.T.V.M. (2001a). Psychiatric problems related to persecution and refugee status. In F. Henn, N. Sartorius, H. Helmchen, & H. Lauter (Eds.), *Contemporary psychiatry, Vol 2: Psychiatry in special situations* (pp. 279–298). Berlin, Heidelberg, New York, Tokyo: Springer.

De Jong, J.T.V.M. (2001b). Remnants of the colonial past: The difference in outcome of mental disorders in high- and low-income countries. In D. Bhugra & R. Littlewood (Eds.), *Colonialism and mental health*. New Delhi: Oxford University Press.

De Jong, J.T.V.M., Komproe, I.H., Van Ommeren, M., El Masri, M., Mesfin, A., Khaled, N., Van de Put, W.A.M., & Somasundaram, D. (2001). Lifetime events and posttraumatic stress disorder in 4 postconflict settings. *Journal of the American Medical Association, 286*, 555–562.

De Jong, J.T.V.M. (2002). Public mental health, traumatic stress and human rights violations in low-income countries. A culturally appropriate model in times of conflict, disaster and peace. In J.T.V.M. de Jong (Ed.) (2002) *Trauma, war, and violence: Public mental health in socio-cultural context*. New York: Kluwer/Plenum.

De Vries, M.W. (1995). Culture, community and catastrophe: Issues in understanding communities under difficult conditions. In S.E. Hobfoll & M.W. De Vries (Eds.), *Extreme stress and communities: Impact and intervention*. Dordrect/Boston/London: Kluwer. In cooperation with NATO Scientific Affairs Division.

Desai, N. (2000, September). *Statement to the General Assembly of the United Nations* (Second and Third Committees), 55th session.

Eitenger, L. (1973). A follow-up study of Norwegian concentration camp survivors: Mortality and morbidity. *The Israeli Annals of Psychiatry and Related Disciplines, 11*, 199–209.

Felliti, V.J., Anda, R.E., Nordenberg, D., Williamson, D.F., Spitz, A.M., Edwards, V., Koss, M.P., & Marks, J.S. (1998). Relationship of childhood abuse and household dysfunction to many of the leading causes of death in adults. *American Journal of Preventive Medicine, 14*, 245–258.

Friedman, M.J., Charney, D.S., & Deutch, A.Y. (Eds.) (1995). *Neurobiological and clinical consequences of stress*. Philadelphia: Lippincott-Raven.

Green, B.L. (1993). Identifying survivors at risk: Trauma and stressors across events. In J.P. Wilson & B. Raphael (Eds.), *International handbook of traumatic stress syndromes*. (pp. 135–144). New York: Plenum.

Green, B.L. (1994). Psychosocial research in traumatic stress: An update. *Journal of Traumatic Stress, 7*, 341–362.

Green, B.L., Goodman, L.A., Krupnick, J.L., Corcoran, C.B., Petty, R.M., Stockton, P., & Stern, N.M. (2000). Outcomes of single versus multiple trauma exposure in a screening sample. *Journal of Traumatic Stress, 13*, 271–286.

Green, B.L., & Kimerling, R. (in press). Trauma, PTSD, and health status. In P.P. Schnurr & B.L. Green (Eds.), *Trauma and health: Physical health consequences of exposure to extreme stress*. Washington, DC: American Psychological Association.

Heise, L., Ellsberg, M., & Gottemoeller, M. (2000). Ending violence against women. In *Population reports*. Published by Johns Hopkins Center for Communication Programs, with support from the US Agency for International Development.

Herman, J.L. (1992). Complex PTSD: A syndrome in survivors of prolonged and repeated trauma. *Journal of Traumatic Stress, 5*(3), 377–391.

Hobfoll, S.E. (1991). Traumatic stress: A theory based on rapid loss of resources. *Anxiety Research, 4*, 187–197.

Holzer, C.E. III, Shea, B.M., Swanson, J.W., Leaf, P.J., Myers, J.K., George, L., Weissman, M.M., & Bednarski, P. (1986). The increased risk for specific psychiatric disorders among persons of low socioeconomic status. *American Journal of Social Psychiatry, 6*, 259–271.

International Federation of Red Cross and Red Crescent Societies (2002). *World disasters report 2002*. Bloomfield, CT: Kumarian Press, Inc.

Kessler, R.C., McGonagle, K.A., Zhao, S., Nelson, C.B., Hughes, M., Eshleman, S., Wittchen, H.U., & Kendler, K.S. (1994). Lifetime and 12 month prevalence of DSM-III-R psychiatric disorders in the United States. *Archives of General Psychiatry, 51*, 8–19.

Kessler, B.C., Sonnega, A., Bromet, E., Hughes, M., & Nelson, C.B. (1995). Posttraumatic stress disorder in the National Comorbidity Survey. *Archives of General Psychiatry, 52*, 1048–1060.

Kessler, B.C., Sonnega, A., Bromet, E., Hughes, M., Nelson, C.B., & Breslau, N. (1999). Epidemiological risk factors for trauma and PTSD. In R. Yehuda (Ed.), *Risk factors for posttraumatic stress disorder* (pp. 23–59). Washington, DC: American Psychiatric Press.

Kirmayer, L.J. (1996). Confusion of the senses: Implications of ethnocultural variations in somatoform and dissociative disorders for PTSD. In A.J. Marsella, M.J. Friedman, E.T. Gerrity, & R.M. Scurfield (Eds.), *Ethnocultural aspects of posttraumatic stress disorder: Issues, research, and clinical applications*. Washington, DC: American Psychological Association.

Levav, I. (1998). Individuals under conditions of maximum adversity: The Holocaust. In B.P. Dohrenwend (Ed.), *Adversity, stress and psychopathology*. New York: Oxford University Press.

Manson, S.M. (1997). Cross-cultural and multiethnic assessment of trauma. In J.P. Wilson & T.M. Keane (Eds.), *Assessing psychological trauma and PTSD* (pp. 239–265). New York: Guilford.

Marsella, A.J., & Yamada, A.M. (2000). Culture and mental health: An introduction and overview of foundations, concepts, and issues. In I. Cuellar & F. Paniagua (Eds.), *The handbook of multicultural mental health: Assessment and treatment of diverse populations*. New York: Academic Press.

Nagengast, C. (1997). Women, minorities, and indigenous peoples: Universalism and cultural relativity. *Journal of Anthropological Research, 53*, 349–369.

Pearlin, L.I. (1982). The social contexts of stress. In L. Goldberger & S. Breznitz (Eds.), *Handbook of stress: Theoretical and clinical aspects*. New York: The Free Press.

Schnurr, P.P., & Green, B.L. (in press). Understanding relationships among trauma, PTSD, and health outcomes. In P.P. Schnurr & B.L. Green (Eds.), *Trauma and health: Physical health consequences of exposure to extreme stress*. Washington, DC: American Psychological Association.

Schnurr, P.P., & Jankowski, M.K. (1999). Physical health and posttraumatic stress disorder: Review and synthesis. *Seminars in Clinical Neuropsychiatry, 4,* 295–304.

Solomon, S. (1986). Mobilizing social support networks in times of disaster. In C.F. Figley (Ed.), *Trauma and its wake: volume II: Traumatic stress theory, research, and intervention* (pp. 232–263). New York: Brunner/Mazel.

Terheggen, M.A., Stroebe, M.S., & Kleber, R.J. (2001). Western conceptualization and Eastern experience: A cross-cultural study of traumatic stress reactions among Tibetan refugees in India. *Journal of Traumatic Stress, 14,* 391–403.

Turner, R.J., Wheaton, B., & Lloyd, D.A. (1995). The epidemiology of social stress. *American Sociology Review, 60,* 104–125.

United Nations Article 1, of General Assembly resolution 48/104 of 20, December, 1993.

Van der Kolk, B. (1987). *Psychological trauma*. Washington, DC: American Psychiatric Press.

Van Ommeren, M., Sharma, B., Thapa, S., Makaju, R., Prasain, D., Bhattarai, R. & De Jong, J. (1999). Preparing instruments for transcultural research: Use of the Translation Monitoring Form with Nepali-speaking Bhutanese Refugees. *Transcultural Psychiatry, 36,* 285–301.

WHO International Consortium in Psychiatric Epidemiology (2000). Cross-national comparisons of the prevalences and correlates of mental disorders. *Bulletin of the World Health Organization, 78,* 413–426.

World Health Organization (1992). *The ICD-10 classification of mental and behavioral disorders: Clinical descriptions and guidelines*. Geneva: Author.

Young, B.H., Ford, J.D., Ruzek, J.I., Friedman, M.J., & Gusman, F.D. (1998). *Disaster mental health services: A guidebook for clinicians and administrators*. Palo Alto, CA/White River Junction, VT: National Center for PTSD.

Chapter 3

Social Deprivation

Ellen L. Bassuk and Brigid Donelan

With Bukelwa Selema, Salma Ali, Adriana Cavalcanti de Aguiar, Evelyn Eisenstein, Panos Vostanis, Elena Varavikova, and Madeleine Tashjian

More than half the global population is extremely poor. Many live in substandard housing, can't read, earn barely enough to feed themselves and their families, and have few opportunities to better their circumstances. Their struggle to survive is often compounded by feelings of helplessness, terror, and despair. Although most of these people are remarkably resilient, exposure to persistent stressors and traumas wears down the spirit and depletes even the hardiest person's resources.

Homelessness, hunger, poor health, illiteracy, and unemployment have high psychological costs. When these are associated with social exclusion, marginalization, and social disintegration, life is filled with even more uncertainty. Marginalized in society without the basic resources to escape, people in these circumstances are vulnerable to further traumatization and must develop unusual coping strategies to survive. Within this context, individuals are more likely to develop physical and mental health problems, and, by extension, families and communities are affected as well.

This chapter describes the context for the social and humanitarian crises that many people in the world experience. Persistent poverty and social deprivation increase the likelihood that many of the traumatic events described in this book will occur. This chapter describes the circumstances in which half the global population lives by defining social deprivation, describing factors that contribute to it, and discussing its varied dimensions. These living conditions translate into individual and societal stress, and eventually to the erosion of social mores. Since the majority of people living in these circumstances are women, special attention will be focused on their plight.

WHAT IS SOCIAL DEPRIVATION?

The economic dimension of social deprivation is easily seen. People struggle daily to eat, clothe, and shelter themselves and their families. *Economic deprivation* is mirrored in a hungry child, a homeless family, or an unemployed man. Extremely poor people face persistent hardships that compromise their physical, social, and mental well-being. *Social deprivation* extends far beyond economic factors, however. People who are socially deprived lack freedom of choice, opportunity, political voice, and dignity. They experience barriers to full participation in community life. Frequently, through a process of oppression and domination, they are denied the most basic human rights to food and housing; education and work, health and safety, and an equal share in the benefits of social progress. Left with minimal opportunity, they struggle to survive and are exposed to a wide range of stressors.

Nobel Prize-winning economist Amartya Sen (1997) summarized social deprivation as **"a deprivation of basic capabilities due to a lack of freedom, rather than merely low income."** In addition to political freedom and economic opportunity, individuals need social opportunities that ensure the substantive freedom to live better. Sen concluded that the lack of freedom experienced by extremely poor people extends beyond economic and political factors to social and interpersonal factors.

It is important to note that economic deprivation (i.e., severe poverty) may occur without its extension into the social arena and without an evident power differential. Similarly, it is possible for social deprivation to occur without poverty. However, for the purpose of this chapter, we are discussing a gradient of experiences of oppression that lead to varying degrees of disempowerment, subjugation, and marginalization. Relationships and cultural/religious traditions may be protective, but oppression can overwhelm these buffers and, in some cases, provide the justification for the continuation of poor conditions. These conditions may range from inherent systemic constraints that isolate a group within the broader community and reduce its opportunities, to outright racism, sexism and, at its extreme, genocidal activities that are socially sanctioned.

Regardless of the cause, social deprivation is often psychologically devastating, and can result in the creation of an underclass. What has been written about some Americans living in ghettos may be true of marginalized city dwellers worldwide:

> Here is a youngster to whom one says, "Why don't you marry the girl you got pregnant? Instead of standing on the street corner hustling, why don't you go to the community college and learn how to run one of those machines in the hospital? You could learn that with a couple of years at the community college instead of being a misfit," and the answer is not, "I have done my sums and the course you suggest simply does not pay." Instead, his answer is, "Who, me?" He cannot see himself thus.
> ... Ghetto dwellers ... are a people apart, susceptible to stereotyping, ridiculed for their cultural styles, isolated socially, experiencing an internalized sense of helplessness and despair, with limited access to communal networks of mutual assistance.... (Loury, 1999, p. 15). In the face of their despair, violence, and self-destructive behavior, it is morally obtuse and scientifically naïve to argue that if "those people" would just get their acts together we would not have such a horrific problem ... (Loury, 1999, p. 16). Social processes encourage the development of self-destructive behavior. This is not to say that individuals have no responsibility for the wrong choices they may make. Instead, it is to recognize a deep dilemma, one that does not leave us with any good choices.... (Loury, 1999, p. 27).

Unequal distribution of opportunities, particularly among social groups, has also been described as "structural violence" (Galtung, 1969; 1975). Such violence is seen to have three interrelated dimensions: poverty (deprivation of basic material needs); repression (deprivation of human rights); and alienation (deprivation of higher needs). These deprivations may be measured in terms of loss of life years, or life expectancy. They may also combine with cultural violence to foster direct interpersonal violence, with injury and loss of life. Cultural violence is evident when a culture teaches and justifies repression or other forms of structural violence until they become part of "how things are" in a given setting (Galtung, 1990). Galtung proposes cultural violence as the third corner of a "violence triangle"—consisting of structural violence (a social process), direct violence (an event), and cultural violence (an ongoing belief or attitude that provides the rationale for the other two). Thus, "with the violent structure institutionalized, and the violent culture internalized, direct violence also tends to become institutionalized, repetitive, ritualistic ... " (Galtung, 1990, p. 302).

Because much of this book focuses on the experiences of direct violence, the concept of structural violence is a useful link to the more general social conditions that may serve as the context for these more direct forms of violence. The elements that make up this social structure, especially poverty and its correlates, are described herein.

WHEN DOES SOCIAL DEPRIVATION OCCUR?

Social deprivation occurs when there is a power differential in which something has been denied or taken away from one party by another. It results in one group being excluded or subordinated, and left with fewer opportunities for advancement and growth, with the dominant group viewing the other group as different and, therefore, inferior. It carries a moral judgment that justifies bias and discrimination and precludes equality—conditions that justify the differential use of power. Social deprivation may occur at an individual level, but social systems that sanction oppression of a group by a dominant group by virtue of race, ethnicity, gender, religion, sexual orientation, disability, or other differences are usually the purveyors. Although individual relationships and cultural customs are often protective against traumatic stressors, which routinely arise under conditions of social deprivation, these relationships and customs may also contribute to social deprivation.

The growing gap between rich and poor worldwide provides the economic context for social deprivation and is often accompanied by colonialism, militarism, racism, and the subjugation of women. Poor, disenfranchised people living in these circumstances are more likely to be subjected to dramatically disruptive events, to chronic hardships and stress, and to repeated violence and trauma. Because this gap carries with it a lack of opportunity and freedom of choice, it extends into the arena of social deprivation.

Studies have shown that people living in poverty experience more violence and other stressors than those with better economic circumstances (e.g., Durkin, Davidson, Kuhn, O'Connor, & Barlow, 1994; McLeod & Kessler, 1990; Turner, Wheaton, & Lloyd, 1995). Sources of stress are multiple and complex: disasters and external enemies, frequently expressed as racism, sexism, and xenophobia; violence from within communities, homes, and families; and bodily threats, including the HIV epidemic. Unrelenting traumatic stress is interwoven into the social fabric of society and the routine of daily life for many people worldwide. The danger is constant, real, and inescapable, with only a remote possibility of change.

When oppression takes the form of violence as a social practice that is tolerated and even sanctioned, people can be victimized because of their membership in a particular group. The *Human Development Report 2000* (United Nations Development Programme [UNDP], 2000) describes how violence against minority groups is "a burning political issue" worldwide. It describes, for example, how immigrants and minorities in the

15 countries of the European Union experience racism and xenophobia—conditions giving rise to violent attacks, intimidation, and discrimination. Minorities live with the "daily knowledge shared by all members of oppressed groups that they are liable to violation, solely on account of their group identity" (Young, 1990, p. 62). Systemic violence at its most extreme can result in extermination of the group. In such a case, society itself is the purveyor of trauma.

In addition to random violence, interpersonal violence among those known to each other is pervasive in poor communities. Interpersonal violence—especially against women—has become a growing public health problem worldwide. Domestic violence is a common form of gender violence (see Chapter 8), and is especially pernicious since it is perpetrated by intimates. Home and close relationships do not provide expected safety, protection, and security; instead, social supports become threatening, betraying, and dangerous. Children trapped in these circumstances often manifest serious post-trauma responses (see Chapter 5).

The specter of catastrophic health problems among economically deprived populations compounds this bleak picture. With the galloping progression of the AIDS epidemic and limited access to health care, especially in places such as Sub-Saharan Africa, one may no longer be safe even from one's own body. For those with no place to turn, living in persistently oppressive conditions that threaten their lives may render them powerless. It may not be possible for them to take charge and make significant changes.

A universal response to acute and persistent threat is to seek help through close relationships, cultural traditions, and community structures. Researchers have established the importance of social supports as a buffer for stressful life events, and as a mediating factor in the development of mental and physical illness. Such supports are a powerful predictor of adjustment and well-being. They include tangible aids such as goods and services, the transaction of empathy and concern within interpersonal relationships, the provision of critical information and advice, and powerful shared beliefs in religion and cultural traditions. Researchers have shown that poor people are more vulnerable to the negative mental and physical health consequences of stress (Kessler, Turner, & House, 1989; McLeod & Kessler, 1990). Obviously, those who are poorer have fewer resources to cope with stressful life events. They often live in unsafe situations and cannot provide adequate protection for themselves or their families—and their support network may be equally stressed. When the societal structures that anchor people, and foster family and community cohesiveness, are eroded or overwhelmed by societal threat, people can no longer rely on these supports to mediate stress and buffer chronic crises.

Similar to individuals, social organizations and cultural groups may become distressed and disintegrate under the pressures of extreme and persistent social deprivation, as well as prolonged and inescapable violence and trauma:

> Culture is supposed to render life predictable. When the cultural defense mechanisms are lost, individuals are left on their own to achieve emotional control . . . Traditional systems break down and a conservative element often takes hold. Ethnicity, nationalism, tribalism, and fundamentalism become means of survival; all of these are regressive moves to release individuals behaviorally and ideologically from an intolerable complexity that cannot be managed in a more productive way. When culture as the identity-giver fails, other models of identity formation and social group formation take its place. The roles and status that had previously organized the system may have no further meaning. (De Vries, 1996, p. 407).

These processes are often reflected by the disempowerment of adult men, the emergence of predatory teenage gangs, and increased violence against women. When communities fragment, elders, mature nonviolent men, and women no longer occupy positions of power and influence. Instead, the community, driven out of its ecological niche, is overtaken by an ethic of male dominance, militarism, and conflict. Within this context, a cycle of increasing violence erodes familiar societal structures, and safe relationships are no longer available.

Journalist Percy Qoboza captured the breakdown in relationships and socially sanctioned roles when he described the effects of fighting against apartheid on the youth of his country—the internalization of violence that can take hold even when fighting a "just war":

> If it is true that a people's wealth is its children, then South Africa is bitterly, tragically poor. If it is true that a nation's future is its children, we have no future and deserve none . . . . (We) are a nation at war with its future . . . for we have turned our children into a generation of fighters, battle-hardened soldiers who will never know the carefree joy of childhood. What we are witnessing is the growth of a generation that has the courage to reject the cowardice of its parents . . . . There is a dark, terrible beauty in that courage. It is also a source of great pride—pride that we, who have lived under apartheid, can produce children who refuse to do so. But it is also a source of great shame . . . that (this) is our heritage to our children: the knowledge of how to die, and how to kill (Qoboza, 1986, p. 1).

The twin legacies of direct and structural violence, both with their roots in apartheid, may underlie South Africa's continuing struggle with high rates of crime.

DIMENSIONS OF SOCIAL DEPRIVATION: POVERTY AND ITS OUTCOMES

The power differential resulting in disparity in the access and distribution of resources, in control over production, and in participation in the economic and political institutions that oversee these processes, are the hallmarks of poverty. This section begins by defining poverty, followed by a review of how the unprecedented worldwide growth of the income gap reflects a growing power differential among groups of people and increasing systemic oppression. The cascading effects of economic deprivation into the social arena are described in the subsequent section. Because poverty limits opportunity disproportionately for women, the devastating consequences on family and children are described in this chapter's final section.

Nature and Extent of Poverty

Income Poverty. Poverty is usually defined in narrow economic terms, most commonly as *income poverty*. This generally refers to cash household income that falls below a certain defined standard. *Extreme poverty* is a form of income poverty in which individuals are unable to meet even basic food needs. An estimated one billion people live in extreme poverty, with many going hungry every day. *Absolute poverty*, often used interchangeably with extreme poverty, is a fixed standard usually used for comparative purposes. Though progress has been made in recent years, income poverty is still a massive problem:

- Almost a quarter of the world's inhabitants—1.3 billion people—live in absolute poverty, surviving on less than US $1 per day. The largest proportion of people living in absolute poverty reside in Africa, where 46% live on less than US $1 per day (World Bank, 1999).
- Over 500 million people in Southeast Asia live in absolute poverty (World Bank, 1999).
- When the poverty line is increased to US $2 per day, 56% of people in developing nations—approximately 2.8 billion people—live in poverty (World Bank, 1999).
- Industrial nations are not immune, with up to 17% of their populations living in income poverty (UNDP, 1998).

Recently, the United Nations Development Programme (1997) coined the term *human poverty* to reflect a broader understanding of poverty that extends beyond pure economics. This definition, consistent with the description of social deprivation presented in this chapter, includes the denial of choices and access to opportunity. It initially consists of three indicators: deprivation of survival; deprivation of knowledge; and lack of a decent standard of living.

Income Gap.   As we enter the new millennium, economic activity worldwide has grown considerably by almost any measure. However, the scale of inequality has reached unprecedented proportions, emphasizing how the rewards of globalization have been inequitably realized:

- The richest top fifth of countries have 86% of the Gross Domestic Product (GDP); the bottom fifth have just 1% (Mandela, 2000).
- The richest top fifth command 82% of the world's export markets and 68% of foreign direct investment; the bottom fifth command just 1% of each (UNDP, 1999).
- Poorer countries, in which nearly four-fifths of the world's population lives, consume only one-quarter of the global yield (Morrison & Tsipis, 1999, p. 139).
- Among Western industrialized nations, the US has the greatest and most rapidly growing income gap: the top 20% of US households receive 50% of the aggregate income, while the bottom 20% receive only 4% (Cook & Brown, 1995).
- Inequalities in consumption are also stark. Globally, 20% of the world's people in the highest-income countries account for 86% of total private consumption, with the poorest 20% accounting for just 1% (UNDP, 1998).
- The richest fifth consume 58% of total energy; the poorest fifth consume less than 4% (UNDP, 1998).

Outcomes of Poverty

Food Insecurity, Hunger, Malnutrition, and Famine.   Poor people are more vulnerable to hunger and malnutrition because they have less diversified sources of income and fewer assets. They are more likely to be affected by weather-related uncertainties, plant disease, and livestock problems that may lead to crop failure as well as to fluctuating food prices. These risks then set the stage for increased vulnerability to other stressors (e.g., illness).

Data documenting the number of hungry and malnourished people vary according to the definition of hunger, the source of the data, and how the numbers are obtained. When hunger is defined as lacking "the basic food intake to provide...energy and nutrients for fully productive and active lives" (UNDP, 1998), an estimated 840 million people worldwide (one-seventh of the world's population) are hungry. Of the 24,000 who die of starvation each day, 75% are children under the age of 5 years. Total deaths each year approach nine million. One-quarter of the global population is malnourished. A majority of these people live in rural areas, particularly in Sub-Saharan Africa, and in Southeast and East Asia. Although the global food supply is adequate, it is not consumed or produced equitably.

Chronic food insecurity, hunger, and malnutrition interfere with how children grow and thrive, emotionally and physically. Recent studies show that inadequate nutrition may lead to restricted brain development, decreased immune function and greater likelihood of disease, nutritional anemia and protein deficiencies, impaired cognitive development and overall ability to learn, loss of school days, and school failure (Eisenstein & Taddei, 1999). In the developing world, the WHO Global Database on Child Growth estimates that 472 million children under 5 years of age are considered underweight, stunted, and wasted (Eisenstein & Taddei, 1999). Worldwide, the prevalence of stunted children is approximately 34% (Center on Hunger and Poverty, 1999; Eisenstein & Taddei, 1999). During adolescence, chronic malnutrition may lead to delayed onset of puberty and of menarche, and loss of final height potential.

Homeless and street children and youth are at increased risk for nutritional deficiencies, a condition that is also associated with their use of drugs and high rates of HIV/AIDS. Institutionalized youth, including those living in orphanages, locked juvenile facilities or so-called "minor prisons," or who reside in slums, "favelas," or isolated rural areas, suffer disproportionately from all degrees of acute and chronic malnutrition, especially throughout the developing world (Eisenstein & Taddei, 1999).

Hunger and malnutrition spare no country. In the US, some 36 million Americans, of whom 14 million are children, live in households where access to nutritionally adequate food is uncertain. Of these, 10 million experience hunger (Center on Hunger and Poverty, 1999). Food insecurity and endemic hunger are far more common in families living below the poverty level. In 1997, almost 10% of low-income American infants under two years were of short stature (Center on Hunger and Poverty, 1999).

Even more extreme are famines. Although acutely devastating and more highly visible than endemic hunger, they affect far fewer people (usually far less than 10% of the population) than endemic hunger, and the amount of food that would reverse famine conditions is much less than that needed to correct hunger worldwide. In addition to ecological issues, famines are largely related to a region's political structure (Sen, 1999). Famines that may kill millions of people within a country or nation somehow spare the rulers, and it is interesting to note that since independence, India has not suffered from a famine. As observed by Sen,

"Famines... thrive on the basis of severe and sometimes suddenly increased inequality. This is illustrated by the fact that famines can occur even without a large—or any—diminution of total food supply, because some groups may suffer an abrupt loss of market power (through, for example, sudden and massive unemployment), with starvation resulting from this new inequality" (Sen, 1999, p. 187).

Hunger ravages the mind as well as the body, as chillingly illustrated by anthropologist Nancy Scheper-Hughes in her work in a shantytown in Brazil:

> A mother stops ... to say that things aren't well, that her children are nervous because they are hungry. Biu, on returning from (the market) says, as she drops heavily into a chair and removes the food basket from her head, that she becomes dizzy and disoriented, made 'nervous' by the high cost of meat. She was so harassed, she says, that she almost lost her way home from the market.... I stop in to visit Auxiliadora, whose body is wasted by the final stages of schistosomiasis, to find her shaking and crying. Her "nervous attack" was prompted, she says, by uncovering the plate of food her favorite son ... has sent her. There in the midst of her beans was a fatty piece of salted charque (beef jerky). It will offend her "destroyed" liver. But to eat her beans ... without any meat at all makes her angry-nervous. And so she explains the "childish" tears of frustration that course freely down her cheeks.... Descending the hill I stop, as always, at the home of Terezinha. She says that Manoel came home from work doente (sick), his knees shaking, his legs caving in, so "weak and tired" that he could hardly swallow a few spoonfuls of dinner. She says that her husband suffers from these "nervous crises" (crises de nervios) often, especially toward the end of the week when everyone is nervous because there is nothing left in the house to eat. But Manoel will recover, she adds, after he gets a glucose injection at Feliciano's pharmacy (Scheper-Hughes, 1992, pp. 167–168).

Fundamentally related to producing or buying food, hunger is interconnected with political and social ruptures, gender inequality, disintegration of the family, violence, unemployment, lack of clean water, sanitation and sewage disposal, slum dwelling, and scarce community support. Its causes are intimately connected to food production and agriculture, and to the nature of a region's economy and political structure, which profoundly shapes each individual's access to food, nutrition, and health.

Substandard Housing, Informal Settlements, and Houselessness. Home is more than a physical structure or space, a set of possessions, and a place to eat or sleep. As expressed by poet Robert Frost (1936), "Home is the place where, when you have to go there, they have to take you in.... Something you somehow haven't to deserve." Losing one's home— where one can feel physically and emotionally safe, accepted and loved— can be a devastating experience in which loss of housing is only part of the experience. Homelessness can become a metaphor for disconnection from relationships, routine family life, neighborhood, and community.

In many countries, homeless people have become outcasts who are excluded and marginalized. For example, in a country as affluent as the United States, one of the world's richest nations, homelessness is an embarrassment. Recent estimates indicate that 13.5 million Americans have been literally homeless in their lifetime (e.g., sleeping in shelters, abandoned buildings, bus stations), a number far greater than previously imagined (Link et al., 1994). Although there is an emerging third world in America, homeless people have become essentially invisible, as reflected by the lack of a national affordable housing policy.

Inadequate housing and homelessness have increased as a function of the rapid expansion of the world's urban population. While the global population has doubled since 1960, the urban population has increased fivefold. During the last 10 years, urban areas have absorbed 80% of world population growth, fueling an unparalleled housing problem that has similarities in both developing and developed nations. For the first time ever, by the year 2005, more than 50% of the world's population will be living in urban areas (UN Centre for Human Settlements, 1999). Because availability of decent, safe, affordable housing has not kept pace with demand, the tragedy of living in informal slums and squatter settlements, shantytowns, shelters, or literally on the streets is a worldwide problem. Once homeless or inadequately housed, a person is more vulnerable to the ravages of poverty, crime and violence, and poor health.

In developing countries, between 50% and 70% of urban populations live in informal slums or squatter settlements located largely on unusable and unused public land, and operating outside the law (United Nations Centre for Human Settlements, 1999). These unplanned settlements remain excluded from the formal regulatory and management system. Whether in the "barrios" of Venezuela, the "favelas" of Brazil, or the Kenyan slums, millions of residents are tenuously housed. In addition to the bleakness of their housing situation, many residents also live in constant fear of forced evictions, since their legal status is vague and they do not have access to institutional credit. Because these settlements lack an urban infrastructure, residents either receive no services or they receive a lower standard of services at higher costs. Generally, they do not have access to drinking water and sanitation systems. Water must be purchased from community-based organizations and NGOs, and may come via tankers, handcart delivery, or kiosks. Many people drink unclean water from springs and streams. Similarly, residents do not have access to conventional sanitation systems; they use primitive sewage and solid-waste disposal systems, placing them at higher risk for waterborne diseases such as malaria or cholera. The poorest households may have no connections to electricity or telephones, and national and local regulations as well as physical restrictions may limit utilities to the settlement periphery.

Across the world, a significant but unknown number of people live on the streets. For example, according to the Census of India, more than 2 million people were houseless in 1991, with approximately one-third located in urban areas (www.censusindia.net/houseless.html). Known as "footpath dwellers," they live outdoors, subjected to the vagaries of the weather and street life; many are single women and children. Recently, India has developed a system of community night shelters with water, toilets, and baths.

Despite steady economic growth in many developed nations, the widening income gap between rich and poor and the relative scarcity of decent, affordable housing has set the stage for an epidemic of homelessness. In the US, 170 central cities in 34 states have poverty rates of 20% or higher, and 30 cities have poverty rates estimated at 30% or higher. In many cities, the lack of new housing stock drives up demand for existing units and results in rent levels beyond the reach of poor families:

- Between 1991 and 1997, the number of affordable rental units in the US decreased by 5% (Housing and Urban Development [HUD], 1999b).
- In 1997, for every 100 households at or below 30% of median income, there were only 36 affordable units available to rent (HUD, 1999b).
- Worst-case housing needs increased the most among the working poor, growing by 24% (HUD, 1999a).

The face and character of homelessness in the US began to change during the 1980s. Homelessness now reflects extremely severe housing deprivation, with many people living on the streets or in emergency facilities, as well as in absolute poverty. In the 1960s, families comprised less than 3% of the overall homeless population; they now comprise almost 40%. Most of these families are female-headed with 2 to 3 young children:

As a parent, you're supposed to be providing a solid base so your children can become outstanding citizens, and, all of a sudden, you don't even have the ability to take care of them anymore, not even have a roof to put over their heads or a bed to put them in at night, let alone what it does to them emotionally to be homeless. At eight and nine, my kids were older than the other kids in the shelter. One of my daughters started wetting the bed again, and my other daughter started sucking her thumb and sleeping in the fetal position and having nightmares. So, they regressed in that way, but in other ways, because they were subjected to people shooting up heroin in the closet— and terms they were using—all of sudden they became adults (Roofless Women & Kennedy, 1996, p. 51).

The European situation has many similarities. Although data sources are limited, understandably inconsistent, and not comparable across nations, it is clear that Europe is coping with increasing numbers of homeless people. Europeans characterize homelessness as "rooflessness" (living rough), "houselessness" (relying on emergency accommodation or long-term institutions), or "inadequate housing" (including insecure housing accommodation, intolerable housing conditions, or involuntary sharing). Recent economic and sociodemographic changes similar to those experienced in the US have resulted in larger numbers of people being socially excluded. Unprecedented levels of unemployment, technological change, growing income inequality, and an increase in single-parent families are among the trends that have contributed to the growth of homelessness. Each year in the United Kingdom, for example, 150,000 homeless children are accommodated by councils, 50,000 young people are looked after by local authorities, and 10,000 leave the care system.

Goodman, Saxe, and Harvey (1991) have described how homelessness may be traumatic and serve as a risk factor for emotional difficulties, as well as being associated with other interpersonal traumas in various ways: 1) many people, especially women, lose their homes as a result of domestic violence; 2) the process of becoming homeless is often extremely traumatic; and 3) once homeless, one's living circumstances are often unsafe, unpredictable, frightening, and violent, leading to additional emotional symptoms. They conclude that an empowering and supportive environment can mitigate post-trauma responses associated with homelessness.

Morbidity, Disability, and Mortality.   Health is a vital asset, especially for the poor, because of its association with employment. When a family member is unable to work due to illness, the pressure increases on other members to obtain work in order to generate income for basic needs and to pay costly medical bills. If this proves impossible, the family may gradually become impoverished and may seek alternative, less costly and, often, less effective treatments, or may not be able to afford treatment at all. Illness may catalyze a chain reaction that leaves a family more vulnerable to the ravages of unemployment, starvation, homelessness, and absolute poverty. Furthermore, poor people are often exposed to more environmental hazards that increase the likelihood of illness both at home and at work—thus creating a vicious cycle.

Between 1970 and 1997, average life expectancy increased by 7.6 years across all populations. However, although life expectancy increased in Africa, over 50% of the population is not expected to live past age 60 and life expectancy in sub-Saharan Africa is only 47 (World Bank, 2001). Life expectancy at birth in developed countries is now 78 years; in contrast, life expectancy in poorer countries is about 59 years (World Bank, 2001). Poor children in China, for example, face about three times the risk of dying before their fifth birthday compared to poor children in the US.

Most life-threatening diseases among infants and young children can be prevented or cured. Diarrhea, acute respiratory conditions, malaria, measles, and perinatal conditions are responsible for 21% of all deaths in low and moderate-income countries. This is true for only 1% in high-income countries. In adults, prevalent life-threatening diseases include HIV/AIDS, tuberculosis, malaria, and maternal conditions (e.g., obstructed labor, sepsis, and unsafe abortion). Antimicrobial resistance has worsened worldwide, making treatment of diseases such as tuberculosis and malaria more difficult. Nearly 300 million people develop malaria each year and more than 1 million die of it. Nearly 90% of these deaths occur in Sub-Saharan Africa. Overall, in Africa, 20% of childhood deaths are directly attributable to malaria. The following case illustrates some of the challenges to providing adequate care for life-threatening illness (in this case, tuberculosis) in a developing country:

> Jean Dubuisson lives in a small village in Haiti . . . where he farms a tiny plot of land. He shares his two-room hut with his wife and their three children. He developed a persistent cough, which he initially ignored (his village has no health clinic). When he developed night sweats and began losing weight, he drank herbal teas, known for their effectiveness for the grippe. Several months later, he had an episode of coughing up blood, so he went to the clinic in the next town. He was given multivitamins for two dollars and was told to "eat well, drink clean water, sleep in an open room away from others, and go to a hospital." He was unable to follow this advice because he had no money. Two months later, Jean had another severe episode of coughing up blood and went to a church-affiliated hospital. He was initially admitted to an open ward for two weeks and then referred to a sanatorium. Jean was charged $4 per day for his bed and was given medications only if he paid ahead of time. The hospital did not serve food, so the only time he ate was when his wife brought meals. The cough persisted, as did night sweats and an intermittent fever. Jean continued to lose weight and discharged himself from the hospital when he ran out of money. He did not go to the sanatorium (Desjarlais, Eisenberg, Good, & Kleinman, 1995, p. 247).

HIV/AIDS has played a pivotal role in interfering with human development, particularly in the developing world. According to a recent report in The New York Times (Thea, Rosen, & Simon, 1999), HIV/AIDS "is poised to become the worst infectious disease disaster recorded in human history." At the close of the century, more than 32 million adults and more than 1 million children had HIV; 90% lived in the developing world, of which two-thirds lived in Sub-Saharan Africa. "By conservative estimates, the cumulative death toll for sub-Saharan Africa alone over the next 15 years will exceed the combined 40 million deaths caused by the bubonic plague of the 14th century and the 1917 flu pandemic. The epidemic is decimating families, communities, and institutions, and is stalling progress in nearly every sector of development" (Thea, Rosen, & Simon, 1999).

HIV/AIDS infection is concentrated in socially and economically productive groups, aged 15 to 45, with slightly more women infected than men. It is estimated that since 1999, 16.3 million people have died from HIV-related illnesses, of whom approximately 13.7 million were from Sub-Saharan Africa (Masland & Nordland, 2000). If one considers the full scale of affected Africans—including spouses, children, and the elderly—the total may approach 150 million, more than one quarter of the population.

Illiteracy.   Literacy is intricately enmeshed with social and economic development. Because of research limitations, these relationships have not been fully elucidated, but there is little doubt that a more literate population contributes more productively to society and experiences fewer adverse outcomes. Because most data in this area are derived by using years of schooling or self-assessment as proxy variables, literacy rates may be overestimated. As in most other areas related to poverty, these data are more likely to be available for industrialized countries.

Illiteracy refers to adults 15 years and older who "cannot with understanding read and write a short, simple sentence about their everyday life" (World Bank, 1998). Colin Power, UNESCO Assistant Secretary-General, expanded this definition: "Literacy is not only an initiation in the three R's but also an apprenticeship in coping with the modern world" (Power, 1990).

- Approximately 948 million adults worldwide are illiterate; 98% live in developing nations (www.sil.org/lingualinks/library/literacy).
- One-half of all illiterate people live in India and China.
- More than 70% of adults in Eastern and Southern Asia are illiterate.
- Two-thirds of all illiterate people are women (Lingualink; www.sil.org/lingualinks/library/literacy).

Literacy rates generally do not distinguish among subgroups and may mask inequities, particularly among women and girls, rural residents, and marginalized minority groups. For example, according to UNICEF (Crosette, 1999), South Asia "has the lowest literacy rates for women in the world, the lowest percentage of girls in school, and, with Sub-Saharan Africa, the lowest prevalence of contraception. The region has more than one-sixth of the world's people . . . but . . . only Sri Lanka and the Maldives show levels of female development on par with industrialized nations." Following closely behind Southern Asia, somewhat more than half of all women in the Arab States and Sub-Saharan Africa are illiterate. Although to a far lesser degree, illiteracy is a problem in developed nations as well:

> *Jenny (the mother) dropped out of school in the seventh grade—as did Big Donny (the father), after repeating it three times. She reports that neither she nor Big Donny "can read a lick." She wants to learn to be able to read well enough to be able to help Donny (her older son) with his school work. Although she has "plainly told" the teacher that neither she nor Big Donny can read, the school continues to send written work home and to penalize Donny for not doing it correctly. Jenny told me that while Big Donny preferred to accept his non-literacy, she wanted to learn to read and had begun attending a neighborhood-based adult education center. She wanted to be able to read children's books to her kids. She also wanted to be able to shop in new places without asking friends to come along to read labels and signs for her. "It's hard not knowing how to read. Some people think it's easy . . . But it ain't"* (Purcell-Gates, 1995, pp. 13–14).

Unemployment. The world labor force is expected to increase by 1.2 billion by 2025 to a projected total of 3.7 billion workers (UNDP, 1995). The majority of these individuals can expect to earn less than US $1 per day and "work in unhealthy, dangerous or demeaning conditions." Many of those who can find work will be underemployed and unable to climb out of poverty. Many others will be unable to find work at all. Those with low skills are most likely to lose their jobs first and to experience absolute poverty. Research has shown that unemployment, independent of poverty, is associated with increased medical and emotional disorders as well as excess mortality (Kessler, Turner, & House, 1989; Morris, Cook, & Sharper, 1994; Ungvary, Morvai, & Nagy, 1999).

Unemployment rates in industrialized nations in 1998 ranged from 4.1% in Japan to 12.3% in Germany (Bureau of Labor Statistics, 1999). Of nine industrial nations considered, only the United States and the UK had lower rates of unemployment in 1998 than in 1990 (Bureau of Labor Statistics, 1999). During those eight years, Sweden's unemployment rate increased from 1.8% to 8.4% (Schwartz, 1998). In Organisation for Economic Co-Operation and Development [OECD] countries, conservative estimates of unemployment set the total at more than 35 million people, with an additional 10 million who have stopped seeking work. Among youth, 20% are unemployed. These rates are considered conservative because they do not include seasonal or part-time employment. Additionally, unemployment rates are uneven among subgroups. For example, unemployment rates for Whites in the US are much lower than for inner-city African-Americans with the same education. Furthermore, once employed, the median income for White families is $37,152, compared to $22,429 for African-American families (Bureau of the Census, 1990). Education and professional status do not close the gap.

In the United States and many other countries, earning power is also defined by gender, with women generally earning less than men at all economic levels regardless of education and professional status. In 1994, women in the US were earning only 72 cents for every dollar earned by men with similar educational backgrounds (Blau, 1998–1999). During the last decade, women's participation in both the formal and non-formal labor market has increased significantly, but this has not always translated into increased economic power. In many circumstances, women are preferred workers because they can be paid less and can be subjected to poorer working conditions.

Unemployment data are difficult to obtain for developing nations in which the informal sector plays a significant role in the economy. Furthermore, with increased blurring of the boundaries between formal and informal employment, and between rural and urban areas, defining and measuring different types of work has become more challenging. In Latin America, the informal sector makes up over 50% of the labor force. In some countries rates are as high as 68%, with 85 of every 100 jobs created in the informal sector (UNDP, 1999). Jobs for the poor and for women especially are primarily in the informal sector and are characterized by small-scale family-owned businesses (e.g., food processing and trading, domestic services, sewing) that are labor-intensive and require skills acquired outside of formal education. Despite hard work, life remains a struggle for survival:

Florence lives in Maragoli, Kenya, a western province located near Lake Victoria. She is the mother of eight living children, five of whom live with her now. Two children have died. Her husband is a digger for other people and rarely comes home. She owns a plot that is a quarter of an acre: "My husband used to drink; now he has stopped and he spreads the word of God. He gives 100 or 150 shillings a month to the home. I give the remainder. I care for a cow. I use the milk and I will get a calf for my trouble. Sometimes I sell green vegetables, but most times we eat (them). Sometimes my sister or my son buy clothes, if they can. I used to be better; now I have a lot of difficulties. There is no proper care for my life these days. The government budget makes things too high (prices). If I can buy sugar, some little tea, soap, it's all right. Sometimes I can manage fish, and once in a month, I like to have meat. Life is difficult. I like when my children feed properly, when they sleep without crying" (Abwunza, 1997, p. 65).

With only 2 to 5% of the world's 500 million poorest people having access to institutional credit (UNDP, 1997), "microcredit" programs have been the most highly touted development strategy in recent years, particularly because these programs focus on women using credit to create their own businesses. For example, the poorest women in a community form a group of 12 to create ideas for businesses, such as buying a hen and selling eggs. The poorest woman in the group receives the first loan (usually less than $20, but the range is large) and must pay it back weekly (usually at 20% interest). The rest of the group is allowed to borrow only if the first woman repays her loan, assuring that the remainder of the group will be invested in her success. This strategy not only provides credit, but also creates a support group for women and teaches them business skills. Nevertheless, such programs reach only about 8 million poor people (UNDP, 1997).

Without specific supports, many women are able to find work and eke out a living that can feed their families. However, the personal cost is extremely high:

> *Josefina Valenzuela lives in a squatter settlement in the northwestern part of Mexico. She arises every day at 5:30 and prepares lunch for her 12-year-old daughter, Teresina. Josefina leaves for work at 6 am...before the flow of secondary-school students who jam the buses and travel the same route between her barrio to the subway. Her commute takes 1½ to 2 hours each way. Josefina works 12 to 13 hours per day, which gives her only 4 to 5 hours to sleep and eat. On the way home, she always stays alert on the bus because she worries that she will be robbed of her day's wages. . . . Josefina cleans two apartments a day—working six hours at each— and works six days per week. To pay for Teresina's schoolbooks, uniforms, and medicine, Josefina also takes in washing and mending to supplement her income. Although she considers factory work "the ultimate form of personal liberation," she can't afford to work in a factory: "Supporting myself, paying the rent, and providing for my mother to cook for herself and Teresina when I am at work absorbs everything I earn" (Hellman, 1994, pp. 63–74).*

THE PLIGHT OF WOMEN

Across the world, women are at the heart of families and communities. As the center of the family, they provide security, physical and emotional nurturance, and whenever possible, the resources for family members to grow and develop in an increasingly urbanized and technological world. Societies that support and honor women and their work are able to establish strong family units that fortify communities. Such communities express values of caring and sharing that ward off the forces that create and feed social deprivation. Such communities also create surplus resources that allow for development and expansion. Unfortunately, gender inequality and bias have contributed to the growing feminization of poverty and the profound subjugation of women. This section summarizes their plight.

Feminization of Poverty

The 1998 United Nations Development Programme Poverty Report described the "feminization" of poverty as having three aspects: women are poorer; their poverty is more severe; the prevalence of poverty among women is increasing.

Women's subordinate position is reflected in nearly every aspect of social deprivation described in this chapter. For example, education and other supports that allow women to work in formal positions are often inadequate, even though it has been shown that educating women, even to only a primary-school level, is the most important predictor of their own and their children's health (Desjarlais, Eisenberg, Good, & Kleinman, 1995).

Seventy percent of people in the developing world live in rural areas dependent on agriculture. Women are the major producers of food that is grown to feed their families. For example, in sub-Saharan Africa, almost 90% of food for local consumption is grown and sold by women. Even with increasing urbanization, jobs are often informal and home-based; they lack critical structure and are not secure. Women work longer hours for lower wages, often in sweatshop conditions, and may be severely isolated. There are few unions or public services, and forced and bonded labor is not uncommon (Bullock, 1997; United Nations, 1995).

Many industrialized countries lack adequate supports, such as child care and transportation, that would help poor women work. For example, low-income American families who are able to find child care pay as much as one-fourth of their overall income for this service, compared to only 7% of income for non-poor families (Bureau of the Census, 1991). Within this economic context, women and female-headed families are extremely vulnerable and often at imminent risk of economic disaster.

As part of, and often head of, a home industry responsible for the production of food and other necessities, women must also take care of their children and other dependents, such as elders. Children are a financial burden, and the demands of mothering may constrain many women's job possibilities and already limited earning power. Studies consistently show the adverse impact of economic insecurity on the increasing number of children worldwide who are now being placed outside of their homes. In Armenia, for example, 70% of the estimated 10,000 children who live in institutions were placed there because of their family's inability to support them (Tashjian, 1999). The impact on children is often devastating. In the US, foster care placement has been shown to predict a multiplicity of adverse outcomes that continue into adolescence and adulthood.

Gender Inequality and Social Deprivation

Women are among the most socially deprived groups worldwide on the basis of sheer numbers. They experience a particularly pernicious form of oppression. Gender inequality perpetuates poverty and social deprivation, and vice versa, creating a cycle of despair and demoralization that may be transmitted to the next generation. The reciprocal impact of this cycle has led the United Nations to recognize that "...to be successful, anti-poverty strategies must deal with issues related to women's low status and lack of empowerment"(UNDP report, 1998, p. 72).

Gender inequality intersects with and relates to subjugation and inequity in economic, social, and political arenas. When women are subordinated, the economic and social well-being of the entire community is compromised. For example, when women have lower status and fewer opportunities than men in education, formal sector employment, and asset ownership, they are less able to support and nurture their families and children, and participate equally in community life. Because of their marginalized position in the work force and in society generally, they are poorer and have fewer resources.

Unfortunately, the domination of women is often more egregious. Worldwide, domestic violence is the most prevalent form of gender abuse. The World Bank has estimated that, depending on the region, rape and domestic violence account for the loss of 5–16% of the healthy years of women of reproductive age—rates comparable to those for diseases such as AIDS, or health problems related to childbirth, cancer, and cardiovascular disease (World Health Organization [WHO], 1996). Quantitative population-based studies conducted in 24 countries on four continents documented that 20%–50% of all women have been physically abused by intimates at some point in their lives; they also reported that more than half of those had been raped by intimates (WHO, 1996).

Poor women fare even worse. In the United States, a recent study documented that 92% of sheltered homeless mothers and 81% of extremely poor housed mothers had suffered from *severe physical and sexual assault over their lifespan* (the average age of the mothers was 27 years). More than 40% of both groups had been sexually molested at least once before adulthood (Bassuk et al., 1996). To determine the full scope of the problem, additional data are necessary, especially from developing countries.

Violence against women is not just interpersonal. It is structurally and socially perpetrated when the domination of women is viewed as the norm and is seen as a natural right. In some countries, women are beaten for not fully covering themselves in public. In other cultures, women belonging to certain religious or ethnic groups are abducted and detained by the dominant militaristic group and used for sexual purposes, sold into prostitution, or brutally murdered. The traditional African practice of female genital mutilation, which may put almost 2 million girls a year at risk, has been condemned by WHO. However, to date an estimated 130 million women and girls have undergone this experience.

CONCLUSION

This chapter describes how human poverty, social deprivation, and structural violence are far more than economic—and they plague fully half the world's people, making them more vulnerable to traumatic stressors, such as violence, crime, and abuse. Women comprise the greatest numbers. The complex interplay of political, cultural, and economic forces profoundly limits physical and mental well-being, denying basic rights to food, housing, education, and work—and, finally, extinguishing individual human rights, dignity, and spirit. By understanding social deprivation as a process that can be disrupted by appropriate interventions, and by generating the popular political will to support these interventions, we can help end the daily nightmare of billions of people crushed by hunger, disease, violence and trauma, and oppression.

ACKNOWLEDGEMENTS: The authors wish to acknowledge John Kellogg, Jodie Fesh, Anna Martin, and Eliza Van Dusen for their work on this chapter.

REFERENCES

Abwunza, J.M. (1997). *Women's voices, women's power: Dialogues of resistance from East Africa*. Ontario, Canada: Broadview.
Bassuk, E.L., Weinreb, L., Buckner, J.C., Browne, A., Salomon, A., & Bassuk, S. (1996). The characteristics and needs of sheltered homeless and low-income housed mothers. *Journal of the American Medical Association, 276*, 640–646.
Blau, F. (1998–1999). Women's economic well-being, 1970–1995: Indicators and trends. *Focus, 20*, 7.
Bullock, S. (1997). *Women and work*. London, England: Zed Books Ltd.
Bureau of Labor Statistics (1999). US Department of Labor. Washington, DC: Author.
Bureau of the Census (1990). *Census of population: Social and economic characteristics*. Washington, DC: United States Department of Commerce, Economics and Statistics Administration.
Bureau of the Census (1991). *National child care survey*. Washington, DC: Author.
Center on Hunger and Poverty (1999). *Childhood hunger, childhood obesity: An examination of the paradox*. Boston, MA: Author.

Cook, J., & Brown, J. (1995). *Asset development among America's poor: Trends in the distribution of income and wealth.* Boston: Center on Hunger, Poverty, and Nutrition Policy, Tufts University.

Crosette, B. (1999, September 12). UNICEF says war affects poor children in the millions. *New York Times*, 19.

De Vries (1996). Trauma in cultural perspective. In B.A. Van Der Kolk, A.C. McFarlane, & L. Weisaeth (Eds.), *Traumatic stress: The effects of overwhelming experience on mind, body, and society* (pp. 398–413). New York: Guilford.

Desjarlais, R., Eisenberg, L., Good, B., & Kleinman, A. (Eds.) (1995). *World mental health: Problems and minorities in low income countries.* New York: Oxford University Press.

Durkin, M.S., Davidson, L.L., Kuhn, L., O'Connor, P., & Barlow, B. (1994). Low income neighborhoods and the risk of severe pediatric injury: A small-area analysis in northern Manhattan. *American Journal of Public Health, 84*, 587–592.

Eisenstein, E. & Taddei, J. (1999). *World hunger.* Unpublished manuscript.

Frost, R. (1936). The death of a hired man. Collected poems. New York: Garden City Publications Co.

Galtung, J. (1969). Violence, peace, and peace research. *Journal of Peace Research, 6*, 167–191.

Galtung, J. (1975, November). Presentation to UNESCO Interdisciplinary Expert Meeting on the Study of the Causes of Violence, Paris, France. As cited in Khan, R. (1978), Violence and socioeconomic development. *International Social Scientist Journal, 30*, 834–857.

Galtung, J. (1990). Cultural violence. *Journal of Peace Research, 27*, 291–305.

Goodman, L., Saxe, L., & Harvey, M. (1991). Homelessness as psychological trauma. *American Psychologist, 46*, 1219–1225.

Hellman, J. (1994). *Mexican lives.* New York: The New Press.

Housing and Urban Development (1999a). *The state of America's cities.* Washington DC: Author.

Housing and Urban Development (1999b). *The widening gap: New findings on housing affordability in America.* Washington DC: Author.

India at a Glance (1991). http://www.censusindia.net/houseless.html

Kessler, R., Turner, J.B., & House, J.S. (1989). Unemployment, reemployment and emotional functioning in a community sample. *American Sociological Review, 54*, 648–657.

Link, B., Susser, E., Stueve, A., Phelan, J., Moore, R., & Struening, E. (1994). Lifetime and five-year prevalence of homelessness in the United States. *American Journal of Public Health, 84*, 1907–1912.

Loury, G. (1999, April). Social exclusion and ethnic groups: The challenge to economics. Presented at the annual World Bank Conference on Development Economics, Washington, DC.

Mandela, N. (2000, January 4). Globalizing responsibility. *The Boston Globe*, A15.

Masland, T., & Nordland, R. (2000, January 17). Ten million orphans. *Newsweek*, 37.

Mathers, C.D., & Scholfield, D.J. (1998). The health consequences of unemployment: The evidence. *The Medical Journal of Australia, 168*, 178–182.

McLeod, J.D., & Kessler, R.C. (1990). Socioeconomic status differences in vulnerability to undesirable life events. *Journal of Health and Social Behavior, 31*, 162–172.

Melnick, S., & Bassuk, E.L. (1999). *Identifying and responding to violence among poor and homeless women: Health care provider's guide.* Newton, Massachusetts: The Better Homes Fund.

Morris, J.K., Cook, D.G., & Sharper, A.P. (1994). Loss of employment and mortality. *British Medical Journal, 308*, 1135–1139.

Morrison, P., & Tsipis, K. (1999). *Reason enough to hope. America and the world of the 21st century.* Cambridge, Massachusetts: The MIT Press.

Power, C. (1990). UNESCO's Assistant Director-General for Education. International Literacy Year. In *ILY: A year of opportunity.*

Purcell-Gates, V. (1995). *Other people's word: The cycle of low literacy.* Cambridge, Massachusetts: Harvard University Press.

Qoboza, P. (1986). *Political constraints and opportunities for youth development.* Unpublished manuscript.

Roofless Women, & Kennedy, M. (1996). A hole in my soul: Experiences of homeless women. In D. Dujon & A. Withorn (Eds), *For crying out loud: Women's poverty in the United States.* Boston, MA: South End Press.

Scheper-Hughes, N. (1992). *Death without weeping: The violence of everyday life in Brazil.* Berkeley, CA: University of California Press.

Schwartz, J.E. (1998). The hidden side of the Clinton economy. *Atlantic Monthly, 282,* 18–21.

Sen, A. (1997). *On economic inequality.* Oxford, England: Oxford University Press.

Sen, A. (1999). *Development as freedom.* New York: Alfred A. Knopf.

Tasjian, M. (1999). *Summary of poverty in Armenia.* Unpublished manuscript.

Thea, D., Rosen, S., & Simon, J. (1999, September 14). AIDS is devastating whole societies. *The New York Times,* A23.

Turner, R.J., Wheaton, B., & Lloyd, D.A. (1995). The epidemiology of social stress. *American Sociological Review, 60,* 104–125.

Ungvary, G., Morvai, V., & Nagy, I. (1999). Health risk of unemployment. *Central European Journal of Occupational and Environmental Medicine, 5,* 91–112.

United Nations. (1995). *Women: Looking beyond 2000.* New York: Author.

United Nations. (1995). *World Summit for Social Development: The Copenhagen Declaration and Programme of Action.* New York: Author.

United Nations. (1999). *AIDS/WHO: Epidemic update.* New York: Author.

United Nations Centre for Human Settlements (1999). *Habitat Debate,* 5(3), 24–26.

United Nations Development Programme (1995). *Human development report.* New York: Oxford University Press.

United Nations Development Programme (1997). *Human development report.* New York: Oxford University Press.

United Nations Development Programme (1998). *Overcoming human poverty.* New York: Author.

United Nations Development Programme (1999). *Human development reports.* (1997–1999). New York: Author.

United Nations Development Programme (2000). *Human development report.* New York: Oxford University Press.

WHO (1996). *Fact sheet: Violence against women* (WHO Fact sheet N128). Geneva: World Health Organization.

World Bank. (1998). World Bank Development Indicators. http://www.worldbank.org/data/

World Bank. (1999). *Poverty trends and voices of the poor.* New York: Oxford University Press.

World Bank. (2001). World Bank Development Indicators. http://www.worldbank.org/data/

Young, M.I. (1990). *Justice and the politics of difference.* New Jersey: Princeton University Press.

Chapter 4

Intervention Options for Societies, Communities, Families, and Individuals

John A. Fairbank, Matthew J. Friedman, Joop de Jong, Bonnie L. Green, and Susan D. Solomon

A traumatic stress perspective sheds a particular light on challenges facing the United Nations system—from poverty and exclusion in peacetime to displacement and deprivation in war or after disaster. It is an ever-evolving perspective or lens, and one that needs adjustment for cultural, gender, age, and other dynamic variables. It also needs adjustment according to the size of the targeted population, be it an entire nation or specific communities, families, or individuals. At its core is a concern for how human beings experience and respond to intolerable or traumatic stressors. From that core concern, a traumatic stress perspective then considers what might be desirable in terms of prevention, practice, and policy to alleviate suffering and improve quality of life. A broad menu of possible interventions is presented throughout this book, each of which must be understood in context and within a continually expanding knowledge base about the nature and consequences of traumatic stressors.

An inverted pyramid (see Chapter 11; De Jong 2002a) is used as an organizing and prioritizing concept throughout this book. Starting at the top and widest level, it targets progressively, and in descending order, ever-smaller groups of people (as shown in Figure 4.1). The target groups and levels of intervention are overlapping and interrelated. At the top of the pyramid are societal interventions designed for an entire population, such as international and national laws, public policy, and public institutions supporting human security, equality, dignity, and participation (Marsella,

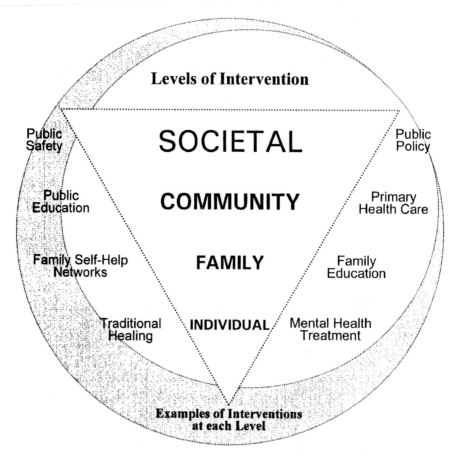

Figure 4.1. Model for Interventions in Social and Humanitarian Crises from a Traumatic Stress Perspective.

1998; De Jong, 2002b). At this broadest level, the aim is to remedy the violence that is inherent in the social structure (structural violence), violence that creates inequality, injustice, and exclusion, as well as interpersonal and collective traumatic stressors that interfere with a safe environment conducive to healthy adjustment. The next layer is community interventions, which include public education, support for community leaders, preservation of social infrastructure, local empowerment, and training and education of local health workers. The next layer from the top is family interventions that focus on the individual within the context of family and clan, as well as on strategies to promote the well-being of the family as a

unit. The bottom layer of the pyramid concerns interventions primarily designed for the individual with psychological symptoms or psychiatric disorders. These include individualized treatments and services provided by
practitioners of traditional methods of healing as well as Western-oriented
psychosocial interventions and psychiatric medication. Because the last are
the most expensive and labor-intensive approaches and require the most
highly-trained staff, they are reserved for the small minority of individuals
who have not benefited sufficiently from the larger-scale interventions at
higher levels of the pyramid.

There is considerable variation worldwide between high- and low-
income countries, and among ethnic, religious, and cultural groups, in
ways of coping with intolerable or traumatic stressors, as can be seen by
the range of examples given throughout the book. Differences exist among
nations and cultures in the kinds of help that are available and perceived as
appropriate to prevent and cope with traumatic stressors (Patel, 2000). In
many low-income countries, traditional healers provide interventions that
are related to the cultural beliefs of communities, families, and individuals, and they far outnumber professional mental health workers trained in
Western-oriented systems of care (Asuni, 1979). In these countries, services
provided by traditional healers are more accessible and more widely used
than professional health services (Leff, 2001). Although there are fewer traditional healers in many high-income countries, there is a growing interest
in many of the methods of traditional medicine (Hopa, Simbayi, & Du Toit,
1998).

High-income countries customarily address traumatic stress responses through psychosocial and/or mental health interventions. Psychosocial interventions address social problems (such as homelessness,
alcoholism, discrimination, or violence in the family) that affect emotional
or psychological well-being, and psychological problems (such as despair
or fear) that undermine social functioning, including a capacity for intimacy, work, and participation in family and communal life. Psychosocial
interventions include public health announcements, self-help and community groups, and school debates (on violence, for example), as well as
counseling services, emotional support, and problem-solving for various
population groups. Programs such as disaster preparedness education,
skills training, school-based violence prevention programs, and long-term
follow-up may be important steps in effectively treating trauma survivors.

Mental health interventions most often target psychiatric disorders,
such as posttraumatic stress disorder (PTSD), diagnosed according to official criteria of the World Health Organization (WHO, 1992) or the American
Psychiatric Association (1994) (see Chapter 2). Mental health interventions

often include psychotherapy and/or medication for the patient as well as education and/or counseling to the patient and his or her family. The majority of mental health professionals in high- and low-income countries have been trained in disease-oriented models of mental health and are frequently most comfortable with this approach. However, people with psychiatric disorders are also vulnerable to psychosocial problems, thereby creating the need to provide psychosocial services to the individual or his or her family or community.

There is a wide disparity across nations in the amount of public and private resources available for psychosocial and mental health interventions, and in the extent to which trauma services are integrated into community health or mental health systems. In the few countries in which trauma prevention and treatment systems are in place, they are often poorly integrated with other health care. Fragmented and ineffective care is often the end result. The United States, for example, is one of the countries that fail to integrate mental health services fully within its public health response to emergency events.

This book—while emphasizing current best practices—also attempts to contribute to an emerging debate on the prevention and remedy of intolerable or traumatic stress. Such stress is being experienced by entire societies worldwide, and within communities, families, and individuals. Our goal is to generate questions, elicit and collect diverse and innovative responses, support communal healing, and cultivate exchange among traditional, psychosocial, and mental health-oriented approaches to the prevention of traumatic stressors and treatment of their consequences. It hopes to support exchanges and collaboration among systems of treating traumatic stress worldwide as well as between mental health and political, economic, and social systems.

LEVELS AND TYPES OF INTERVENTION

Level 1: Societal Interventions

Policy/Public Safety. International and national laws, public policy, and public institutions can all influence the prevalence and impact of exposure to traumatic circumstances. A first line of prevention is the provision for the basic human needs of water, food, safety, shelter, education, and employment; these self-evidently reduce environmental stressors and empower populations to manage their affairs. Thus, national development plans and, relatedly, national health care, employment, welfare, and other systems are all critical to the prevention and treatment of adverse consequences in the wake of large-scale traumatic stressors. Governments play a key role in establishing public safety through the development of policies and systems that prevent or ameliorate the stresses of wars, disasters, and the abuse of women, children, the elderly, and persons with disabilities. Establishing public safety in the aftermath of civil strife and violence, political instability, and natural disasters is an essential element for building an environment conducive to reducing the impact of traumatic stress. Unfortunately, few national systems are adequately prepared for large-scale social or humanitarian crises. The World Health Organization emphasizes the role of disaster preparedness and response through training, assessment of health situations and needs, and coordination among agencies involved in trauma prevention and response operations (De Girolamo, 1993). For example, nations prone to earthquakes may prevent or diminish the traumatic consequences of these natural disasters by developing, implementing, and enforcing building safety codes and standards, and by establishing plans for emergency preparedness and public safety (Abdo, Al-Dorzi, Itani, Jabr, & Zaghloul, 1997).

Official recognition and acknowledgment of the presence of traumatic stressors by the United Nations, national governments, and NGOs is a viable form of societal intervention. Using an interpersonal-level traumatic event as an example, the United Nations' definition of torture has brought considerable recognition to that form of traumatic stressor. The World Health Organization's definition similarly highlighted the problem of torture and gave it greater visibility internationally and, in particular, among health care providers. Coupled with the efforts of Amnesty International, which investigates and estimates the prevalence of torture across all nations, these international efforts have shed valuable light on a common traumatic event plaguing contemporary society.

Efforts to define and measure the many forms of intolerable stress in populations can lead to an assessment of their prevalence, a process that itself raises public awareness, which in turn may reduce the frequency of these events and lead to the development of intervention strategies. In this respect, the ongoing refinement of indicators throughout the UN system—regarding hunger, homelessness, unemployment, lack of schooling, the flow of migrants and refugees, and the status of women, disabled persons, older persons, and youth, among others—begins the process of prevention of traumatic stress exposure.

Ensuring social justice by addressing basic human rights, discrimination, exclusion, and powerlessness can remove enormous individual, familial, and communal stressors. Laws and the use of the criminal justice system can be both preventative and curative. The manner in which a country's criminal justice system interacts with victims of crime can influence psychological outcomes for an individual. Systems that place exclusive emphasis on the perpetrator and his/her punishment may ignore those whose lives have been adversely affected by the victimization. Placing the victim at the center of the legal system, and focusing conjointly upon justice, punishment, reparation, and rehabilitation, may achieve a greater sense of social justice for all those affected by crime. The United Nations' *Declaration of Basic Principles of Justice for Victims of Crime* and the establishment of an International Criminal Court are important international efforts to delineate for countries those policies that, if implemented, would enhance the mental health of victims within countries.

Level 2: Community Interventions

In many communities worldwide, concerns about the social and psychological effects of traumatic exposure, and the treatment and care of those so exposed, are a lower priority than compelling physical health needs (Leff, 2001). However, the two aspects are interrelated (see Chapter 2), and attention to one will positively affect the other. Furthermore, programs to treat the consequences of exposure to traumatic stressors that are based upon local systems, values, and priorities are more likely to be successful than programs that neglect such realities in communities (Jacob, 2001). Community ownership of interventions is critical, and may be achieved by involving all population segments—women as well as men, elders as well as youth, local professional and health workers, and community leaders—in the development and implementation of interventions (Siriam, 1990).

Public Education.   Public education through poster and leaflet campaigns, radio and Internet announcements, and workshops and discussion groups facilitates wide and rapid distribution of important information about, for example, safety, aid and resources, self-help, and legal rights in the aftermath of a traumatic stressor. It can inform people in communities affected by stressful events about the scope of those events and the range of normal or common reactions, as well as those that are more unusual or severe that might require extra attention. In humanitarian crises, when normal modes of communication with the outside are damaged, public education can be used to quell rumors and help the community to have a more realistic view of the situation. It can also assist communities in addressing alcohol or drug abuse in the aftermath of traumatic stressors. In individual or interpersonal level trauma, public education can heighten public awareness about types of behavior that are not well known or understood, such as abuse of the elderly, or abuse of physically or mentally disabled individuals. With regard to preventing violence of all types—toward children, spouses, the elderly, persons with HIV/AIDS, and the disabled—public education can train key individuals or entire communities in peaceful methods of conflict resolution as a way of settling disagreements. Educational material that promotes positive local values, morals, and self-help can be presented in novel ways, such as drama and storytelling, that have the capacity to engage a larger or specialized audience.

Maintaining Local Structures. Activities such as meetings, rallies, or religious ceremonies that are conceptualized and implemented by leaders and individuals in the affected communities can generate a sense of healing and recovery. Some communities have structures for doing this. The Shraddhanjali mass grieving ceremony in Sri Lanka, for example, promotes unity and collective action within grief-stricken communities. In response to crises, such activities can be organized to occur more often initially, perhaps weekly, and then gradually decrease in frequency. Group meetings allow the community to participate as a unit. This kind of collective participation can stimulate brainstorming about methods for rebuilding the community as well as collective action in doing so. Folk and devotional songs about a tragedy can help the mourning process, and help to gather people in a common place to share their grief. Organizing a rally may help to sensitize officials regarding delays in the implementation of restoration, rebuilding, and relocation after a humanitarian crisis, or may heighten their awareness of ongoing community problems which have gone unacknowledged or unaddressed, such as the abuse or exploitation of children. Similarly, national advocacy groups can provide a focal point for education, public awareness, and service development.

Oftentimes, community cohesion can be sparked by simply encouraging adults and children to get back to their normal routines, or by making experiences possible that are likely to promote self-esteem, such as income-generating activities, training opportunities, or sports. Sports, for example, can encourage the constructive use of free time, which is particularly useful for dislocated communities such as those in temporary shelters or in refugee camps. They also provide a venue for children to talk about their experiences with others, a component vital for healing in many cultures. Youth workers or volunteers who facilitate such activities can be taught relevant listening skills, since children may choose to talk to youth workers rather than to teachers or parents (see Chapters 10 and 11).

Prevention and treatment may target the community as a whole, or may focus on vulnerable subgroups such as single and teenaged parents, low socioeconomic or isolated families, the elderly or disabled, or children—as well as vulnerable housing units, neighborhoods, or entire villages. Representatives of the target group must be involved in decision-making that affects them. Volunteers can be recruited and trained to visit with isolated elders or those with disabilities. Community "gatekeepers" who are advocates for the elderly or disabled can be trained to identify abuse and to reach out to isolated elders on the one hand, and community religious, business, and other leaders on the other. A proactive coordinated community approach to investigating cases of abuse also helps prevent abuse and facilitates early detection, when intervention may be more effective.

Enhancing Primary Health Care and Traditional Healing Systems. In many developing countries and rural regions of the world, primary health care workers provide most mental health services to trauma survivors, and traditional healers and religious leaders provide most psychosocial services to survivors. This can easily be seen as a necessity due to lack of trained professionals and resources to provide specialty services (Leff, 2001). However, "train-the-trainer" models provide a useful method for expanding outreach and for integrating and sustaining elements of the traumatic stress perspective into indigenous healing and primary health systems of care, a model that is re-emerging in the West. It also helps to embed knowledge within communities for the long-term, promoting community resilience. Up to five or more years may be required for train-the-trainer systems to take root, with local trainers in a position to continue interventions with minimal assistance from the original trainers. Monitoring and evaluation should be built into the system from the start, facilitating periodic adjustments at the end of a program cycle for each level and stage of intervention (De Jong, 2002b).

Schools. As respected members of the community, local teachers frequently play a critical role in assisting traumatized children, as demonstrated, for example, in the former Yugoslavia, Sri Lanka, and Mozambique. To be effective in complex human emergencies, teachers need training both in the curriculum and in classroom management in order to address the changed behavior of traumatized pupils. They also need to be trained to recognize the behavioral and emotional needs of the children. This training might include skills in talking with children about emotionally difficult matters in a way that helps them cope with their stress reactions, as well as training in how (and to whom) to refer the selected children for further help. Teachers have a pivotal role when most of the affected children are in school. However, community nurses and physicians also have vital roles to play both in helping identify children in need and in organizing services to meet those needs, especially in more chaotic situations.

Level 3: Family Interventions

Interventions at the level of the family make use of informal support systems of family, friends, neighbors, peers, and local community organizations. Relying on natural helping networks, these interventions promote the capacity of family and/or a network of supporters to help family members cope with and recover from traumatic experiences. Interventions at the family level may include organizing "self-help" groups of families who share similar experiences, such as having a family member disappear, be murdered, or be abducted. Self-help groups are also helpful for families who are caring for members with disabilities. Interventions at this level may also assist families in generating income and obtaining other resources necessary for caring for a member who has survived a devastating traumatic experience. It is generally presumed useful to provide family members with accurate information about the nature and consequences of traumatic stress, and how they can best help survivors.

Where there is little social service infrastructure, reliance on social networks may be the most viable option. In some developed countries, interventions for child abuse and neglect emphasize family education and guidance, in a format that is flexible and responsive to the needs of children and families. For example, treatment of physical abuse may help parents and children to understand and re-focus anger, to develop communication and collaboration skills, and to examine distorted beliefs, such as low self-esteem, which often underlie family violence. Similarly, treatment for child neglect focuses on parenting skills and expectations, coupled with training in social competencies that may include home safety, family hygiene, finances, medical needs, drug and alcohol counseling, marital counseling, and other skills needed to manage family resources and to attend to children's needs.

Although family level interventions frequently focus on the needs of the individual within the context of the family, these interventions may also promote the psychosocial well-being of the family itself. Numerous studies indicate that traumatic experiences have effects on family members as well as on survivors and victims. For example, studies of the families of Holocaust survivors, survivors of the atomic bombing of Japan during World War II, refugees and internally displaced persons, and veterans of armed conflicts point to the transgenerational effects of traumatic stressors on their children (Danieli, 1998). Family level interventions may therefore take into account the needs of not only the survivor, but also his or her family members. For example, one approach to the treatment of families of trauma survivors emphasizes the development of a shared understanding of the problem and the joint development and acceptance by the family of a "healing theory." However, when family members themselves are the perpetrators of trauma, as is often the case in abuse of children, the elderly, and the disabled, additional sets of complexities are introduced that are examined in specific chapters of this volume.

Level 4: Individual Psychosocial and Mental Health Interventions

People have coped with traumatic stress in ways unique to individual and culture-specific resources. For much of history, coping has been intuitive. That is, neither the individuals themselves nor the healing professions consciously analyzed the innate or inherited methods employed to see what worked and why (or didn't work and why not). Throughout centuries, traditional health-care systems, such as those of China and India, have developed approaches to treating the problems of survivors of traumatic experiences that include herbal remedies, meditation, exercise, and massage.

Western medicine has adopted a scientific approach—that is, a detached observation of cause and effect, together with testing, measuring, comparing, replication, and peer review—and this has also shaped its approaches to mental health. Today, Western analytic approaches to treating traumatic stress responses have largely examined three areas: cognitive behavioral therapy (CBT), psychodynamic and interpersonal therapies, and pharmacotherapy. These are typically provided by individuals with formal professional training and are usually indicated only under certain circumstances, such as the existence of a ICD-10 (World Health Organization [WHO], 1992) or DSM-IV (American Psychological Association [APA], 1994) diagnosis such as PTSD or major depression. These approaches are likely to have differing degrees of applicability across and within countries, both for cultural reasons and because resource constraints may render them inaccessible.

Additional approaches used internationally—for prevention and treatment—include various forms of meditation, deep muscle relaxation, acupuncture, and exercise adopted from traditional medicine, as well as psychological debriefing and supportive forms of psychotherapy, such as crisis counseling. Decisions to use individual psychosocial and mental health interventions should consider the empirical evidence for a treatment's efficacy as well as the capacity of the intervention to accommodate the relevant cultural premises of communities and individuals (see Chapter 13; Tanaka-Matsumi & Higgenbotham, 1996).

PTSD is not the only formal psychiatric diagnosis associated with exposure to traumatic events (see Chapter 2). Major depression is an especially common outcome, and one that often co-occurs with PTSD. Anxiety disorders other than PTSD are also relatively common following trauma. Since PTSD is often the most common outcome, however, and since it is specifically linked with traumatic exposure, it will be the focus for the rest of this chapter. More detailed information can be found elsewhere (Foa, Keane, & Friedman, 2000).

Cognitive-Behavioral Therapy (CBT). CBT techniques for treating psychological distress in survivors of traumatic experiences include exposure therapy, cognitive therapy, cognitive processing therapy, stress inoculation training, systematic desensitization, assertiveness training, biofeedback, and relaxation training (Foa et al., 1999). Some of these are administered in a group format. To date, exposure therapy is the most rigorously evaluated individual intervention. Exposure treatment methods involve confronting fearful memories within the context of a safe therapeutic relationship. The process involves intentionally experiencing and maintaining the distress associated with the traumatic event until the distress diminishes.

Exposure therapy has been found to be effective in treating the symptoms of PTSD in war veterans and female sexual assault survivors (e.g., Rothbaum, Meadows, Resick, & Foy, 2000). It has also achieved widespread use in the treatment of child and adult victims of crime, child abuse, disasters, torture, and motor vehicle accidents. One form of CBT—cognitive processing therapy—alleviates the symptoms of depression and PTSD among rape survivors (Resick, Nishith, Weaver, Astin, & Feuer, 2002). Another useful CBT approach is stress inoculation training, which involves teaching individuals specific coping skills for reducing or managing symptoms and/or alternative responses to fear and anxiety. Skills include relaxation training, anger management training, thought stopping, assertiveness training, self-dialogue, problem-solving skills training, and relapse prevention (Meichenbaum, 1974). Relaxation techniques and self-dialogue through the repetition of a meaningful word, phrase, or verse to oneself is practiced in cultural and religious systems worldwide. Although CBT has extended the range of effective mental health treatments for PTSD in some developed nations, the generality of treatment efficacy to persons with PTSD in other cultures is just beginning to be evaluated (Paunovic & Ost, 2001).

Psychodynamic Therapy. The psychodynamic formulation views traumatic stress as characterized by two alternating psychological states: one typified by intrusive thoughts, and the other by denial and numbing (avoidance). Psychodynamic interventions tailor treatment to the symptoms associated with the patient's current psychological state. Once intrusive and avoidance symptoms are within manageable limits, the full meaning of the event can be explored. From a psychodynamic perspective, posttraumatic symptoms represent an adaptive attempt to manage the trauma. If the meanings of these symptoms, as well as the meaning of the event, are understood and worked through, the patient will be able to cope more effectively. Psychodynamic treatment of PTSD is primarily an expressive therapy that seeks to increase the patient's understanding of material outside his or her awareness and to improve coping in the context of a strong therapeutic alliance. In comparison with CBT, psychodynamic therapy for traumatic stress has been subjected to much less empirical validation, although initial studies have demonstrated benefits, especially in the long-term (Brom, Kleber, & Defares, 1989). In recent years, psychodynamic techniques have begun to be adapted for use with patients from different cultures (e.g., Nathan, 1989). Interpersonal approaches that are similar conceptually and theoretically, but that focus more on the impact of trauma on current relationships, are also being developed (e.g., Krupnick, 2002).

Pharmacologic Approaches. A substantial body of research has demonstrated abnormalities in the psychobiological systems of persons with PTSD. Many medications have been used to treat specific PTSD symptoms, separately or in combination with psychotherapy. Pharmacologic treatments for PTSD include antidepressants, inhibitors of adrenergic activity, and mood stabilizers (Friedman, 2000). Among these drugs, the most carefully studied and most widely prescribed are the antidepressants. Of the antidepressants, the selective serotonin reuptake inhibitors (SSRIs) are currently regarded as the most efficacious drug treatment for PTSD. The US Food and Drug Administration has recently approved two SSRIs (sertraline and paroxetine) for use in PTSD (Friedman, Davidson, Mellman, & Southwick, 2000), the first medications so designated. Most developing countries have access to tricyclic antidepressants, but not SSRIs, through the *WHO List of Essential Medicines* (World Health Organization, 2001).

Crisis Counseling. Crisis counseling is a supportive intervention that provides traumatized individuals with an opportunity to express feelings about the event within a nonjudgmental context. Crisis counseling is frequently provided to victims of violent crimes, such as rape or sexual assault, as well as to survivors of natural and manmade disasters. General characteristics of crisis counseling are: (a) it is time-limited and issues-oriented; (b) the counselor responds to the crisis requests of the victim; (c) the counselor responds to crisis-related problems and not to other problems; and (d) the counselor takes an active role in initiating follow-up contacts. This approach is often carried out by peer counselors who offer support, information, and empathy to the victim, as well as by trained mental health professionals through such programs as the Disaster Response Network (DRN) established by the American Psychological Association in collaboration with the American Red Cross. Over 1,500 DNR volunteers provide free on-site mental health services to disaster survivors and relief workers (APA, 2002).

Because provision of crisis counseling and psychotherapy to trauma survivors can be stressful for providers, training programs need to incorporate information about secondary traumatic stress (e.g., Pearlman & Saakvitne, 1995) and self-care for trauma professionals (see Chapter 15).

SUMMARY GUIDELINES

The following distillations will help to guide the selection of interventions for the prevention or remedy of traumatic stress in societies, communities, families, and individuals.

- In the aftermath of traumatic collective and individual-level social stressors, self-healing and self-correction occur at all levels. Yet downward spirals can also occur, making careful and timely intervention important. Timely intervention has the capacity to break cycles of distress and deprivation that may be "contagious," spreading outward to family and community or inward from the broader society to individuals and families, and frequently also to the next generation.
- The problems of those exposed to traumatic stressors show some universal characteristics across cultures, perhaps owing to the biological and cognitive dimensions of the nature of the threat, and to responses to traumatic events.
- Those experiencing traumatic stress, and those developing interventions for its prevention or remedy, are all conditioned to varying degrees by innate, experiential, and cultural differences, including gender, age, and other factors. In other words, not everyone experiences or sees traumatic stressors in the same way, making dialogue and openness essential for its

prevention and treatment. It is particularly crucial for interventions to be culturally and developmentally appropriate, as well as gender-appropriate.

- Interventions based on education and training are nearly universally accepted as appropriate—even as these interventions evolve through assessment and feedback from clients and practitioners working in new situations.
- Indigenous and traditional healing systems are the most widely used and accessible worldwide—applied variously by local traditional healers, primary health care workers, wise men and women, and community or religious leaders. There is a need to find creative methods to bridge the gap between traditional, national, and private health systems to better manage the care of survivors of traumatic stressors.
- As illustrated throughout this volume, a variety of psychosocial and mental health interventions exist. They may be neutral, beneficial, or even harmful. Timely, sensitive, and culturally-appropriate interventions can reduce the severity of reactions to traumatic stressors, lend hope for recovery, and prevent a deterioration of psychological status. Inappropriate interventions, however, can exacerbate traumatic conditions. Some may have no effect, however costly they may have been to implement. In short, the interrelationship of condition, intervention, and outcome is complex and needs continued study. Only thus can we help decision-makers devise suitable policies for prevention and treatment of traumatic stress, in war or peacetime situations, and at the levels of societies, communities, families, and individuals.

REFERENCES

Abdo, T., Al-Dorzi, H., Itani, A., Jabr, F., & Zaghloul, N. (1997). Earthquakes: Health outcomes and implications in Lebanon. *Le Journal Medical Libanais*, 45, 197–200.

American Psychiatric Association (1994). *Diagnostic and statistical manual of mental disorders* (4th ed.). Washington, DC: Author.

American Psychological Association (2002). Disaster Response Network: A pro-bono service of the American Psychological Association and its members. American Psychological Association Web site: http://www.apa.org/practice/drn.html.

Asuni, T. (1979). The dilemma of traditional healing with special reference to Nigeria. *Social Science and Medicine*, 13B, 33–39.

Brom, D., Kleber, R.J., & Defares, P.B. (1989). Brief psychotherapy for post-traumatic stress disorders. *Journal of Consulting and Clinical Psychology*, 57, 607–612.

Danieli, Y. (Ed.) (1998). *International handbook of multigenerational legacies of trauma*. New York: Plenum.

De Girolamo, G. (1993). International perspectives on the treatment and prevention of post-traumatic stress disorder. In J. Wilson & B. Raphael (Eds.), *International handbook of traumatic stress syndromes* (pp. 935–946). New York: Plenum.

De Jong, J.T.V.M. (Ed.) (2002a). *Trauma, war and violence: Public mental health in socio-cultural context*. New York: Kluwer/Plenum.

De Jong, J.T.V.M. (2002b) Public mental health, traumatic stress and human rights violations in low-income countries: A culturally appropriate model in times of conflict, disaster and peace. In J.T.V.M., De Jong (Ed.) (2002), *Trauma, war and violence: Public mental health in sociocultural context.* New York: Kluwer/Plenum.

Foa, E.B., Dancu, C.V., Hembree, E.A., Jaycox, L.H., Meadows, E.A., & Street, G.P. (1999). A comparison of exposure therapy, stress innoculation training, and their combination for reducing posttraumatic stress disorder in female assault victims. *Journal of Consulting and Clinical Psychology, 67,* 194–200.

Foa, E.B., Keane, T.M., Friedman, M.J. (Eds.) (2000). *Effective treatments for PTSD: Practice guidelines from the International Society for Traumatic Stress Studies.* New York: Guilford Press.

Friedman, M.J. (2000). A guide to the literature on pharmacotherapy for PTSD. *PTSD Research Quarterly, 11,* 1–7.

Friedman, M.J., Davidson, J.R.T., Mellman, T.A., & Southwick, S. (2000). Pharmacotherapy. In E.B. Foa, T.M. Keane, & M.J. Friedman (Eds.), *Effective treatments for PTSD: Practice guidelines from the International Society for Traumatic Stress Studies* (pp. 84–105). New York: Guilford Press.

Hopa, M., Simbayi, L.C., & Du Toit, C.D. (1998). Perceptions on integration of traditional and Western healing in the new South Africa. *South African Journal of Psychology, 28,* 8–14.

Jacob, K.S. (2001). Community care for people with mental disorders in developing countries: Problems and possible solutions. *British Journal of Psychiatry, 178,* 296–298.

Krupnick, J. (2002, May). Group IPT for PTSD after interpersonal trauma in low-income women. In *New applications of IPT* (Panel conducted at the meeting of the American Psychiatric Association, Philadelphia, PA).

Leff, J. (2001). Mental health services and barriers to implementation: Background information document. In *World Health Organization Ministerial round tables 2001: Mental health.* London: Institute of Psychiatry.

Marsella, A.J. (1998). Toward a "Global-Community Psychology": Meeting the needs of a changing world. *American Psychologist, 53,* 1282–1291.

Meichenbaum, D. (1974). Self-instructional methods. In F.H. Kanfer & A.P. Goldstein (Eds.), *Helping people change* (pp. 357–391). New York : Pergamon Press.

Nathan, T. (1987). Amenagement de la technique psychoanalytique dans les situations inter-culturelles. *Information Psychiatrique, 63,* 781–785.

Patel, V. (2000). The need for treatment evidence for common mental disorders in developing countries. *Psychological Medicine, 30,* 743–746.

Pearlman, L.A., & Saakvitne, K.W. (1995). *Trauma and the therapist: Countertransference and vicarious traumatization in psychotherapy with incest survivors.* New York: W.W. Norton.

Paunovic, N., & Ost, L-G. (2001). Cognitive behavior therapy vs. exposure therapy in the treatment of PTSD in refugees. *Behaviour Research and Therapy, 39,* 1183–1197.

Resick, P.A., Nishith, P., Weaver, T.L., Astin, M.C., & Feuer, C.A. (2002). A comparison of cognitive-processing therapy with prolonged exposure and a waiting condition for the treatment of chronic posttraumatic stress disorder in female rape victims. *Journal of Consulting and Clinical Psychology, 70,* 867–879.

Rothbaum, B.O., Meadows, E.A., Resick, P., & Foy, D. (2000). Cognitive-behavioral therapy. In E.B. Foa, T.M. Keane, & M.J. Friedman (Eds.), *Effective treatments for PTSD: Practice guidelines from the International Society for Traumatic Stress Studies* (pp. 60–83). New York: Guilford Press.

Siriam, T.G. (1990). Psychotherapy in developing countries: A public health perspective. *Indian Journal of Psychotherapy, 32,* 138–144.

Tanaka-Matsumi, J., & Higginbotham, H.N. (1996). Behavioral approaches to counseling across cultures. In P.B. Pedersen, J.G. Draguns, W.J. Lonner, & J.E. Trimble (Eds.), *Counseling across cultures* (4th ed.) (pp. 266–292). Thousand Oaks, CA: Sage.

World Health Organization (1992). *The ICD-10 classification of mental and behavioral disorders: Clinical descriptions and guidelines.* Geneva: Author.

World Health Organization (2001). *WHO Model List of Essential Drugs (EDL)* 11th Edition (Nov, 1999), World Health Organization Web site: http://www.who.int/medicines/organization/par/edl/infed11group.html

Part II

Abuse and Torture

THE ASCENDANT ETHICAL SELF

Historically, one can discern that humankind has habitually exhibited cruelty toward its weakest members, notably women, children, and the elderly, as well as members of conquered groups, be they slaves or prisoners of war. In most cases, the cruelty has been perpetrated by the strongest members of society (or strongest societies): able-bodied better armed men—and less often, but nevertheless remarkably so, women—who have grown to physical adulthood, but are not yet disabled by age, i.e. who are in the prime of life. On a purely biological basis, one could argue that such cruelty serves to weed out the weaker members of the human group. Humankind's "inhumanity" to humankind is natural and characteristic of *homo sapiens*. We know, however, that humankind has historically sought to overcome the reflex of cruelty. Protection of the vulnerable and innocent has been held up as virtuous by a range of moral philosophies for several thousand years. What now characterizes human thought and behavior is the tension between cruelty and protection rather than simple barbarism. The question then arises whether we are in transition to a new, ethical order, and whether we are capable of vanishing brutality.

The impulse to violence is self-sustaining. Yesterday's victims are today's perpetrators, and today's victims are tomorrow's perpetrators. Not all persons live out such predictions, but new recruits are brought into the cycle of violence by serendipity and hazard, while others are finally exhausted by the hardship, or are rehabilitated.

The potential for violence is also widespread. We have good reason to suspect that child abuse, wife-beating, and abuse of the elderly are underestimated, and that their prevalence may be largely additive. Taking account of both victims and perpetrators, even in times of peace, and even

73

with formal abolition of slavery, the part of any population touched by abuse of any kind is large.

The vista is compelling. Brutality is a daily occurrence among receivers and givers of violence, and continues to be visited on each generation to greater or lesser degree. Every person alive today may carry a history of abuse or violence, may have had a grandparent or a parent touched by harm. Such widespread experience of violence assures a large reservoir of pent-up resentment and anger, waiting to erupt into violence should it be triggered. It is likely that the latent reserve of violent energy is larger at given points of history than at other times, and particular settings may favor more or less violence. What is not clear is whether, left untriggered, the charge diminishes over time, or whether it remains ever ready to erupt if not continually controlled and regulated.

Still, humankind has gained remarkably in its short history. Religious teaching and moral exhortation, the rule of law, and enforcement have served to dampen brutality, with greater or lesser success depending on time and place. To a large extent, also, most people touched by violence do cope, and the proportion that survives to be psychologically hobbled by the experience is not large. Efforts to make our ethical selves ascendant are ever-intensifying in contemporary societies, and it is clear that we are driven now by a vision of the world that could be free of inhumanity.

This will require sustained efforts in science and knowledge, to comprehend human behavior and how we regulate ourselves; in actions to disarm, establish rules of law, and enforce compliance to non-violent treatment of conflict; and to deepen understanding of how to diagnose, treat, and prevent the sequelae of traumatic abuse and violence visited on individual human beings.

ODILE FRANK
Chief, Social Integration Branch
Division for Social Policy and Development
Department of Economic and Social Affairs
United Nations
September 2002

Chapter 5

Child Abuse in Peacetime

David A. Wolfe and Madhabika B. Nayak

Maltreatment of children rarely raised concern prior to the mid-20th century, because many societies viewed harsh forms of discipline and corporal punishment as inconsequential and a parent's right and responsibility. Sexual abuse remained hidden, as did the exploitation of children through the sex trade and child labor. Children who witnessed violence between their parents remained silent victims, seemingly unaffected by the unpredictable and frightening outbursts.

Fortunately, counter-efforts to value the rights and needs of children, and to recognize their exploitation and abuse, began to take root during the latter part of the 20th century in many developed countries, spurred by the *Convention on the Rights of the Child* (United Nations, 1989). Article 19 of the Covenant states:

> States Parties shall take all appropriate legislative, administrative, social and educational measures to protect the child from all forms of physical or mental violence, injury or abuse, neglect or negligent treatment, maltreatment or exploitation, including sexual abuse, while in the care of parent(s), legal guardian(s) or any other person who has the care of the child.

Although still in its infancy, the growing recognition of widespread child maltreatment has brought worldwide interest in public health strategies to document and reduce the incidence of child maltreatment. Today, 32 countries have an official government policy regarding child abuse and neglect, and about one-third of the world's population is included in countries that conduct an annual count of child abuse and neglect cases (Bross, Miyoshi, Miyoshi, & Krugman, 2000). Such efforts provide the critical first steps to identifying the scope of the problem, and justify the implementation of important societal, community, and cultural changes to combat it.

Child abuse deserves special consideration among all of the perils faced by children in countries around the world, because it is largely preventable and has long-lasting and pervasive consequences. Unlike other forms of childhood stress and trauma, child abuse typically occurs within ongoing relationships that are expected to be protective, supportive, and nurturing. Rather than receiving consistent and appropriate guidance, children from abusive and neglecting families are placed in jeopardy of physical and emotional harm. Yet, their ties to their family—sometimes even to the abuser—are very important to their emotional and physical well-being, so child victims may feel torn between a sense of belonging and a sense of fear and apprehension. Other children may be abused outside of their homes, and may be victimized by multiple abusers. What these children have in common, however, is a sense of fear, loss of protection, and feelings of hopelessness in escaping circumstances well beyond their control.

This chapter considers various forms of child abuse and neglect, including physical and sexual abuse, exploitation, and female genital mutilation. Prevalence estimates of these forms of abuse are described on the basis of available national statistics from several countries, as well as research studies and less formal reporting sources. The chapter discusses the definition and scope of maltreatment (physical abuse, emotional abuse, neglect and negligent treatment, sexual abuse, exploitation), its impact on development, and contributing factors (individual and family, societal and cultural). This discussion is followed by examples of prevention and treatment initiatives, including prevention priorities, community-based approaches, and individual-based approaches.

This chapter recognizes that each culture has problems of child maltreatment associated with unique causes, as well as approaches to prevention. Prevention is generally shaped by an interaction of historical perspectives, ratified United Nations, goals, and a country's current resource capabilities. Most research and observations of child abuse have been made in the developed countries; nonetheless, these countries still struggle with the many issues involved, including recognizing the importance of cultural diversity in determining the needs of children and families. Although not yet tested worldwide, several community-based and individual- and family-based strategies are highlighted that may be of benefit to other communities in their efforts to find solutions to child maltreatment.

Programs to prevent child abuse and neglect that are community-based are considered most promising, since they reach more families and are designed to address problems before they become severe. Programs that offer a personalized approach (such as home visits by an individual who is familiar to the recipient) stand out as most successful in helping high-risk families and children, who may be eligible for such services due to their economic circumstances, living conditions, or similar factors identified by local communities. Parental need for support, parenting instruction, and resource linkage seem to be fulfilled by the more personalized, outreach nature of the home visitor approach. Program development should focus on providing child development and parenting information that is easily understood, practical, and accessible to all present and potential parenting populations.

Attention must be particularly directed to societal influences that play a role in child abuse and neglect, especially in circumstances where families are exposed to major effects of poverty, health risks, and environmental conflict. The underlying and contributing causes of poverty need to be exposed and remedied, whether historical or current inequalities, and whether within or between countries (UNICEF, 2000). Such a cross-cultural perspective on child abuse and neglect prevention would re-direct the focus away from individuals and families, and explore societal and cultural conditions that attenuate or exacerbate these problems. These larger systemic factors are not explored here, though they provide an ever-present backdrop to the discussion (see also Chapter 3).

Community-based programs to end sexual abuse and exploitation need to expand their focus beyond the potential child victims. In particular, few programs or existing laws target adults who come into contact with children, whether these adults are potential abusers (such as tourists seeking child prostitutes) or potential resources for child protection and safety (such as teachers and parents). Recommendations are offered concerning additional resources for programs targeting parents and other adults through places of employment, churches, and community service groups, as well as through small discussion groups in local homes. In addition, public media should be used to provide information about safety, to increase community awareness, and to offer helpful advice on locating services.

Child sexual abuse prevention must also turn its attention toward some of the underlying social and cultural issues that are suspected to be at the root of such exploitation and abuse. To date, little research has been conducted on the motivating factors involved in child sexual abuse. Because the majority of the offenders are male, a long-term strategy should be developed that addresses some of the sociocultural roots of such behavior. More responsibility for prevention should be directed at community agencies and cultural institutions that can heighten society's awareness of the problem and attack the roots of sexism that exist at all levels.

DEFINITION AND SCOPE

Abused children suffer a wide variety of physical, emotional and developmental problems which can hamper their ability to live healthy and productive lives. In addition to health consequences, abused children have difficulty in school, problems with substance abuse and problems with the law. It is a public health issue of vital importance for WHO, and it represents a challenge for the next millennium (World Health Organization, 1999).

Child maltreatment is a generic term referring to four primary acts: **physical abuse, emotional abuse, sexual abuse, and neglect.** It cuts across all lines of gender, national origin, language, religion, age, ethnicity, disability, and sexual orientation. However, as shown below, girls suffer predominately or exclusively from specific types of harm both because they are female, and because of the historically unequal power relations between men and women (United Nations Division for the Advancement of Women, 1997).

Defining child maltreatment is not straightforward, due to geographical, cultural, legal, and theoretical considerations. A World Health Organization report (WHO, 1999) states that child abuse **"constitutes all forms of physical and/or emotional ill-treatment, sexual abuse, neglect or negligent treatment or commercial or other exploitation, resulting in actual or potential harm to the child's health, survival, development or dignity in the context of a relationship of responsibility, trust or power"** (p. 15). UNICEF (2000) considers victims of child maltreatment to be persons under age 18 who suffer **"occasional or habitual acts of physical, sexual or emotional violence, be it in the family group or in social institutions."** A common element of all definitions of child maltreatment is that it includes not only acts of aggression and exploitation, but also acts of omission (such as abandonment or failure to provide) as well as acts that serve to suppress individual and collective rights.

Estimating the scope of child maltreatment in various countries worldwide is also a daunting task. In general, there is a lack of information from developing countries, which may be due to the overwhelming nature of poverty affecting many, requiring priority attention to the basic survival needs of water, food, and shelter. As well, many countries are reluctant to challenge existing structures of family authority in such areas as physical discipline, resulting in a high threshold for reporting child abuse. Consequently, apathy regarding physical child abuse, particularly when it occurs within the family, is widespread. In contrast, different forms of "societal" child abuse have commanded more attention in developing countries, such as child prostitution, maiming, and the selling of children for beggary.

Based on current estimates, child maltreatment is found in all societies and is almost always a highly guarded secret wherever it occurs. In North

America (where the most comprehensive statistics are available), studies estimate that about one in every five girls and one in nine boys will experience some form of sexual abuse (Finkelhor, 1994; Finkelhor, Hotaling, Lewis, & Smith, 1990), and each year about one of every ten children is the victim of severe physical violence by a parent or other caregiver (Straus & Gelles, 1986). Countless other children suffer the effects of emotional abuse and neglect, which, like physical and sexual abuse, can cause known harm to their psychological development (Trocme & Wolfe, 2001).

Worldwide, the World Health Organization estimates that each year 40 million children aged 0–14 are victims of child abuse and neglect (WHO, 1999), confirming suspicions that childhood is not a peaceful time for many. Although it is difficult to draw comparisons between countries because of differences in defining and reporting child maltreatment, what little is known about the prevalence of maltreatment suggests, unfortunately, that physical and sexual abuse are at epidemic proportions in many societies worldwide.

The following definitions of the types of child maltreatment are based on a recent consensus meeting by WHO (1999). Due to the lack of comparable incidence studies, the scope of each type of maltreatment is estimated from a variety of sources.

Physical Abuse

WHO (1999) defines physical abuse of a child as **"that which results in actual or potential physical harm from an interaction or lack of an interaction, which is reasonably within the control of a parent or person in a position of responsibility, power or trust. There may be a single or repeated incidents."** Some of the more prominent, acute physical signs for children who have been physically abused include external signs of physical injury, ranging from bruises, lacerations, scars, and abrasions to burns, sprains, or broken bones. As well, internal injuries may be present, such as head injury (from violent shaking or contact with a hard object), bone fractures, and intra-abdominal injuries (e.g., ruptured liver or spleen).

Population-based studies (i.e., those that rely on adult self-report rather than officially reported cases) estimate that physical abuse is quite common, affecting between 10% (Straus & Gelles, 1986) and 25% (MacMillan et al., 1997) of all adults at some point during their childhood. Whereas most acts of physical abuse involve bruises and cuts, WHO (1999) estimates that as many as 1 in 5,000 to 1 in 10,000 children under the age of 5 die each year from physical violence.

Female genital mutilation (FGM) is also included in the current discussion of physical abuse, because it is a deeply rooted traditional practice that has serious health consequences for girls and women, especially in its more severe forms. In addition to physical and sexual abuse worldwide, over 130 million girls and women have undergone some form of FGM, with two million girls being at risk each year. These women live primarily in African countries and a few countries in the Middle East and Asia, but FGM is also becoming a concern in Australia, Canada, Europe, New Zealand, and the United States due to its practice in immigrant communities (Barstow, 1999).

Emotional Abuse

WHO (1999) defines emotional abuse as **"the failure to provide a developmentally appropriate, supportive environment, including the availability of a primary attachment figure, so that the child can establish a stable and full range of emotional and social competencies commensurate with her or his personal potentials and in the context of the society in which the child dwells. There may also be acts towards the child that cause or have a high probability of causing harm to the child's health or physical, mental, spiritual, moral or social development. These acts must be reasonably within the control of a parent or person in a position of responsibility, power or trust. Acts include restriction of movement, patterns of belittling, denigrating, scapegoating, threatening, scaring, discriminating, ridiculing or other non-physical forms of hostile or rejecting treatment."**

Some countries, such as the US and Canada, have also begun to include children's exposure to domestic violence as a form of emotional abuse or neglect, since it is known that such experiences have a pronounced effect on children's adjustment (Trocme & Wolfe, 2001). Despite considerable agreement that emotional abuse is harmful and widespread, efforts to document the incidence of this type of maltreatment have not as yet overcome the difficult challenges posed by this broad definition.

Neglect and Negligent Treatment

WHO describes neglect as **"the failure to provide for the development of the child in all spheres: health, education, emotional development, nutrition, shelter and safe living conditions, in the context of resources reasonably available to the family or caretakers, and causes or has a high probability of causing harm to the child's health or physical, mental, spiritual, moral or social development."** This includes the failure to properly supervise and protect children from physical harm and to provide the emotional security of being cared for. Child neglect typically emerges as the most common form of maltreatment in nationwide incidence studies in North America (Sedlak & Broadhurst, 1996; Trocme & Wolfe, 2001).

Given that the US and Canada are among the world's wealthiest countries, these figures may be higher among poorer countries. On the other hand, countries that have maintained open and cohesive community structures may have *less* neglect, despite the stress of poverty. That is, some wealthier countries may have achieved economic success at the expense of social inclusiveness, resulting in some individuals living emotionally isolated lives, which is a significant risk factor for child neglect (Thompson, 1994). Unfortunately, neither official nor unofficial estimates from developing countries are currently available on the incidence of child neglect.

Sexual Abuse

WHO (1999) defines child sexual abuse as **"the involvement of a child in sexual activity that he or she does not fully comprehend, is unable to give informed consent to, or for which the child is not developmentally prepared and cannot give consent, or that violates the laws or social taboos of society. Child sexual abuse is evidenced by this activity between a child and an adult or another child who by age or development is in a relationship of responsibility, trust or power, the activity being intended to gratify or satisfy the needs of the other person."** This may include but is not limited to the inducement or coercion of a child to engage in any unlawful sexual activity, the exploitative use of a child in prostitution or other sexual practices, and the exploitative use of children in pornographic performances and materials.

International studies conducted in 19 countries, from different world regions including, for example, South Africa, Sweden, and the Dominican Republic, have reported prevalence rates for sexual abuse ranging from 7% to 34% among girls, and from 3% to 29% among boys (WHO, 1999). Estimates of sexual abuse for African, Middle Eastern, or Far Eastern countries, however, are not currently available (for recent discussion of the realities of sexual abuse disclosure in the Arab world, see Shalhoub-Kevorkian, 1999). Information compiled in the US over the past decade similarly indicates that sexual abuse occurs among children and adolescents of all ages, that girls are abused 1.5 to 3 times more frequently than boys, and that approximately 15% of substantiated cases of child maltreatment involve sexual abuse (Sedlak & Broadhurst, 1996; Trocme & Wolfe, 2001).

Exploitation

WHO (1999) describes commercial or other exploitation of a child as **"the use of the child in work or other activities for the benefit of others. This includes, but is not limited to, child labor and child prostitution. These activities are to the detriment of the child's physical and**

mental health, education, and spiritual, moral or social-emotional development." Countless children worldwide are pressed into dangerous work for long and exhausting hours, putting them at risk for death. If they survive, the work they are forced to perform turns them into adults long before their time. According to estimates from the International Labour Organization (ILO), there are close to 15 million child workers under the age of 15 in Latin America and the Caribbean, and 250 million worldwide. The ILO estimates that well over half of all working children in the world are girls, and that the vast majority of these perform "invisible" tasks that are not valued, let alone accounted for in official statistics (International Labor Organization, 2001).

An especially pernicious form of work forced on many children is sexual. Every year, an estimated one million children worldwide are lured and forced into child prostitution. Globally, as many as 10 million children may be victims of child prostitution, the sex industry, sex tourism, and pornography, although accurate statistics are not available (WHO, 1999). A UNICEF supported study by the 1996 World Conference against Sexual Exploitation of Children revealed that 47% of sexually exploited girls in Central American countries were victims of abuse and rape in their homes. Almost half of them had begun commercial sexual activity between the age of 9 and 13, and the majority had used drugs to sustain such exploitation (UNICEF, 2000). Rates of child prostitution tend to be higher in Asia and Latin America, but an alarming growth has been recorded in Africa, North America and Europe, with Eastern Europe emerging as a new market in the sexual exploitation of children. Poverty is the greatest factor in the child prostitution explosion, as migration of families from the rural areas into cities creates unemployment, the breakdown of family structures, homelessness and, inevitably, an increase in child prostitution.

EFFECTS OF CHILD ABUSE IN PEACETIME

Maltreated children experience ongoing, uncontrollable events that challenge their successful development and adaptation in a pervasive manner and pose a threat to their core psychological well-being. They not only have to face acute and unpredictable parental outbursts or betrayal; they also have to adapt to environmental circumstances that pose developmental challenges. These influences include the more dramatic events, such as marital violence and separation of family members, as well as the mundane but important everyday activities that may be disturbing or upsetting, such as unfriendly interactions, few learning opportunities, and chaotic lifestyle. Children who are sexually and physically abused undergo pronounced interruptions in their developing view of themselves and the world, resulting in significant emotional and behavioral changes indicative of their attempts to cope with such events (Kendall-Tackett, Williams, & Finkelhor, 1993; Wolfe, 1999).

Because the source of stress and fear is often centralized in their families, children who are maltreated are challenged on a regular basis to find ways to adapt that pose the least risk and offer maximum protection and opportunity for growth. Like other forms of adversity and trauma during childhood, however, child maltreatment does not affect each child predictably or consistently. The impact of maltreatment depends not only on the severity and chronicity of the events themselves, but also on how such events interact with the child's individual and family characteristics.

Finally, it is worth noting that child abuse by family members has received the most scientific and professional attention, whereas knowledge on the impact of abuse committed by perpetrators in (non-familial) community organizations and institutions is lacking. Educational and vocational institutions, religious and spiritual institutions, sporting, cultural, and recreational organizations, and special needs facilities are part of every community, and in the vast majority of cases they operate in a safe and caring manner. Nonetheless, media reports, public lawsuits, and survivors' accounts of such experiences have brought attention to the need for more research and prevention initiatives in this area (Wolfe, Jaffe, Jette, & Poisson, *under review*).

Maltreatment destroys a child's sense of personal safety and ability to trust others, which often includes those persons to whom the child is closest. As a result, child maltreatment can have a profound effect on development, disrupting the normal course of growth and adaptation. Child physical abuse or neglect, for example, may interfere with the important process of infant-caregiver attachment, which normally provides the child with a secure base from which to explore his or her environment. In the absence of such a secure base, a child may become more difficult to manage, which in turn causes the caregiver to react with even more withdrawal or abuse. A damaging, interactive pattern may develop which, over time, places the child's development in further jeopardy (Wolfe, 1999). In contrast, children may be protected in part from the harmful effects of maltreatment if they have a positive relationship with at least one important and consistent person in their lives who provides support and protection (Cicchetti & Rogosch, 1997).

Some of the major developmental consequences identified among physically abused and neglected children include a poorly developed understanding of the effect of their behavior on others, leading to the reliance on aggression to solve conflicts with peers. Similarly, they may form a view of the world as made up of victims and victimizers, based on their own experiences (Dodge, Pettit, & Bates, 1994). One of the most far-reaching effects of child maltreatment is the loss or disruption of children's ability to regulate the intensity of their emotional feelings and impulses (Van Der Kolk & Fisler, 1994). As they grow older and are faced with new situations involving peers and other adults, this inability to regulate emotions can lead to emotional disorders, such as depression and anxiety (Brown, Cohen, Johnson, & Smailes, 1999), as well as behavioral problems such as hostility, aggression, self-injury, substance abuse, and criminal and antisocial behavior (Wolfe, Scott, Wekerle, & Pittman, 2001).

Child sexual abuse affects children's ongoing development in ways that are somewhat distinct from other forms of maltreatment. The initial effects of sexual abuse often include symptoms of distress, confusion, and fear, depending on the child's age, available supports, and other factors. Common concerns among children and younger teens include age-inappropriate sexual behavior and knowledge, fearfulness, nightmares and sleep disorders, depression, anger and hostility, behavior problems, and somatic complaints (Browne & Finkelhor, 1986). By late adolescence and young adulthood, prior experiences of child sexual abuse may have a profound effect on one's ability to form close, trusting relationships, and lead to more pervasive and chronic psychiatric disorders such as anxiety and panic disorders, depression, eating disorders, sexual problems, and personality disturbances (Brown, Cohen, Johnson, & Smailes, 1999; Flisher et al., 1997; Kendler et al., 2000).

Contributing Factors

Concerted efforts to understand the causes and consequences of child maltreatment have led to immense gains in knowledge and resources, while at the same time pointing out the complex nature and unknown elements of the problem. It is widely accepted today, for example, that the context of child maltreatment includes societal, cultural, and socioeconomic factors, as well as those closest to the child's social world—the parent-child relationship and the nuclear and extended family.

Notwithstanding the critical role of the offender, child maltreatment is rarely caused by a single risk factor. Various risk signs are usually present, but these risk signs may be common to many families under stress who do not harm their children. Because child maltreatment is a series of events (rather than a "disorder"), it is necessary to consider multiple interactive causes. These causal conditions stem largely from the interaction of individual, familial, and cultural influences, described below.

Individual and Family. Physically abusive and neglecting parents have often experienced similar problems in their families of origin, where they were exposed to traumatic or harmful events such as family violence, instability, alcoholism, and maltreatment. Although abusive and neglecting parents share many common psychological and situational problems, they typically do not suffer from specific psychiatric disorders that account for such behavior. As adults, they often are incapable of managing the levels of stress found in their environment. Women in particular face multiple environmental stressors—poverty, discrimination, and traditional expectations that they bear innumerable children, remain at home to serve their families and, increasingly, also work in the wage sector.

Often, stress and limited resources can make someone avoid social contacts and choose to remain isolated, in an effort to reduce additional stress. Inadequate or inappropriate exposure to positive parental models and supports (in both the present and the past), coupled with limited intellectual and problem-solving skills (i.e., the ability to make appropriate judgments during childrearing situations), may serve to make childrearing a difficult and aversive event. Consequently, maltreating parents may report symptoms indicative of health and coping problems, which further impair their ability to function effectively as parents (Wolfe, 1985).

Child sexual abusers come from many walks of life, and they are seldom discernible on the basis of personality traits, occupation, or age. Individual and situational conditions affecting sexual abuse have been described by Finkelhor (1984) as involving four offender characteristics as necessary pre-conditions to sexual abuse: 1) the motivation to sexually abuse, 2) overcoming internal inhibitors, 3) overcoming external inhibitors, and 4) overcoming the child's resistance. The first two conditions are necessary for abuse to occur—i.e., the perpetrator must be inclined to abuse and be uninhibited about it. The background of sexual abusers likely contributes to this pattern. Past experiences of physical or sexual maltreatment, in particular, may set in motion a cautious, distrustful approach to intimate relationships (Marshall, Serran, & Cortoni, 2000). Sexual offenders, as a group, are more likely to have significant social and relationship deficits, including social isolation and difficulty forming emotionally close, trusting relationships (Smith & Saunders, 1995). The pressures of modern urban living further contribute to social isolation, with boys and men being most at risk.

Family circumstances, most notably conflict and marital violence, also contribute to child maltreatment. In close to half of families where adult partners are violent toward one another, one or both parents have also been violent toward a child at some point during the last year (Edleson, 1999). Incestuous abuse is also more likely in a family where domestic violence occurs and, in fact, spousal rape may be part of the pattern. Domestic conflicts and violence against women most often arise during disagreements over childrearing, discipline, and each partner's responsibilities in childcare, in which children may be caught in the "cross-fire" between angry adults. An escalating cycle of family turmoil and violence begins, whereby children's behavioral and emotional reactions to the violence create additional stress on the marital relationship, further aggravating an already volatile situation.

Family factors may also increase children's vulnerability to sexual abuse. Low income and social isolation, in particular, are related to increased risk of sexual abuse because parents may lack resources or opportunities for suitable childcare and safety precautions (Finkelhor, 1984). They often lack significant social connections to others in their extended families, neighborhoods, and communities, as well as to social assistance agencies. Unfortunately, maintaining family privacy and isolation may come at the cost of restricted access to healthier childrearing models and social supports. Neglecting families are especially prone to such isolation and insularity, which may be tied to the parents' significant interpersonal problems (Polansky, Gaudin, & Kilpatrick, 1992).

Societal and Cultural.   Family childrearing practices and community care of children are influenced by numerous cultural and situational factors that determine the level of conflict or cooperation in the emerging parent-child relationship. Such practices are made up of community and societal norms of acceptable or tolerable behavior toward children, which are shaped by past and current expectations and experiences. Many of these expectations are passed along from generation to generation with little outside influence and education. Cultural values, historical precedent, and community standards, such as endorsement of corporal punishment, may indirectly contribute to the rate of child maltreatment, especially if accompanied by limited cultural opportunities to learn about alternative childrearing practices and receive necessary education and supports.

The context of child maltreatment often includes social and economic deprivation, cultural expectations, and gender inequality, which contribute to a belief that physical force or sexual intrusiveness is harmless or inconsequential. In addition, some adults may rely on abusive methods or neglecting withdrawal to control the irritating, daily events that they experience, or turn to child exploitation in an effort to support the family. Coupled with prevailing cultural traditions, abusive behavior is seen as justifiable because children are considered "parents' property" and as such should obediently submit to their parents' decisions in matters of education, discipline, behavior, personality development, and so forth (UNICEF, 2000). Such cultural and economic influences are illustrated in the following case:

> *Dr. Duong Quynh Hoa, director of a pediatric hospital in Ho Chi Minh City,*
> *Vietnam, treats child prostitutes in her hospital. The doctor often asks parents why*
> *they sell their children. One father came in with his 12-year-old daughter. Dr. Hoa*
> *recalled, "She was bleeding from her wounds and as torn as if she had given birth."*
> *[The father] told me: "We've earned $300, so it's enough. She can stop." Another*
> *parent, accompanying his 11-year-old daughter who was in terrible pain explained,*
> *"First of all, we are very poor. And this is a good age to do it. She is still too young*
> *to get pregnant." When Dr. Hoa asked about the child's future, the father said, "She*
> *is very young now. She will grow up and she will forget it." (Simons, 1993).*

Therefore, although child maltreatment is certainly not limited by the boundaries of socioeconomic status, the problem must be considered in the context of poverty, environmental stress, and cultural traditions. Poverty is associated with severe restrictions in the child's expectable environment, such as lack of adequate emotional support, daycare, safety, and housing, which often impair or impede the development of healthy parent-child relationships. As well, adults below poverty level suffer more individual and family problems, such as substance abuse and emotional disorders (Lung & Daro, 1996). Just the same, many materially impoverished rural communities can be emotionally rich and supportive while, conversely, materially rich urban communities are often emotional sterile and unhealthy for children.

Cultural norms and practices influence the prevalence of sexual abuse and exploitation as well. The erotic portrayal of children not only in pornography but also in mainstream advertising raises concerns about boundaries and appropriate messages. Existing criminal sanctions are inadequate at deterring offenders, since they rely heavily on child victims' testimony. The recent explosion of child prostitution in Asia, moreover, may be a function of the worldwide increase in AIDS, because some adults believe that the younger the child, the less likely the risk of HIV infection. Unfortunately, such fear may increase the exploitation of younger and younger children. Abuse of children in developing countries is seen as a lucrative trade in which several family and non-family factors work together to subject the child to various types of exploitation. An illustration is provided in the *Report on The National Consultation on Child Prostitution* (1995):

> *Young girls are beaten, raped, and starved, and thus pressured into receiving cus-*
> *tomers. A 14-year-old in a Mumbai brothel resisted all pressure for three weeks.*
> *Consequently she was put in a small room with a live cobra. She sat there numb,*
> *unable to move or sleep for two days, and eventually gave in to her captors.*

There is also grave concern stemming from the quantity of child pornography circulating on the Internet, where child pornography has become accessible and child sexual abusers share information, exchange pornography, and make contact with potential child victims. Because particular geographic areas or nation-states cannot be isolated, the Internet poses a real challenge to the protection of minors from illegal or harmful influences (Akdeniz, 1997). Furthermore, children who have been exposed to pornography may be desensitized and socialized into believing that pornographic activity is normal for children (McCabe, 2000). Preliminary studies suggest that children who have been used in the production of pornography show psychological symptoms such as emotional withdrawal, antisocial behavior, mood swings, depression, fear and anxiety, and disorders such as posttraumatic stress disorder (PTSD; Rosenberg, 1997).

PREVENTION AND TREATMENT

This section describes the state of prevention and treatment methods for various forms of child abuse, followed by descriptions of community-based programs and ideas that can be adapted for other cultures and communities. Based on the current state of the art, it is reasonable to assume that a large proportion of abusive incidents and their associated outcomes are preventable. Nonetheless, retooling from a detection and protection approach to a more prevention-oriented model of family assistance and support poses considerable challenges that require long-term strategies (Melton & Barry, 1994). There are no short-term or inexpensive solutions to child maltreatment—only gradual, meaningful steps that lead to progressive and lasting change.

Efforts to enhance positive experiences at an early stage in the development of the parent-child relationship hold considerable promise for the prevention of child maltreatment and its consequences. Similarly, programs that instruct children and their parents on how to avoid and report sexual abuse improve children's response to victimization, although relying on child-focused prevention alone is not sufficient (Finkelhor, Asdigian, & Dzuiba-Leatherman, 1995). Formal treatment efforts also increase the chances of overcoming the harmful effects of abuse and neglect. Examples of such prevention and treatment strategies for different forms of child abuse follow.

Prevention Priorities

As noted previously, child maltreatment occurs most often in conjunction with the day-to-day stress of childrearing, the pressures of poverty, and the cultural expectations that allow parents and others to exploit children for financial gain. For example, toddlerhood poses particular challenges to parents, who are expected to provide careful supervision and guidance to the child at all times, regardless of other pressures and demands. Similarly, times of family instability and disruption, such as migration, divorce, or job loss, require additional social supports and services for families, especially those who have learned to fear or hide from authorities. The elimination of poverty and the fostering of open and cohesive communities are necessary for preventive measures to be sustainable in the long term.

Fortunately, many of the risk factors associated with child abuse are recognizable today, which is why prevention and early intervention approaches make considerable sense for building resistance against many of the unavoidable pressures acting upon high-risk families. Prevention can also involve actions that enhance something positive for children, especially an improved parent-child relationship (Wekerle & Wolfe, 1993).

The primary goals of prevention involve the development of strong, positive childrearing abilities. This is accomplished by strengthening the early formation of the parent-child relationship, improving the parent's abilities to cope with stress through exposure to a mental health or social services support system, and strengthening the child's adaptive behaviors, which will contribute to his or her further emotional and psychological adjustment. Approaches to prevention, early intervention, and treatment emphasize education and guidance in a format that is flexible and responsive to the needs of families and individuals. Moreover, intervention must be re-directed toward the important issues that families face during each of the emerging developmental stages that the child and parent must endure, as opposed to attempting to repair the difficulties in the relationship later on. A major challenge to prevention programs, however, is the identification and selection of appropriate, desirable, and attainable goals that can be addressed through community action programs, individual skills-training efforts, and similar activities.

Far-reaching programs aimed at preventing child abuse focus on increasing the general public's awareness and understanding of child maltreatment, as well as ways to access important community resources. These methods include a variety of delivery formats, such as media campaigns, home-based services for families, and community networks that provide support and feedback to families. For example, strategies used to prevent child abuse were recently surveyed among member countries of the International Society for Prevention of Child Abuse and Neglect (Bross et al., 2000). Based on reports from 58 countries worldwide, those strategies believed to be most effective involved *public education*, such as awareness and media campaigns to inform the public of the signs of abuse and how to respond to suspected child abuse and neglect; *environmental improvements* for families, such as housing; *professional education;* and enhanced *methods of case identification,* such as screening tools and inter-agency communication.

Due to the secretive and often commonplace nature of many forms of child maltreatment, active detection should be the first step of any intervention strategy. To avoid posing further risk to the child (especially when abuse involves other family members), reporting mechanisms must be developed that are efficient and easily accessed, and enable action that is as quick as the situation requires. Community level networks should be created for the detection and rapid reporting of maltreatment. At the same time, training of educators, social service providers, and all others whose work puts them in contact with maltreated children is essential (UNICEF, 2000).

Prevention and intervention efforts may also target vulnerable populations, such as single and teenaged parents, low socioeconomic level or isolated families, and parents undergoing crises, to offer assistance to these sub-groups during pre- and post-natal periods and times of excessive stress. For example, local programs may assist identified high-risk families during transitional periods, offering help from parent aides who model effective parenting methods in the home, providing childrearing assistance, and involving trained health visitors that sensitize parents to the health and psychological needs of their children. Below are some concrete examples of these approaches.

Community-Based Approaches

Various community-based programs hold promise for preventing the occurrence of child abuse, or assisting children who are at risk or who are known victims. Due to the rapid expansion of Internet resources, many community programs can now be located relatively simply, and information about the programs can be widely disseminated. Many of the programs and resources described below were located from Internet sites due to the lack of more formal outlets for such resources. While they are illustrative of promising community efforts to prevent child abuse, we urge caution in drawing any firm conclusions concerning their effectiveness, due to lack of evaluation findings. Moreover, these programs have not often been attempted in other locales, and would likely require adaptation to be effective in other cultures and settings. Nonetheless, these state-of-the-art programs provide a good starting point for diverse communities worldwide that are interested in preventing child abuse at its broadest level.

Child Physical Abuse and Neglect.   Model programs in the area of physical abuse and neglect have developed from the field of public health and nursing, and involve efforts to provide education and support for new parents by home-visiting programs. At the individual and family level, the need for support, instruction, and resource linkage among new parents is best met by a personalized outreach strategy, such as home visitation, which is relatively adaptable to different cultures and locations.

The Prenatal/Early Infancy Project developed by Olds and colleagues at the University of Colorado Health Sciences Center is a strong illustration of effective home visitation (Olds et al., 1997). This team targeted first-time parents who displayed one or more child abuse risk factors, such as being teenaged, single, or having a low income. Childcare services and pre- and post-natal home visits from a nurse were offered to establish resource linkages and offer education in child development. Notably, individuals receiving this intervention were seen in terms of their strengths and abilities rather than their deficits, which translates into an empowerment strategy. Women were assisted in understanding and meeting their own needs and those of their newborn children, and were taught skills necessary to enhance this relationship as well as their own self-development.

The encouraging findings from this community-based prevention program support these methods of influencing major psychological determinants of healthy parent-child relationships. Mothers who received the program developed or changed their understanding of child health and development, their expectation for their own development, and their personal strengths (i.e., self-efficacy). In particular, 15 years following their completion of the program, the participants showed better family planning concerning number and spacing of children, less need for welfare, less child maltreatment, and fewer arrests of their children during adolescence. Although this program uses trained nurses, it would likely meet with similar success if neighbors or para-professionals were used to deliver the support services, especially in locales where professionals are in short supply.

Healthy Families America is another promising example of home visitation programs that emphasize child abuse prevention in the context of family assistance and support. This network of programs, currently being evaluated in 29 of its 270 sites across the US, offers a comprehensive assessment of the strengths and needs of families at the time of birth, outreach to build trust relationships and acceptance of services, teaching of problem-solving skills, expansion of support systems, and promotion of healthy child development and positive parent-child relationships (Daro & Harding, 1999). Current findings indicate that home-based intervention promotes a more nurturing environment in which mothers are more involved and sensitive to children's cues and use less punishment. Again, these services may be offered in the home by local residents or trusted community members (e.g., teachers, childcare providers) who can assist families in learning important childrearing basics.

The Kempe Community Caring Program in Denver, Colorado is an example of community-based services delivered to all expectant and new parents. The service involves a free home visitation program for two populations: a low-risk population served by trained community volunteers, and a high-risk population served by trained parenting consultants. The low-risk population consists of parents who are generally able to recognize the frustrations and insecure feelings that can arise as part of having a newborn, and who require only the reassurance of another adult. The high-risk population, on the other hand, consists of parents who need more intensive support and assistance in increasing their sensitivity and strengthening their emotional bond with their infants, building self-esteem and confidence as parents, and recognizing and accessing community resources. The developers report that the program has led to a lower rate of child abuse reports for the participants (compared to the general population), that the program is well received by parents, and that families have become more confident in their parental role (for more information: http://www.calib.com/nccanch.htm).

Some communities have chosen to offer a wide range of services to families in an effort to meet their diverse needs and prevent maltreatment. Family Focus, for example, promotes non-physical forms of discipline and strives to strengthen parent-child relationships to prevent and stop child abuse and neglect. The program provides a broad range of community services to parents of children from birth to age 10: advocacy, case management, childcare, counseling/therapy, home visitation, information/referral, parent-aide services, a school-based prevention curriculum, support groups, transportation, parent education, a resource library, a 24-hour crisis line, and volunteer opportunities. The program reports that participants show increases in knowledge and improved attitudes and behaviors (for more information: http://www.calib.com/nccanch.htm). Although such programs require considerable coordination and initial investment, they reflect the comprehensive needs of this diverse population of children and families. Furthermore, this approach can be adapted to other cultures, since it relies on teachers, neighbors, and other volunteers.

Another community-based program is the Child Abuse Prevention Program, which empowers children, professionals, and parents to recognize, resist, and report abuse and neglect. Elementary school workshops use life-sized puppets in skits that explore a variety of potentially abusive situations for the purpose of creating a safe atmosphere in which children can discuss their views and concerns about physical and sexual abuse. Children are also given the opportunity to speak individually with an adult to express personal concerns. If child abuse is disclosed, staff members provide appropriate social service referrals and monitor the progress and outcome of each case. This program also provides training to community agencies and assists in the development of long-term strategies for preventing child maltreatment (for more information: http://www.calib.com/nccanch.htm).

Female Genital Mutilation. Efforts to curtail FGM are very recent, but valuable insights from governmental and non-governmental sources warrant consideration. As with efforts to fight diseases, the health sector may be crucial for establishing a national policy on FGM in the countries involved, coordinating actions with relevant governmental and non-governmental organizations. An initial step may involve educating health care providers themselves about the harmful effects of FGM and providing the necessary information and skills to carry out the task. In addition, the elimination of FGM involves teamwork among different UN agencies, both within the countries where female genital mutilation is practiced and at the regional and global levels (Barstow, 1999).

Child Sexual Abuse. Community-based programs to prevent or treat child sexual abuse often address such topics as teaching children about the exploitative nature of sexual abuse, in an effort to increase children's awareness of possible abusers and emphasize their right to control their own bodies. Formats usually include descriptions of a variety of "touches" that children can experience, focusing on actions that children can take in a potentially abusive situation (e.g., saying "No," or leaving or running away), educating children that some secrets should not be kept and that children are never at fault for sexual abuse, and stressing that children should tell a trusted adult if touched in an inappropriate manner until something is done to protect them. Although they are promising, matching such efforts in a culturally sensitive and beneficial manner remains challenging. Furthermore, such child-focused educational strategies must be backed up with careful professional training and community awareness programs for adults.

The School Project, coordinated by Interventions for Support, Healing, and Awareness (1999) in New Delhi, exemplifies a community prevention program that uses child-oriented, indigenous methods to raise awareness about child sexual abuse. The project targets children between 12 and 16 years within the school setting and involves teachers, school counselors, parent groups, and the media in protecting children's rights. The focus is on providing children with skills for self-articulation and increasing body awareness. The school project uses various media formats to communicate these concepts, such as puppet shows, street theatre, films/documentaries, discussions, and other creative exercises and games. This approach is well suited to developing nations, since it can be implemented through schools and community organizations.

Telephone helplines offer accessible prevention resources for many developed and developing countries. For example, the *Kids Help Phone* was launched in Canada by the Kids Help Foundation in 1989, and it became Canada's only national, toll-free, bilingual, confidential helpline for troubled and abused children. The accompanying manual provides a compelling rationale for the benefits of phone counseling and provides a clear outline of how to operate such a service, which is directed at a range of counselors and community professionals, such as child protection workers, social workers, youth workers, therapists, clergy, and others. Helplines are often aided by public education initiatives, which enhance public education and awareness through brochures, videos, and TV spots that highlight key issues in corporal punishment, teacher education, and child safety. Although the preventive benefits of helplines have not been formally evaluated, they have been well received in various developed countries, and they provide a grassroots beginning to removing the barriers to child abuse reporting.

Exploitation.   Recently, intergovernmental efforts have begun in an effort to curb child exploitation and the sex trade worldwide. The World Congress Against Commercial Sexual Exploitation of Children, held in Sweden in 1996, led to a list of principles and directions, which are being developed by leading nations through legislation, improved law enforcement, and/or attempts to boost public awareness.

For child victims of the sex trade, assistance can take many forms, such as counseling, education, training, and protection to ensure the child is not forced back into prostitution. The Kamla Project, for example, was launched by the Bangkok-based Foundation for Women as part of its program to combat child prostitution by educating people at the source. *Kamla* is a book for children that relates the tragic story of a young girl from northern Thailand who was one of the child prostitutes killed in the fire in Phuket in 1984. The book has been used in many primary schools in northern Thailand, which is an area vulnerable to the procurement of children for prostitution. After a workshop with teachers, a second book was produced, together with audio-visual materials suitable for rural youth (for more information: http://www.jubileecampaign.demon.co.uk/children/cpr1.htm).

Similarly, the Rainbow Project in Taipei (Taiwan) concentrates on the provision of alternative employment, training, and counseling for young girls seeking to escape from prostitution. The project has also been very active in advocacy work, such as organizing protests (for more information:

http://www.scfa.asn.au/porn.htm). Organized coalitions and religious organizations have also assisted grassroots efforts to curb sexual exploitation by calling on the strength and ability of their large, international memberships. One such religious-affiliated coalition is End Child Prostitution in Asian Tourism, a campaign focused on enacting legal and policing methods to end the abuse of children in Sri Lanka, Thailand, the Philippines, and Taiwan (for more information: http://www.scfa.asn.au/porn.htm).

Individual- and Family-Based Approaches

Physical Abuse and Neglect.   Treatment of child abuse and neglect can be delivered in a number of ways: to individual parents, children, parents and children together, or to the entire family. No matter how it is delivered, treatment of physical abuse usually attempts to change how parents teach, discipline, and attend to their children, often by training parents in basic childrearing skills accompanied by cognitive-behavioral methods to target specific anger patterns or distorted beliefs. Similarly, treatment for child neglect focuses on parenting skills and expectations, coupled with training in social competence that may include home safety, family hygiene, finances, medical needs, drug and alcohol counseling, marital counseling, and similar efforts to manage family resources and attend to children's needs (Azar & Wolfe, 1998).

Because abusive and neglectful parents place too much emphasis on control and discipline, as well as ways to avoid contact and responsibilities, they seldom know how to enjoy their child's company. Family-based treatment, therefore, often begins with efforts designed to increase positive parent-child interactions and pleasant experiences. Moreover, such services can be provided by individuals other than mental health professionals, such as neighbors (who have been properly trained), public health nurses, religious counselors, and many other community members with knowledge of healthy childrearing methods and a comfort level with families undergoing stress.

Therapists demonstrate for parents how to do things with their child that serve to strengthen the child's areas of weakness (such as language development) and to promote healthy, adaptive functioning (such as learning to follow simple commands). The activities are behaviorally and developmentally specific, such as stimulating appropriate language and social interaction (Wolfe, 1991), and are selected to maximize the child's attention and provide ample opportunity for pleasant interchanges.

Once parents learn a more flexible, adaptive teaching style that suits their child's development and their own cultural beliefs, efforts are begun to strengthen the child's ability to follow directions and establish self-control. Parents observe while the therapist models positive ways to encourage the child's attention and appropriate behavior, followed by practice and feedback. Therapists model for the parent how to express positive affect—smiles, hugs, physical affection, praise—and also how to show dismay or concern when necessary, such as appropriate facial expression, firmer voice tone, and similar cues that express disapproval. Therapists also model how to express frustration and annoyance without becoming abusive and harsh, and parents are then encouraged to discuss and rehearse how they can handle the situation. Gradually, parents learn to replace physical punishment or apathy with more positive approaches. Realistically this takes time, and parental frustration and impatience are to be anticipated.

Cognitive-behavioral approaches have received support with this diverse population, based on controlled studies as well as numerous clinical reports (see Hansen, Warner-Rogers, & Hecht, 1998; Kolko, 1996; Wekerle & Wolfe, 1993). These methods are effective (relative to standard protective service intervention involving brief counseling and monitoring) in helping parents learn to use appropriate methods of teaching and discipline, while aiding parents in controlling anger and abuse. Parents may be taught ways to control and manage anger and arousal (such as breathing techniques), ways to attend positively to their child when he or she deserves attention, and what to expect from their child as he or she develops. These skills can be taught to parents in small, supportive groups or tailored individually to their particular needs. In addition to learning new ways to encourage child development and structure child activities, neglecting parents, in particular, require very basic education and assistance in managing everyday demands, such as financial planning and home cleanliness. Programs such as Project 12-Ways provide multi-component interventions that address the various needs of neglecting and multi-problem families, such as marital counseling, financial planning, cleanliness, and similar concerns, using para-professionals such as students, neighbors, and childcare workers (Lutzker, Bigelow, Doctor, Gershater, & Greene, 1998).

Treatment services aimed specifically at the needs of abused or neglected children are less common than parent-oriented interventions, largely because parental behavior is often the primary concern. However, some important inroads have been made by creatively combining the benefits of daycare activities with structured peer activities. For example, withdrawn children with maltreatment histories can be paired with non-maltreated peers who are exceptionally strong at positive play activities (Fantuzzo et al., 1996; Fantuzzo, Weiss, & Coolahan, 1998). As they learn to play together, the competent players are encouraged to interact with less competent children in special play areas where adults have only a minimal role. A strength of this intervention is that it can be conducted in community settings that offer comprehensive services for disadvantaged children and their families.

In brief, successful interventions for child abuse and neglect to date often include methods to provide parents or other caregivers with ways of improving and expanding their childrearing abilities and motivation. In turn, these parent-focused efforts help maltreated children to gain important developmental milestones and skills, and to enhance the overall parent-child relationship. Many communities are also developing specialized preschool programs for younger maltreated and disadvantaged children, which provide added guidance and opportunities to learn important interpersonal skills.

Sexual Abuse. Sexually abused children have usually experienced a world of secrecy, silence, and isolation. Once they have broken that silence by disclosing the abuse, or it was discovered by accident, the path toward healing can be difficult. They must access not only unpleasant memories, but buried feelings such as guilt, confusion, fear, and low self-worth. Because of the diverse manner in which sexual abuse may affect a particular child, interventions have to match the needs of a wide age range of children, who may show all kinds of symptoms or even no symptoms at all. Moreover, the impact and treatment of sexual abuse is affected by its diverse context, including individual, family, and cultural dimensions. That is, the child's recovery may depend strongly on the responses of other important factors, such as the nature of maternal support, cultural reaction, and legal intervention.

Treatment programs for children who have been sexually abused usually provide several crucial elements to restore the child's sense of trust, safety, guiltlessness, and self-worth (Finkelhor & Berliner, 1995). One major element involves education and support to help them understand why this happened to them and how they can learn to feel safe once again. Information and education about the nature of sexual abuse helps to clarify false beliefs that might lead to self-blame, and feelings of stigma and isolation are often addressed through reassurance or group therapy involving other child victims. Animated films and videos offer ways for child victims to acknowledge and validate their feelings, help them talk about their feelings, and move them toward the future with a sense of hope and empowerment. Children are also taught ways to prevent sexual abuse and restore their sense of personal power and safety, again using animated films and behavioral rehearsal to learn how to distinguish appropriate from inappropriate touches and how to disclose such actions to proper authorities (Wurtele, 1990).

Cognitive behavioral methods are also valuable in achieving these goals, especially when education and support is provided not only to the child victim, but to (non-offending) parents as well. The secretive betrayal that underlies the nature of sexual abuse causes some parents to feel ambivalent about whether to believe their child or how they feel about the alleged perpetrator, who they often trusted. Parents may need advice on ways to understand and manage their child's behavior, which may include regressive or sexual behaviors due to the abuse. Understandably, they often experience their own fears and worries as a result of the disclosure, and discussion with other parents and therapists can provide valuable support. In conjunction with education and support, sexually abused children need to express their feelings about the abuse and its aftermath—anger, ambivalence, fear—within a safe and supportive context. This can often be achieved through ongoing group therapy involving other children with similar experiences.

In brief, interventions for sexually abused children seek to help them understand that what happened to them was abuse, that it was wrong, and that it may have caused them some temporary problems (Berliner, 1997). Importantly, children should have supportive relationships in place, especially with parents and other caregivers who have received adequate knowledge and assistance to understand the possible impact the abuse may have on their child's behavior and adjustment. Finally, a successful treatment outcome would be for the child to regain a normal course of development as he or she recovers from the effects of maltreatment. The level of evidence supporting successful interventions for sexually abused children, however, is based at present primarily on anecdotal and uncontrolled group studies, due largely to the inherent ethical conflicts in maintaining a no-treatment control group as well as the diversity and range of symptoms expressed by child victims.

RECOMMENDATIONS

At the most basic level, prevention of the various forms of child abuse and neglect should encourage diversity and opportunities for the development of unique resources among children and parents. Societal influences that play a role in child abuse and neglect, especially in circumstances where families are exposed to major effects of poverty, health risks, and environmental conflict, require concerted efforts. The special risks and strengths of diverse cultural and ethnic groups need to be addressed, along with greater sensitivity to ethnic and cultural issues in the planning of services. Such a cross-cultural perspective on child abuse and neglect intervention and prevention would re-direct the focus away from individuals and families, and explore societal and cultural conditions that worsen or improve these problems.

Several conclusions and recommendations are drawn from the previous overview of prevention and intervention initiatives:

Community-Based Prevention[1]

- Strengthen neighborhood environments (urban, suburban, and rural) for children and families, and promote neighborhoods and residents as valuable resources.
- Reorient the primary health care and delivery of services so that it is easier to provide services to assist families in *preventing* child maltreatment, rather than responding after the fact.
- Capitalize on the use of documented public health and health promotion approaches to the prevention of child abuse and neglect, such as home visitation.
- Provide child development and parenting information that is easily understood, practical, and accessible to all present and potential parenting populations.
- Involve women's groups, local governments, and non-governmental organizations in intervention and prevention at the grass-roots level. Such groups are crucial in developing countries, where a large portion of the population resides in underserved rural areas.

Gather Incidence Data[2]

- Increase the careful monitoring of the incidence of child abuse and neglect in developed and developing nations. Recent work by the International Society for Prevention of Child Abuse and Neglect (Bross et al., 2000) reveals the limited state of such critical first steps in some nations, and provides a starting point for others.
- Collect data on the incidence of all forms of child maltreatment (sometimes described as "surveillance"). This task involves the systematic collection, analysis, and dissemination of data relating to children's health and safety. Incidence data informs officials at all levels of government of possible risks

---

[1] Based on conclusions from the US Advisory Board on Child Abuse and Neglect (1993); Wolfe (1999).

[2] See Wolfe and Last (2000), A Conceptual Framework for a Child Maltreatment Surveillance Capacity, available from Health Canada, Child Maltreatment Division, LCDC, Ottawa, Ontario.

and trends affecting children's health and safety, and assists in program development and prevention initiatives.
- Collect routine information related to particular health and safety outcomes, risk factors, and intervention strategies, which supports research, public health planning, and program development.

Combating Child Exploitation[3]

The elimination of child exploitation must involve measures to improve family and community living conditions, law enforcement, and inter-governmental cooperation, such as:

- Generate worldwide awareness of the prevalence of poverty and powerlessness, and mobilize forces to address these conditions as the breeding ground for physical and sexual abuse of children.
- Enforce strict and wide-sweeping measures to combat corruption. Recognize the criminality of the sexual exploitation of children and that methods to combat child prostitution will not be effective if corruption prevents law enforcement.
- Ensure that every child has a government-issued birth certificate, to confirm if a child is under the legal age of consent.
- Although challenging, legislation should be introduced in tourist-sending countries that confers extra-territorial jurisdiction. This would make it an offense in that country for its nationals and residents to commit sexual offenses against children abroad.
- Increase cooperation between law enforcement agencies of tourist-sending and tourist-receiving countries, especially in countries where tourism supports and increases child prostitution.
- Encourage countries to punish foreigners who commit sexual offenses against children in their jurisdiction. Mere deportation is ineffective and enables the offender to re-offend elsewhere, or even to attempt to return at a later date.
- Confiscate profits from the sexual exploitation of children and of premises used for such purposes, to diminish the profitable image of the sex-slave trade and prevent its continuation. Such assets can be used for the benefit of the victims of the trade.

[3] Some of these recommendations were based on a report from the Jubilee Campaign (for more information: http://www.jubileecampaign.demon.co.uk/children/cpr1.htm). See also: The Senate of Canada (1999), Report on the 1997–98–99 Activities of the Canadian Strategy Against Commercial Sexual Exploitation of Children and Youth as a Follow-up to the First World Congress in Stockholm (1999). Ottawa: Author.

- Increase law enforcement priorities to deal with the sexual exploitation of children. Governments should allocate more resources to ensure that police forces are adequately trained to deal with child abuse and related issues such as child pornography.
- Monitor pedophile organizations, which contribute significantly to the sexual exploitation of children. Making information available as to where child prostitutes can be obtained should be treated as a crime.
- Involve the local community and its leaders in detecting pedophile activity. Self-policing enhances the chances of catching offenders and helps to sensitize the community to the issue.
- Where a pedophile or suspected pedophile is expelled, improve communication between the country in which the offense took place, neighboring countries, and the suspect's country of origin.
- Reform existing laws that are inadequate or too lenient in dealing with child prostitution. Laws should facilitate the prosecution of those who sexually exploit children (and not the children themselves).
- Develop special teams of police officers trained in working with violence against children in each country. Such teams would work with child advocacy and protection groups to minimize secondary trauma associated with the reporting of child abuse.

Child Sexual Abuse[4]

- Expand prevention programs beyond the focus on potential child victims to include parents, other adults children may tell, and males at risk to abuse children.
- Implement public awareness programs designed to alert parents to potentially abusive situations (such as babysitting) and to increase adult supervision of children.
- Increase support to families under stress or in transition through family support programs.
- Extend program content beyond a discussion of "good touch-bad touch" to include topics such as personal safety, assertiveness, and problem-solving, based on active child involvement.
- Implement strategies that improve adult supervision and reduce children's exposure to possible risk situations.
- Direct greater responsibility for prevention at community institutions such as schools, churches, clubs, and so forth, in an effort to heighten society's awareness of the problem.

[4] Based on Wolfe, D.A., Reppucci, N.D., & Hart, S. (1995). Child abuse prevention: Knowledge and priorities. *Journal of Clinical Child Psychology, 24*, 5–22.

- Increase the important role of the media in public education directed toward the awareness and prevention of all forms of child maltreatment.

ACKNOWLEDGEMENTS: The authors wish to express their sincere gratitude to Anna-Lee Pittman and Paula Meunier for their assistance is preparing this report.

REFERENCES

Akdeniz, Y. (1997). The regulation of pornography and child pornography on the Internet, 1, *The Journal of Information, Law and Technology*. http://elj.warwick.ac.uk/jilt/internet/ 97_1akdz.

Azar, S., & Wolfe, D. (1998). Child physical abuse and neglect. In E.J. Mash & R.A. Barkley (Eds.), *Treatment of childhood disorders* (2nd ed.; pp. 501–544). New York: Guilford.

Barstow, D.G. (1999). Female genital mutilation: The penultimate gender abuse. *Child Abuse & Neglect, 23*, 501–510.

Berliner, L. (1997). Trauma-specific therapy for sexually abused children. In D.A. Wolfe, R.J. McMahon, & R. Dev. Peters (Eds.), *Child abuse: New directions in prevention and treatment across the lifespan* (pp. 157–176). Thousand Oaks, CA: Sage.

Bross, D.C., Miyoshi, T.J., Miyoshi, P.K., & Krugman, R.D. (2000). *World perspectives on child abuse: The fourth international resource book.* Denver, CO: Kempe Children's Center and the International Society for Prevention of Child Abuse and Neglect.

Brown, J., Cohen, P., Johnson, J.G., Smailes, E.M. (1999). Childhood abuse and neglect: Speci- ficity of effects on adolescent and young adult depression and suicidality. *Journal of the American Academy of Child and Adolescent Psychiatry, 38*, 1490–1496.

Browne, A., & Finkelhor, D. (1986). Impact of child sexual abuse: A review of the literature. *Psychological Bulletin, 99*, 66–77.

Cicchetti, D., & Rogosch, F.A. (1997). The role of self-organization in the promotion of resilience in maltreated children. *Development and Psychopathology, 9*, 797–815.

Daro, D., & Harding, K. (1999). Healthy Families America: Using research to enhance practice. *The Future of Children, 9*, 152–176.

Dodge, K.A., Pettit, G.S., & Bates, J.E. (1994). Effects of physical maltreatment on the devel- opment of peer relations. *Development and Psychopathology, 6*, 43–55.

Edleson, J.L. (1999). The overlap between child maltreatment and woman battering. *Violence Against Women, 5*, 134–154.

Fantuzzo, J., Sutton-Smith, B., Atkins, M., Meyers, R., Stevenson, H., Coolahan, K., Weiss, A., & Manz, P. (1996). Community-based resilient peer treatment of withdrawn maltreated preschool children. *Journal of Consulting and Clinical Psychology, 64*, 1377–1386.

Fantuzzo, J., Weiss, A.D., & Coolahan, K.C. (1998). Community-based partnership-directed research: Actualizing community strengths to treat child victims of physical abuse and neglect. In J.R. Lutzker (Ed.), *Handbook of child abuse research and treatment* (pp. 213–237). New York: Plenum.

Finkelhor, D. (1984). *Child sexual abuse: New theories and research.* New York: Free Press.

Finkelhor, D. (1994). The international epidemiology of child sexual abuse. *Child Abuse & Neglect, 18*, 409–417.

Finkelhor, D., & Berliner, L. (1995). Research on the treatment of sexually abused children: A review and recommendations. *Journal of the American Academy of Child and Adolescent Psychiatry, 34*, 1408–1423.

Finkelhor, D., Asdigian, N., & Dzuiba-Leatherman, J. (1995). The effectiveness of victimization prevention instruction: An evaluation of children's responses to actual threats and assaults. *Child Abuse & Neglect, 19*, 141–153.

Finkelhor, D., Hotaling, G., Lewis, I.A., & Smith, C. (1990). Sexual abuse in a national survey of adult men and women: Prevalence, characteristics, and risk factors. *Child Abuse & Neglect, 14*, 19–28.

Flisher, A.J., Kramer, R.A., Hoven, C.W., Greenwald, S., Alegria, M., Bird, H.R., Canino, G., Connell, R., & Moore, R.E. (1997). Psychosocial characteristics of physically abused children and adolescents. *Journal of the American Academy of Child & Adolescent Psychiatry, 36*, 123–131.

Hansen, D.J., Warner-Rogers, J.E., & Hecht, D.B. (1998). Implementing and evaluating an individualized behavioral intervention program for maltreating families. In J.R. Lutzker (Ed.), *Handbook of child abuse research and treatment* (pp. 133–158). New York: Plenum.

International Labor Organization (2001). Reports on facts, pros and cons of child labor. http://www.ilo.org/public/english/230actra/child/index.htm.

Interventions for Support, Healing, and Awareness (1999). *Communication and the art of self expression: A project for children and adolescents.* IFSHA, New Delhi, India.

Kendall-Tackett, K.A., Williams, L.M., & Finkelhor, D. (1993). Impact of sexual abuse on children. *Psychological Bulletin, 113*, 164–180.

Kendler, K.S., Bulik, C.M., Silberg, J., Hettema, J.M., Myers, J., & Prescott, C.A. (2000). Childhood sexual abuse and adult psychiatric and substance use disorders in women: An epidemiological and co-twin control analysis. *Archives of General Psychiatry, 57*, 953–959.

Kolko, D.J. (1996). Clinical monitoring of treatment course in child physical abuse: Psychometric characteristics and treatment comparisons. *Child Abuse & Neglect, 20*, 23–43.

Lung, C.T., & Daro, D. (1996). *Current trends in child abuse reporting and fatalities: The results of the 1995 annual fifty state survey.* Chicago: National Committee to Prevent Child Abuse.

Lutzker, J.R., Bigelow, K.M., Doctor, R.M., Gershater, R.M., & Greene, B.F. (1998). An ecobehavioral model for the prevention and treatment of child abuse and neglect. In J.R. Lutzker (Ed.), *Handbook of child abuse research and treatment* (pp. 239–266). New York: Plenum.

MacMillan, H.L., Fleming, J.E., Trocme, N., Boyle, M.H., Wong, M., Racine, Y.A., Beardslee, W.R., & Offord, D.R. (1997). Prevalence of child physical and sexual abuse in the community: Results from the Ontario Health Supplement. *Journal of the American Medical Association, 278*, 131–135.

Marshall, W.L., Serran, G.A., & Cortoni, F.A. (2000). Childhood attachments, sexual abuse, and their relationship to adult coping in child molesters. *Sexual Abuse: Journal of Research and Treatment, 12*, 17–26.

McCabe, K.A. (2000). Child pornography and the Internet. *Social Science Computer Review, 18*, 73–76.

Melton, G.B., & Barry, F.D. (1994). Neighbors helping neighbors: The vision of the US Advisory Board on Child Abuse and Neglect. In G.B. Melton & F.D. Barry (Eds.), *Protecting children from abuse and neglect: Foundations for a new national strategy* (pp. 1–13). New York: Guilford.

Olds, D., Eckenrode, J., Henderson, C.R., Kitzman, H., Powers, J., Cole, R., Sidora, K., Morris, P., & Pettit, L.M. (1997). Long-term effects of home visitation on maternal life course and child abuse and neglect: Fifteen-year follow-up of a randomized trial. *Journal of the American Medical Association, 278*, 637–643.

Polansky, N.A., Gaudin, J.M., & Kilpatrick, A.C. (1992). Family radicals. *Children and Youth Services Review, 14*, 19–26.

Report on The National Consultation on Child Prostitution (1995). *Child Prostitution: The Ultimate Abuse.* New Delhi.

Rosenberg, D.A. (1997). Unusual forms of child abuse. In M.E. Helfer, R.S. Kempe, & R.D. Krugman (Eds.), *The battered child (5th ed., pp. 431–447)*. Chicago: The University of Chicago Press.

Sedlak, A.J., & Broadhurst, D.D. (1996, September). *Third national incidence study of child abuse and neglect: Final report*. Washington, DC: USDHHS.

Shalhoub-Kevorkian, N. (1999). The politics of disclosing female sexual abuse: A case study of Palestinian society. *Child Abuse & Neglect, 23*, 1275–1293.

Simons, M. (1993, April 9). The sex market: Scourge on the world's children. *The New York Times*, pp. A3.

Smith, D.W., & Saunders, B.E. (1995). Personality characteristics of father/perpetrators and nonoffending mothers in incest families: Individual and dyadic analyses. *Child Abuse & Neglect, 19*, 607–617.

Straus, M.A., & Gelles, R.J. (1986). Societal change and change in family violence from 1975 to 1985 as revealed by two national surveys. *Journal of Marriage and the Family, 48*, 465–479.

Thompson, R.A. (1994). Social support and the prevention of child maltreatment. In G.B. Melton & F.D. Barry (Eds.), *Protecting children from abuse and neglect: Foundations for a new national strategy* (pp. 40–130). New York: Guilford.

Trocme, N., & Wolfe, D.A. (2001). *Child maltreatment in Canada: Selected results from the Canadian Incidence Study of Reported Child Abuse and Neglect*. Ottawa: Minister of Public Works and Government Services Canada.

United Nations (1989). *Convention on the Rights of the Child*. General Assembly resolution 44/25.

UNICEF (2000, April 12). *Report of the Executive Director: Progress and achievements against the medium-term plan*.

United Nations Division for the Advancement of Women (1997). *Gender-based persecution: Report of the Expert Group Meeting*.

Van Der Kolk, B.A., & Fisler, R.E. (1994). Childhood abuse and neglect and loss of self-regulation. *Bulletin of the Menninger Clinic, 58*, 145–168.

Wekerle, C., & Wolfe, D.A. (1993). Prevention of child physical abuse and neglect: Promising new directions. *Clinical Psychology Review, 13*, 501–540.

Wolfe, D.A. (1991). *Preventing physical and emotional abuse of children*. New York: Guilford.

Wolfe, D.A. (1999). *Child abuse: Implications for child development and psychopathology (2nd Edition)*. Thousand Oaks, CA: Sage.

Wolfe, D.A. (1985). Child abusive parents: An empirical review and analysis. *Psychological Bulletin, 97*, 462–482.

Wolfe, D.A., Jaffe, P., Jette, J., & Poisson, S. (under review). Child abuse in institutions and organizations: Advancing professional and scientific understanding. *American Psychologist*.

Wolfe, D.A., Scott, K., Wekerle, C., & Pittman, A. (2001). Child maltreatment: Risk of adjustment problems and dating violence in adolescence. *Journal of the American Academy of Child and Adolescent Psychiatry, 40*, 282–298.

World Health Organization (1999, March). *Report of the consultation on child abuse prevention*. WHO, Geneva: Author.

Wurtele, S.K. (1990). Teaching personal safety skills to four-year-old children: A behavioral approach. *Behavior Therapy, 21*, 25–32.

Chapter 6

Abuse of Older People

Rosalie S. Wolf, Gerry Bennett, and Lia Daichman

The focus of this chapter is on abuse of elderly people as a traumatic event. For many of the world's elders, whose psychological well-being has been compromised by poverty, illness, war, and famine, abuse can have a devastating effect. Although there is conflicting evidence concerning the susceptibility of older persons to severe stress (they may be no more, and possibly even less, vulnerable to the psychological effects of severe trauma or negative life events than younger persons), anecdotal reports show that late-life stressors can cause a recurrence of symptoms related to early traumatic experiences. Unfortunately some conditions, like forgetfulness, anxiety, and depression, are often mistakenly considered to be the inevitable consequences of aging.

This discussion will include sections on domestic and institutional elder abuse and socio-structural factors that victimize older people. Most of the studies it is based on were conducted in developed countries, though studies from developing countries were also used when available. Elderly people are defined as *persons aged 60 years and older.* **Among some populations with shortened life expectancies, such as persons who are developmentally disabled or who are living in developing countries, the age limit might be lowered to 50 or 55 years.**

The mistreatment of older persons is not a new phenomenon; accounts of intergenerational conflict can be found in ancient texts and the myths and legends of all lands. However, as a recognized social problem in developed countries, elder abuse only dates back to the mid-1970s, the result of public disclosures about family violence and concern about the increasing numbers of older persons who no longer were able to care for themselves and whose families were not available or able to give them care. Among developing countries, the concept of elder abuse is slowly emerging, influenced by the rapidity of socioeconomic change; weakening of the extended family; rising elderly populations; and growing concern for human rights, equality, and justice. Today, concern about elder abuse has driven a worldwide effort to increase awareness of the problem and encourage development of treatment and prevention programs. It is predicated on the belief that elders are entitled to live out their advancing years in peace, dignity, good health, and security.

> Mrs. Smith was an 88-year-old widow who owned a single-family home in a pleasant middle-class US neighborhood. She shared her home with her only child, Michael, 55 years old, who had lived with his mother all of his life. He had worked in a steel mill for many years, but the plant had closed about 5 years previously and he had been unemployed ever since. Though a deeply religious woman, Mrs. Smith was unable to attend church services, so her pastor often came to visit her. At one of his monthly visits, the pastor noticed that her legs were swollen and badly bruised, and that there were lacerations around one ankle and foot that were obviously infected. Her injury had occurred a few days before when her son became irritated that the food she had cooked for him was not hot enough, and he threw a heavy iron pot at her. She conceded that there had been other such instances. He was often "mean" and used foul language when she suggested that he find a job or criticized him for leaving her alone all day. She admitted that she was sometimes fearful when he came home late at night, and often barricaded her bedroom door. While his pattern of behavior seemed clearly to indicate a drinking problem, Mrs. Smith steered clear of any mention of alcohol. She protested that she did not want to "cause trouble" or be a "bother," and became quite agitated when medical treatment or the police were mentioned. She was informed that she could file charges of assault and battery against her son or seek an order of protection that would enjoin him from further harming her, including a requirement that he vacate the premises. Mrs. Smith was not interested in taking any action against her son. She tried to discount the seriousness of the abuse and seemed much more worried about the "disgrace of the family."

NATURE AND SCOPE OF THE PROBLEM

Traditionally, older people were to be respected and to be provided with comfort and leisure. This reverence for the aged was reinforced through major philosophical traditions and public policy. For Western countries, it could be traced to the biblical exhortation to "honor thy father and thy mother." In Chinese society it was embedded in a value system that emphasized "filial piety." Asian countries also stressed family harmony, which meant that the individual's well-being was secondary to the good of the group.

As the world becomes more sensitized to issues of family violence and human rights, some long-held traditions, such as property confiscation from widows in African countries, forced levirate marriages (based on an ancient Hebrew law that requires, upon the death of a husband, that the widow marry his brother), and abandonment of South Asian widows, are being viewed as abusive acts requiring not only action against individuals, but also changes in community and societal values. Every year in Tanzania, an estimated 500 women accused of witchcraft are murdered, with many more driven from their homes and communities. The problem is especially acute in northern Tanzania, where the murders represent 40% of all homicides. Research by HelpAge International cites social and economic problems including poverty, pressure on land, inadequate or inaccessible health services, and poor education as underlying causes. Not able to explain illnesses, crop failures, or dried-up wells, the people look for a scapegoat. Although men are sometimes accused of witchcraft, the situation of women and their low status in society has made them more vulnerable (Till & Clark, 2000). Even in countries where the family is the central institution and filial obligation is strong, elders are being displaced as heads of households and deprived of their autonomy. As described in a Costa Rican study, this "overprotection," or "infantilization," has left the older person feeling depressed and demoralized (Gilliand, & Picado, 2000).

Definitions

The definition of elder abuse approved by the UK charity, Action on Elder Abuse, is representative of the meaning used in most developed countries: **a single or repeated act or lack of appropriate action occurring within any relationship where there is an expectation of trust, which causes harm or distress to an older person.** The behavior can be intentional or unintentional and of one or more types: physical, psychological (emotional), financial, sexual, and neglectful. Whether it is labeled abusive, neglectful, or exploitative may depend on its frequency, duration, intensity, severity, and consequences. Questions have been raised about the usefulness of statutory and professional definitions, since the older person's perception of abuse and the cultural context may be the salient factors in identification and intervention. Abusive behavior is wide-ranging, including such acts as striking, burning, threatening, humiliating, isolating, abandoning, starving, and taking property without consent.

Recently, to determine the level of knowledge and understanding of elder abuse in South Africa, focus groups were held with older persons from three historically "Black" townships. They cited acts of physical, verbal, financial, and sexual abuse and neglect but, in addition they included loss of respect for elders, which they paired with neglect, accusations of witchcraft and consequences of being a witch, and systemic abuse, which they described as the dehumanizing treatment given older persons at health clinics and pension offices, and as marginalization by the government. These lay definitions (as classified by the researchers) were the first attempt to elicit information directly from older persons in South Africa (Keikelame & Ferreira, 2000). A similar assessment, "how elders perceive mistreatment," was carried out in four states in Brazil. Among the abuse reported, 35% was psychological, physical and/or financial, but 65% was social violence; that is, the result of how society and specifically the government regulations treated the respondents. Older people's perceptions of abuse were researched in five developing countries (India, Lebanon, Argentina, Kenya, and Brazil) as well as three developed nations (Canada, Sweden and Austria), again using focus group methodology (WHO/INPEA, 2002). Analysis of the major themes revealed remarkable similarities across participating countries. Older people perceived abuse under three broad areas:

Neglect—isolation, abandonment, and social exclusion
Violation—of human, legal, and medical rights
Deprivation—of choices, decisions, status, finances, and respect

In addition, two key factors emerged as underpinning virtually all forms or contexts of abuse: gender and socioeconomic status.

Prevalence

So far, prevalence studies have been restricted to the developed nations. Five community-based prevalence surveys have been conducted in five countries using different methods of data collection. Two, from Canada and the UK, were national in scope (Podnieks, 1992; Ogg & Bennett, 1992); a third encompassed the retired population of a small Finnish town (Kivelä, Köngäs-Saviaro, Kesti, Pahkala, & Ijäs, 1992), and the other two utilized representative samples from Boston (Pillemer & Finkelhor, 1988) and Amsterdam (Comijs, Pot, Smit, Bouter, & Jonker, 1998). Interestingly, although the methodologies were different and the proportion of abuse types varied among the five, the prevalence for all types ranged between 4–6%. In one study, a member of the household was interviewed if the designated person was unable to answer the questions. The other four only interviewed persons who could respond to the telephone or be present for a face-to-face interview. Consequently, the prevalence figures are considered to be a minimal estimation. In the Boston and Canada studies, men and women were found to be mistreated equally; in the Finnish and Amsterdam surveys, female victims outnumbered male victims.

A later national Canadian survey on family violence found that in the previous five years, 7% of older adults had experienced some form of emotional abuse from adult children, partners, or caregivers (paid or unpaid); 1% had experienced financial abuse, and 1%, physical abuse or sexual assault. Men (9%) were more likely than women (6%) to report being victims of emotional or financial abuse. Because of the difference in the time frame and survey questions, these findings cannot be compared to the earlier Canadian study, which found a much smaller proportion of emotional abuse (1%) and a larger proportion of financial abuse (3%).

Although there is no systematic collection of abuse statistics or prevalence surveys in the developing world, crime records, journalistic reports, social-welfare records, and small-scale studies contain evidence that abuse, neglect, and financial exploitation of elders are occurring. For example, a survey of three selected villages in Andhra Pradesh, India found that 40 out of 1000 older persons had experienced physical violence; verbal abuse was even more prevalent. Of 50 respondents to a survey conducted in Baroda, a city in one of the western states of India, 10 persons aged 70 years or older reported being neglected in their households; 2 of the 10 had been abandoned (Shah, personal communication, 1999).

> Tulsbai is an 80-year-old widow in India suffering from arthritis, hypertension, and incontinence. She also has complained of diminishing eyesight. In her younger years, she was financially self-sufficient. In addition to her husband's income, she managed lunch services for the working population of the community. She also managed a poultry business. However, as a self-employed entrepreneur, she had no social security.
>
> Her family consisted of her husband and one son. After her husband's death, her son and his family continued to stay with her. He had a good job in the fire brigade and earned a respectable amount of money. However, he was addicted to alcohol, and his health was deteriorating. His wife was suffering from chronic illness. The grandchildren were developing behavior problems; the eldest granddaughter was not attending school.
>
> Tulsbai's savings were gone, spent on the needs of the family. She was totally dependent on them for her needs. The family, instead of providing support, was harassing her. She was not given adequate nutrition or medical care and was physically abused by her daughter-in-law and at times teased by the grandchildren. Her life depended on the kindness of neighbors, who gave her money to buy food. She was reluctant to report the situation to the police or to move into an institution.

A random sample study of elders' perceptions of abuse in three Argentinean towns was conducted. Almost half (45%) of the elders reporting admitted that they had been mistreated; the highest incidence was psychological abuse. Using a similar protocol, residents were sampled in four Chilean cities. The percent of mistreatment ranged from 25% to 36%. Psychological abuse occurred in 31–64% of the four city samples; physical abuse, in 14–35%. A more comprehensive picture of prevalence and incidence is expected with the completion of a national survey of primary care consultants in the public health system that is being conducted by the National Ministry of Health and the School of Medicine of Universidad de Concepción.

Theoretical Explanation

Using various theoretical models, researchers in the developed countries have viewed elder abuse as a problem of an overburdened caregiver (situational model), a dependent elder (exchange theory), a mentally disturbed abuser (intra-individual dynamics), or learned behavior (social learning theory) (Bennett, Kingston, & Penhale, 1997). Others have used the imbalance of power within relationships (feminist theory) and the marginalization of elders (political economic theory) to explore this issue (Whittaker, 1997). Most recently the lack of fit between the organism and the environment (ecological theory [Schiamberg & Gans, 1999]) has been used to explain why elder abuse occurs.

Early on, elder abuse researchers realized that a single theory could not accommodate such a complex, multifaceted phenomenon. For child abuse, and more recently domestic violence, a similar realization has led to the adoption of the ecological model as a means of explaining interactions across systems (Schiamberg & Gans, 1999). In its initial formulation, the ecological model was conceived as a nested arrangement of four levels of environments. According to this conceptualization, violence results from individual, interpersonal, social-contextual, and societal factors. This framework for elder abuse may be helpful not only in understanding the causes of the problem, but also in promoting interventions that address all levels of the environment.

Risk Factors

Without data to support the theories, the emphasis in research and practice has been on risk factors, attributes, or characteristics that increase the probability of victimization but are not necessarily causal agents.

Individual Determinants. Although early researchers in child abuse and battered woman syndrome renounced individual personality disorders as reasons for abusive behavior in favor of socio-psychological factors, more recent research has shown that abusers who are the most aggressive are more likely to have personality disorders and alcohol problems than the general population. Similarly, in elder abuse, abusers are more apt to have mental/emotional and substance abuse problems than non-elder abuse cases.

The influence of cognitive or physical impairment of the victim as a causal agent is not as clear-cut as was originally proposed. A comparison of abuse and non-abuse cases from the caseload of a social service agency revealed that the abused elders were not more impaired than the non-abused elders and in some situations, especially cases of physical abuse by adult children, were less so. Several comparative studies of abuse and non-abuse in families with a member with Alzheimer's disease found that degree of impairment was not a significant factor.

The low status of women may also be a determinant, especially in those countries where culturally sanctioned beliefs about the rights and privileges of husbands have led to their domination. Feminist theorists contend that power and gender are key elements leading to intimate partner violence, but the relationship may be more complex than these factors alone can explain. Unfortunately, little is known about the prevalence and impact of abuse in older men.

Interpersonal Factors. Early reports about domestic elder abuse focused on caregiver stress and victim dependency as important predictors of mistreatment. Today, there is evidence that neither dependency of the care recipient on the caregiver nor caregiver stress differentiates between abuse and non-abuse cases. Investigations into elder abuse situations involving families dealing with Alzheimer's disease suggest that the pre-existing relationship between caregiver and care recipient may be the important predictive factor: problems in a relationship prior to the illness may be perpetuated in the caregiving situation. Without a reservoir of good feelings and affection toward the older person, the caregiver may respond angrily or violently when confronted with the difficulties of caregiving, especially if the care recipient is aggressive. The current wisdom is that stress may be a contributing factor in cases of abuse, but it does not explain the phenomenon. On the other hand, the dependency of the abuser, particularly adult sons, on the victim for housing and finances continues to be an important distinguishing characteristic between abuse and non-abuse cases.

Social Context. Social isolation, or the lack of social supports, has been a consistent risk factor in many elder abuse studies. Similar to findings among battered women, social isolation can be both a cause and a consequence of elder abuse. Abuse may be the result of poor health and infirmities that inhibit the ability of the older person to leave the home setting or the lack of opportunity because of the loss of family members and friends. Even if localities have a strong community support network, victims may not avail themselves of the services that would provide relief from a home setting laden with conflict. Studies have shown that victims of abuse tend not to make use of community centers or day-care programs.

Many elders live in societies whose cultural traditions are rooted in ageism, sexism, and violence. The picture of older persons as weak, frail, and dependent has made them appear to be less worthy of governmental investment than other groups and ready targets for exploitation. Economic difficulties and rapid changes in customs regarding respect for the older person and the caregiving responsibilities of the family are also common factors. Some cultural and superstitious practices have abusive tendencies often directed at isolated older women: mourning rites, for instance, and accusations of witchcraft.

Sociostructural Factors. While most research on elder abuse has dealt with individual and family attributes as predictors of elder mistreatment, systemic, structural features of society have been cited as creating an abusive environment for older persons, though there has been no empirical support for these claims. It has been suggested that the period of political transformation affecting the eastern European post-communist countries has provided a milieu that increases the risk of abuse. The pauperization of significant parts of society, the lack of stability, the loss of pensions and health and welfare services, the increase in aggressive behavior, especially among young people, and unemployment are viewed as affecting the psychosocial and physical health of the whole population and, in particular, elderly persons.

In Chinese societies, a lack of respect from young people for the older generation, the state of tension between traditional and new family structures, a restructuring of the basic support networks for elderly people, and the migration of young couples to new towns, leaving older persons in deteriorating residential areas in town centers, have also been said to contribute to an environment that fosters abuse and neglect (Kwan, 2000).

Describing the societal forces in Africa that are conducive to elder mistreatment, one writer lists the following: patrilineal and matrilineal inheritance systems and land rights that affect the political economy of relationships and the distribution of power inherent in them; the social construction of gender, which places older women at risk; rural-urban migration and formal education, which has reduced the interdependency of generations within the family unit; and the forces of modernization that have caused a loss of tradition, ritual, and arbitration roles for elders within the family (Argyryko, personal communication, 2000). Members of the South African focus groups stated that most abuse took place in the context of social disorganization, specifically domestic violence exacerbated by crime, alcohol, and drugs.

The following report from India includes many of the same risk factors noted above (Shah, 1999):

—changes in family values that have weakened family ties
—reduction in family size, which affects the caretaking role
—education of children, which places heavy demands on young parents in terms of financial resources, energy, and physical space
—lack of government programs to assist the sizable population of elders engaged as agricultural laborers
—loss of shelter, particularly for older women, who have no rights to their parents' homes or who have given over custody of their homes to children
—migration of young people in search of jobs, leaving older persons to fend for themselves
—relationship of mothers-in-law and daughters-in-law who have lived together
—policies of age segregation, which leaves elders without opportunities for employment
—absence of a pension system, which leaves the elderly population at greater risk

The ecological framework, which incorporates the individual, interpersonal, social-contextual, and socio-structural factors, appears to be a much more appropriate theoretical framework for viewing elder abuse from a worldwide perspective, at least until knowledge based on sound research can validate which factors are most relevant. Because of its application to all forms of family violence, it may suggest some common approaches.

THE EFFECTS OF ABUSE

Domestic Abuse

Clinical and case-study data from developed countries have documented the severe emotional distress experienced by older persons as a result of mistreatment, but empirical evidence is often lacking. Several studies have reported a higher proportion of older victims with depression/psychological distress in an abuse sample than in a non-abuse sample. Since these were cross-sectional in design, there is no way of knowing whether the condition was an antecedent or a consequence of the abuse. Other suggested symptomatology includes feelings of learned helplessness, alienation, guilt, shame, fear, anxiety, denial, and posttraumatic stress disorder [PTSD]; research on these conditions still remains to be done. Emotional effects, along with health problems, were also cited by the South African focus group participants; one member called these "illnesses of the heart."

In a seminal study in the United States, Lachs and colleagues (1998) combined data from an annual health survey of 2,812 elders with reports of elder abuse and neglect made to the local adult abuse agency over a nine year period. When they compared the mortality rates of the non-abused and the abused, they found that by the 13th year following the study's initiation, 40% of the non-reported (i.e., non-abused, non-neglected) group were still alive and only 9% of the physically abused or neglected elders. After controlling for all the possible factors that might affect mortality (e.g., age, gender, income, functional status, cognitive status, diagnosis, social supports, etc.) and finding no significant relationships, the researchers speculated that mistreatment causes extreme interpersonal stress that may confer an additional death risk.

Institutional Abuse

Although the emphasis in the past quarter of a century has been on interpersonal abuse within the family setting, ethnographic studies, media exposés, license reports, and anecdotal information since the 1960s have consistently confirmed the existence of abuse, neglect, and exploitation in nursing and residential care homes. From 4% to 7% of elders in developed nations reside in long-term care facilities. Older persons in Africa can be found in long-stay hospital wards, homes for the destitute and disabled and, in the sub-Sahara countries, in witches' camps. The current rate for nursing home utilization in South Africa is 5%. In Latin American countries, 1–4% of the older population is in institutional settings that are no longer viewed as unacceptable places for an older relative but are now seen as an alternative by their families. The government-sponsored *asilos* in Latin America, originally large institutions resembling English workhouses, have been converted to smaller facilities with professional staff representing many disciplines. Other homes are sponsored by religious and immigrant organizations. The social, economic, and cultural changes underway in the developing countries will mean families will be less able to provide care for frail elders, thus portending an increase in residential care.

Abusive and neglectful behavior toward elders in institutions has been attributed to the marginal place assigned to elders in society (structural), the lack of properly trained staff, adequate facilities, and management expertise (environmental), and staff who are ill-suited by temperament or history to be caregivers to dependent elders (individual) (Clough, 1999). In the developing world, institutional abuse is said to be perpetuated by staff through unquestioning regimentation (in the name of discipline or imposed protective care) and exploitation of the elder's dependence, exacerbated by the lack of professionally trained management.

Despite the amount of research and investigation that has centered around institutional facilities, little is known about the incidence of abuse. In interviews with a sample of nursing home personnel from one state in the United States, 36% of the staff reported having seen at least one incident of physical abuse in the preceding year by other staff members, and 10% admitted having committed at least one act of physical abuse themselves. A total of 81% of the sample had observed at least one incident of psychological abuse against a resident in the preceding year, and 40% admitted to having committed such an act themselves (Pillemer & Moore, 1989).

Staff-to-resident abuse is most prevalent, but mistreatment can also occur at the hands of visiting family members and other residents. Reports from Sweden, Israel, South Africa, and Brazil provide clear evidence that mistreatment in long-term care institutions, whether narrowly or broadly defined, is a worldwide reality.

Large-Scale Emergencies

The types of emergencies affecting older persons are many, varied, and seemingly increasing. In times of war, civil strife, conflict, and natural disasters, older persons are more likely to become victims of physical harm than younger people. They are physically weaker, their bones more brittle, and their rate of convalescence from bodily injury is slower. Even a relatively minor injury can cause serious permanent damage. When forced to flee from their homes, older people are less able to find food or live without shelter. Some elders refuse to leave. Yet remaining behind in a war-torn area when younger people have moved out, as happened in Eastern Slavonia, is likely to leave an older individual isolated and fearful. The downward-spiraling economic condition of some eastern and central European countries has robbed elders of their pensions and adequate health and welfare services. Older people comprise as much as 35% of communities of refugees and displaced persons (HelpAge International, 2002).

In the presence of violence, such as the uncontrolled gang warfare that has occurred in Jamaica and in South African townships, older persons may become virtual prisoners in their own homes, afraid to venture out on the streets. Still another catastrophe, the HIV/AIDS epidemic, has forced older women in several African countries who are living under the most dire circumstances to take on the added burden of caring for children and grandchildren with AIDS or grandchildren orphaned by the death of their parents from AIDS.

Following natural disasters, older people do exhibit adverse psychological symptoms, including anxiety, depression, and PTSD, according to studies in the US (e.g., Phifer & Norris, 1989). Whether the psychological impact is greater among the elderly population in comparison to younger people is still open to question (see Chapter 13). Elders have been thought to be at special risk in times of natural disaster because they are more reluctant to evacuate their homes, more disturbed by altered patterns of life, and more likely to live in dwellings susceptible to damage. On the other hand, age is believed to bestow some advantages. Experience with disasters early in life may create a repertoire of successful coping skills that can be called upon in old age.

While both these perspectives have validity, it is also true that individual differences, exposure to massive trauma that may overwhelm predisposition and previous experience, and post-trauma environmental factors may play a role in adaptation (Danieli, 1997). As some of the studies of World War II veterans and Holocaust survivors have shown, time may not heal. When the latter were "liberated" after the war, they were not offered opportunities to speak about the atrocities they had endured. If they did talk, their experiences were often misunderstood, and hence a "conspiracy of silence" developed between the traumatized person and the professional helper (Danieli, 1997). They carried their emotions inside without any outlet for their pain, and so it has stayed with many of them into old age (Hassan, 2002; also see Chapter 12).

The aging process itself is said to contribute to a re-emergence of traumatic memories. While involvement in the past through memory may be part of normal aging, a bereavement, retirement, or illness may also reactivate the "unfinished business" of earlier losses.

INTERVENTION STRATEGIES

Domestic Abuse

Principles of Intervention. Interventions for older adults receiving care have been guided by a set of global principles that espouse dignity, choice, freedom, safety, least disruption of lifestyle, and least restrictive care alternative. Other sets of principles are contained in various professional codes of behavior. At the core of all of them are the ethical values espoused in varying ways by different religions and cultures, which are now part of basic human rights: autonomy (the right to make choices), beneficence (the right to receive care from others that maintains or enhances one's welfare), justice (the right to be treated equitably), nonmaleficence (the right to expect others to do no harm), fidelity (the right to have others show loyalty when assistance is needed), accountability (the right to expect others to tell the truth and be responsible for their actions), and privacy (the right to maintain privacy regarding information about oneself). These concepts guide decision-making when conflicting goals and interests, especially evident in cases of elder abuse, seem to defy resolution.

Levels of Intervention

Social Policies.   Social policies that guarantee the rights and dignity of all people and provide for the basic necessities of life are the underpinnings of a violence-free society. Changes in cultural values and norms may be necessary to overcome aging and gender stereotypes that have contributed to the vulnerability of older persons. For many countries, efforts to promote human rights have been thwarted by inequalities in gender, class, region, tribe, and ethnic background. The most disadvantaged—children, adult women, and the aged—have received low priority. Heretofore, gerontology as a field of practice, policy, and research has received very little attention in the developing economies. To call attention to the aging of the global population, the United Nations General Assembly designated 1999 as the International Year of Older Persons. The United Nations Secretariat, in collaboration with States, experts, and the NGO Committee on Ageing, conducted a series of aging-related events and research in support of the Year. Two forums on aging held that year, as well as several questionnaires that were distributed to States, the UN agencies and bodies, and 2500 aging-related organizations produced a series of proposed actions. Of particular interest here was the call for programs "to address the victimization of older persons which result from crime, homelessness/inadequate housing, inability to access needed health/social services, and physical/psychological/financial abuse" (NGO Committee on Ageing, 2000).[1]

Using the legal system as a tool for identification, prevention, and treatment of abuse is most closely associated with the system of adult protective services established in the United States. Each state has passed legislation

---

[1] Also relevant is General Comment No.6, "The economic, social and cultural rights of older persons," adopted in 1995 by the Committee on Economic, Social and Cultural Rights as a guide for States. The General Comment referred back to the 18 UN Principles for Older Persons of 1991 and the earlier 62 recommendations of the 1982 International Plan of Action on Ageing.

that designates an adult protective services unit with responsibility for receiving reports of suspected elder mistreatment, screening for potential seriousness, conducting a comprehensive assessment if indicated, and developing a care plan. In 43 states, the law makes it mandatory for certain categories of individuals (e.g., physicians, social workers, nurses, etc.) to report a case to the authorities "if there is reason to believe" that abuse, neglect, or exploitation has taken place. Only the four eastern Canadian provinces and Israel have adopted similar legislation. So far, other countries have rejected mandatory reporting.

Critics maintain that while it may be appropriate for child abuse, the underlying assumptions of mandatory reporting are not applicable to elders. The method infantilizes the elder's position in society, fosters negative stereotypes of the aged, and limits older persons' ability to control their own lives. In addition, communities are apprehensive about implementing such a system without a fully developed 24-hour, 7 day-a-week reporting system and the requisite health and welfare services to respond.

Despite growing concern about the problem, most countries have not passed specific elder abuse legislation. An act that criminalizes elder abuse and provides for mandatory reporting of suspected cases has been proposed for South Africa, but no action has been taken on it. The delay has been attributed to the great amount of other legislation needed to meet the transformation needs of that country. Similarly, a proposed public law protecting vulnerable adults in Britain is not going forward; rather, changes to existing law relative to capacity and care standards have been suggested.

Other laws not specific to elders can be applied to elder abuse cases, such as mental health and disability statutes, domestic violence legislation, and criminal codes. Contract law can provide some safeguards against financial exploitation, and the law of tort or civil wrongs can be applied under "trespass of the person" in situations of assault, battery, and false imprisonment and when duty of care is breached.

Community Efforts. Providing information and educational sessions about rights of older people, supporting older people or their representatives to pursue their rights and to stop the abuse, and assisting with strategies to plan for future protection are part of community advocacy efforts. The advocacy model recognizes that victims of elder abuse are adults in a vulnerable position, and advocates act on their behalf to guarantee their rights and to obtain needed services. It assumes that existing family supports, legal mechanisms, and community services can be used to assist abused older persons and their families. Training professionals who work with older persons to recognize the signs and symptoms and to make referrals to community resources is an ongoing effort. Such activities have been reported by elder abuse projects in Canada, Australia, Britain, South Africa, Germany, New Zealand, Norway, and Costa Rica. A national helpline for elder abuse is operating in Britain, and local demonstration projects are under way in Japan, France, Spain, and Germany.

Elder abuse cases often involve a myriad of problems of a medical, psychological, legal, social, environmental, criminal justice, and financial nature. One of the ways of dealing with the array of agencies and professionals needed to resolve a case is with either a formally established multidisciplinary team or a group called together on an as-needed basis. Some teams limit their activity to consultation on difficult cases; others have an expanded agenda that includes education, training, technical assistance, outreach, advocacy, and public policy.

Without question, the press and electronic media have played a critical role in increasing awareness of the issue around the world and in motivating policy-makers to take action. The participants in the South African focus group referred to earlier also called attention to the importance of the media in increasing public awareness: "It must be in the news. Everybody must hear about it."

Neighborhood Networks. The social-network model makes use of the informal support systems of family, friends, neighbors, peers, and local community organizations. Using natural helping networks, service providers can disseminate information, increase community awareness, identify cases, and inform victims about services. Even isolated elders may have neighbors who are aware of or suspect that abuse and neglect may be occurring. Where there is little social service infrastructure, reliance on this approach may be the only alternative. In Guatemala, blind older people who were being ejected from their homes by their families formed a committee, created a safe house for themselves, and developed handicrafts and income-producing projects in the community.

Family and Individual Interventions. Within developed countries, interventions in cases of elder abuse have focused on the individual victim within the context of the family. If the case involves some degree of caregiver stress, it may be necessary to help the caregiver by providing formal services in the home, placing the elder in adult day care, or educating the caregiver about helping a physically and cognitively impaired client. When it is advisable for the victim to leave the home temporarily, emergency shelters can be used. Legal remedies, such as protective orders or temporary commitment papers, may be necessary if the abused and abuser have to be separated or a medical or psychiatric assessment has to be carried out. If the victim lacks the capacity to make decisions, then the court must be approached to assign a guardian or conservator. For victims unable or unwilling to leave an abusive situation, support groups are an option if the elder is able to function in a group setting. In cases of abusive adult children who are dependent on their elders, services to encourage independence, such as housing and financial assistance, job training, and substance abuse and mental health counseling may be appropriate.

Care management is a key component of this approach. It is defined as "a process of coordinating a range of support services into flexible packages of care to meet the assessed needs of the older person and caregiver" (Biggs, Phillipson, & Kingston, 1995, p. 111). Protocols are used to collect medical, functional, social, psychological, environmental, and socio-demographic data on the victim and information on the circumstances leading to the mistreatment. On the basis of the comprehensive assessment, a plan for managing services can be developed. There is a municipally established program in Oslo, Norway that follows this pattern. If necessary, a referral is made for psychiatric consultation.

> Julia is single, 76 years old, and living in Argentina. She has no known relatives. To recover from a bad case of the flu, at the suggestion of Maria, her house porter, she was admitted from her own flat to a private nursing home for a two-week period. As soon as she felt better, she began to ask to return home, but she was always given "no" as an answer. Occasionally she would have visitors. She was never left alone and never allowed to leave the nursing home, even at Christmas-time. Almost a year passed, and she remained in the nursing home for no medical reason. Martha, the nursing home manager, who is a close friend of Maria, had taken all of Julia's pension ($600 US) as payment, leaving Julia with no cash.
>
> On behalf of Julia, an old neighbor, Rosa, appealed to the government, claiming illegal deprivation of freedom and emotional abuse. A couple of days later, Julia was visited by a social worker from the Buenos Aires Government Program on Elder Abuse, who tried to remove her from the nursing home. She encountered opposition from the nursing home owners, who also asked that their own physician examine Julia and provide a written report that she had no signs of physical mistreatment. After several hours had passed, and with great perseverance on the part of the social worker, Julia was able to go home.
>
> On top of the emotional shock and the traumatic situation that she had had to endure, Julia found upon returning home that her jewelry and money, which she had been keeping in a safety box, had been removed. It appears that they had been taken by Maria, who had a key to the flat. The following day, Julia and the social worker went to the police station to report the theft and the situation. The case is now in court.
>
> Julia, who always was a fairly happy person, independent, polite, educated, and self-confident, is now, after being held against her will, distressed, frightened, and insecure. Currently, she has a helper who comes to her home to assist her with daily activities. She is also receiving, psychological assistance and a weekly follow-up session with a social worker.

Institutional Abuse

The ethical values of autonomy, beneficence, justice, nonmaleficence, fidelity, accountability, and privacy that guide treatment in other settings are also applicable to institutional life. Even in cases where an elder is extremely frail, the staff must be able to offer care that allows for maximum autonomy and minimum dependence without placing unrealistic demands on the patient at the same time.

Over the years, governments have responded to reports of neglect and abuse of nursing home residents with formal inquiries and study commissions. In some instances, the findings have been so detrimental to the authorities that they have never been disclosed. A rich research literature already exists on quality-of-care measures; the question is whether the political will exists to implement them. Certification of providers, standards of care, staffing requirements, and periodic inspections have the potential of improving care and decreasing the possibility of elder mistreatment, but often additional resources are needed. Advocacy groups can play a role in educating the public and policy-makers about conditions in nursing homes, while resident councils, family committees, and ombudsman programs are important mechanisms for bringing concerns to the attention of management. The situation in the developing countries is exacerbated by the scarcity of funds.

An abuse prevention training program for long-term care staff is under way in several states in the US (Hudson, 1992). The curriculum is designed to address issues that can precipitate abusive or neglectful behavior, with emphasis on staff participation in sharing their own experiences of day-to-day problems and working together to create solutions. It includes such topics as an overview of abuse in nursing facilities, identification and recognition of abuse, possible causes, understanding feelings about caregiving, cultural and ethnic perspectives, abuse of staff by residents, ethical and legal issues, and strategies for prevention. However, the success of the program depends on the commitment of management to quality care, good working conditions, and creative problem-solving. It also requires that staff recruitment practices screen out persons who have had previous records of abuse, who have little empathy for frail elders, and who are unable to handle stress and conflict. Some US states now maintain registries of persons who have been found guilty of abusing elders and/or who have police records.

Large-Scale Emergencies

For victims of natural disasters, research in the US suggests that after basic needs are met, mental health intervention should take place soon after the disaster, before more severe, chronic psychopathology develops (Phifer, 1990). Assisting older victims with practical problems that may arise, such as difficulties with medical care, housing, material aid, and social services, rather than providing help for "mental problems," appears to be more acceptable to older persons. Similarly, the outreach efforts are more satisfying to the elders if provided by "natural helpers" such as clergy or community volunteers.

Contrary to what might be expected, a highly structured, sophisticated service model may not be the most appropriate way to provide for large numbers of people, as the example below depicts. In developing countries with little social service infrastructure, such an approach may also be unrealistic.

> *Following a bomb incident within London's docklands in 1996, hundreds of people living in state housing were traumatized by the extensive structural damage and the death of two men running a newspaper kiosk. The hospital in charge of the psychiatric and psychology services put its major incident plan into operation immediately. The initial advice to all social and health care workers in the area was to encourage clients to talk about their personal stories related to the blast as much as possible. This preventive approach also allowed time for the identification of those people who would need to receive the next level of input—counseling.*
>
> *It was expected that up to 10% of this population would need such help and that following this level of intervention a subgroup, probably another 10%, would require formal psychiatric help. In fact, very few people were deemed in need of counseling or further intervention, though those so deemed had significant problems. In effect, the community coped with a traumatic event using an inexpensive social support model framework. Key social and health care workers were guided as to the best course of action to advocate for large numbers of people and were advised what symptoms indicated early and severe psychological trauma. A line network was available which, at its end, would have a trained professional. However, by using the human resources available, a sophisticated network of professionals screening large populations was not needed, even if such a model could have been established.*
>
> *In this particular situation, much was made of the older citizens in the community. They had lived through the Blitz, and the late-middle-aged had been children during the war. A long-lost spirit of cooperation and helpfulness was quickly reestablished as emergency shelters were utilized, and the oldest became invaluable as guides through the rigors of enforced group living. Following the "talk about it" advice, adults as well as children were channeled for further treatment through their general practitioners. For the community support staff that functioned through the emergency, there were debriefing sessions (Millar, 1996).*

Research on the experiences of older people in different types of emergencies in Bangladesh, Bosnia, the Dominican Republic, and Rwanda found a gap between their concerns and the main activities of the relief agencies. The older people gave priority to receiving income so that they could become self-sufficient, while the relief agencies focused on delivering health and welfare services. The older people in the study asked that in situations resulting from conflict or natural disasters that they be "seen, heard and understood, that they have equal access to essential support services, and that their potential and contributions be recognized and supported" (HelpAge International, 1999).

According to the head of a London program that offers Holocaust survivors the model of a social center next door to a specialist service where they can talk of their experiences, listening to survivors has been the key to developing meaningful responses to their needs. Some survivors wish to confront the "dark shadow" of the atrocities they have been through, while others wish to find strategies to deal with the present. At the core of the program is the principle of empowerment: reinforcing coping abilities and emphasizing issues of survivorship rather than victimization. The key to therapeutic work is its meaningfulness to the people receiving the service. For those who have been severely traumatized, the importance of mutual support and self-help groups cannot be overstated.

This experience with the World War II Holocaust survivors has helped the program develop services for a group of Bosnian refugees who were also World War II Holocaust survivors. Because of displacement, problems with the language, increasing physical frailty, and isolation, they were particularly vulnerable. A social program and support group, with staff as facilitators, have given them a sense of dignity and a feeling that they have not been forgotten. In this last phase of their lives, this elderly group of refugees was thus given an opportunity to deal with "unfinished" business and also to provide testimony about events in the former Yugoslavia as a service to their new community (Hassan, 2002).

Virtually none of the approaches and programs presented above have undergone rigorous evaluation using randomized experimental-control designs or quasi-experimental methodology. Even though the US adult protective services programs have been in operation since the late 1970s, it was not until 1999 that one county-based program was able to analyze its performance in terms of client outcomes. A few states use a risk assessment tool that measures client outcomes in terms of future risk. Most states in the US, although they are handling thousands of cases annually, do not have the capacity or resources to evaluate their programs. With regard to these programs and those in other countries, the level of empirical evidence could be best described as "based on recently developed treatment that has not been subjected to clinical tests."

Types of Costs

Although there have been efforts to estimate the annual cost of child abuse and domestic violence in the US, no similar computation has been done with elder abuse. This omission is due partly to the state of elder abuse research and partly to the association of social-cost analysis with productivity. Erroneously, elders have been viewed as non-contributors to their nation's gross national product. Yet it is elders in the rural areas of many developing countries who are left to work the fields and care for grandchildren while sons and daughters go to the cities to find work. In fact, economic circumstances in the poorest countries, which have no pension systems, require older persons to continue to work.

Costs of intervention can be direct (those associated with the provision of treatment and services), and indirect (those resulting from reduced productivity, diminished quality of life, and decreased ability to take care of oneself or others). A model for determining the social and economic costs of abuse in later life (Spencer, 1999) includes as direct costs health/medical care; community social services; criminal and civil justice procedures; institutional care; employment and volunteer services; taxes and transfers; costs to business; and prevention, education, and research programs. Trying to capture the intangible costs of mistreatment, such as premature mortality, suffering, emotional pain, distrust, and loss of self-esteem, is even more difficult than estimating direct costs.

GAPS AND INFORMATION NEEDED

As noted at the outset, few empirical studies have been reported on the psychosocial consequences of abuse and other forms of violence experienced by older people. Even after 20 years of activity, little is known about the nature, scope, and causes of interpersonal abuse against elderly persons or the outcome and effectiveness of prevention and intervention strategies. The complexity of the problem hinders efforts to define researchable questions. Outcome measures are elusive, in that separation of the abuser and the abused may not be an alternative; mistreatment may be preferable to institutionalization. Confidentiality of data, mental competency of victims, and government bureaucracy are often insurmountable obstacles for the researcher. Lack of interest on the part of established investigators in such fields as psychology, sociology, gerontology, medicine, and law has also been a factor in the paucity of solid studies. Further, research has been limited to the developed world, although descriptive reports are available from the Latin American countries, South Africa, and India.

With knowledge about the impact of abuse on older persons barely in its infancy, the need for research on all aspects is paramount. Greater understanding of the theoretical underpinnings will be required to design effective interventions. Efforts to reduce or eliminate abuse will mean greater attention not only to individual factors but also to family, community, and societal conditions. At the heart of this challenge is the older person, whose voice has been absent from the discourse. To abolish the ageism and sexism that have been associated with abuse, older people must be involved in defining the issues and in planning and developing the services.

RECOMMENDATIONS

The abuse of older persons cannot be addressed without at the same time ensuring that the basic needs of all people for food, shelter, economic security, and access to health care are met and, additionally, for older persons, that there be opportunities to continue in roles that are not only beneficial to society but also crucial to communities and family relationships. With this goal in mind, a list of recommendations to reduce and prevent abuse of older persons within the family, the institution, and the community are presented below. Following the pyramid described in Chapter 4, the listing for each section (domestic, institutional, socio-structural) begins with the most cost-effective interventions in terms of the numbers of persons reached, the amount of money spent, and assumed impact (direct or indirect) on reducing abuse.

Domestic Abuse

- Establish laws to guarantee the human rights of older persons; as one example, name older women as a target group in domestic violence laws
- Use the media to increase public awareness of abusive behavior toward older persons and where help may be received
- Organize a national advocacy group to provide a focal point for education, public awareness, and service development
- Encourage the development of social networks to promote solidarity and social support among peer elders within villages, neighborhoods, and housing units
- Establish a helpline to receive calls and to make referrals
- Add a module on elder abuse to all professional training curricula (e.g., medicine, psychology, nursing, social work, law)
- Promote linkages between programs serving mistreated elders and the mental health service system so that counseling services to treat the mental health consequences of abuse are more accessible

Institutional Abuse

- Allocate to residential care institutions the necessary funds to maintain a pleasant, caring environment with adequate staffing
- Establish a "zero tolerance" statement for abuse within the institution, including a commitment by management to provide staff training on the nature of abuse and neglect, ways to prevent it, and ways to report it
- Redesign nursing homes so that they are more home-like
- Offer more choice and control to residents of institutions: for example, include elders and their families in decision-making about their care
- Provide opportunity for staff to participate in institutional decision-making so they have more control over their working arrangements
- Promote institutional-community partnerships that will bring programs such as child day care, support groups, and intergenerational activities into the institution to improve its image and provide diversion for the residents
- Offer psychiatric services to residents of the nursing homes

Large-Scale Emergencies

- Use media and other means of communication to educate society about human rights for older persons, especially older women
- Combine efforts with other international groups that share similar interests
- Promote the concept of productive aging by including older persons in literacy, education, and income-generating programs
- Pass legislation that will encourage employment of older workers who wish to work
- Organize "self-help" groups or grass-roots organizations with older persons and provide the start-up funding to encourage self-sufficiency
- Open information and referral centers to advocate for older persons with governmental agencies
- Establish socialization and support groups for elders to reduce isolation
- Provide mental health counseling programs

The case described below illustrates the power of non-violent collective action against societal abuse in its most virulent form.

> *This story is one of the many stories about the Buenos Aires "Mothers of Plaza de Mayo." Following the military coup in 1976, men, women, and children of all ages began to disappear without reason or explanation. The mothers and grandmothers, because they could do it more "safely" than male members of the family, began to seek news of their relatives at the Ministry of Internal Affairs, the police, and from representatives of various churches and banned political parties. Undertaking this desperate search together, they became a group with a mission looking for a new way to act in the midst of bloody repression and people's unexpected indifference.*

Among the women was Azucena Villaflor, a 55-year-old homemaker. One of her four children had been kidnapped in November 1976 from his place of employment, a garage in Villa Dominico, Buenos Aires. She had looked for him in all the police stations, government offices, hospitals, and even the morgue without success.

One day when meeting with the other mothers, realizing that they had been unsuccessful in their inquiries, she proposed that they go to the Plaza de Mayo square at the Town Hall and ask for an audience to obtain information about their children. That particular march on April 30, 1977 was the first of thousands that the mothers and grandmothers carried out in the following years, demanding to know the fate of their loved ones. Six months following the first march, Azucena Villaflor was kidnapped at her home, tortured, and killed.

The mothers of the Plaza de Mayo are a leading example of the nonviolent spirit in Latin America. After 20 years, several former military officials have begun to talk about the tortures and killings, admitting what the mothers have known all along. This admission is partly attributed to the mothers and grandmothers who are still walking about the squares.

REFERENCES

Bennett, G., Kingston, P., & Penhale, B. (1997). *The dimensions of elder abuse: Perspectives for the practitioner.* London: MacMillan Press.

Biggs, S., Phillipson, C., & Kingston, P. (1995). *Elder abuse in perspective.* Buckingham, UK: Open University Press.

Clough, R. (1999). Scandalous care: Interpreting public enquiry reports of scandals in residential care. In F. Glendenning & P. Kingston (Eds.), *Elder abuse and neglect in residential settings* (pp. 13–27). Binghamton, NY: Haworth Press.

Comijs, H.C., Pot, A.M., Smit, J.H., Bouter, L.M., & Jonker, C. (1998). Elder abuse in the community: Prevalence and consequences. *Journal of the American Geriatrics Society, 46,* 885–888.

Danieli, Y. (1997). As survivors age: An overview. *Journal of Geriatric Psychiatry, 30,* 9–26.

Gilliand, N., & Picado, L. (2000). Elder abuse in Costa Rica. *Journal of Elder Abuse & Neglect, 12,* 73–87.

Hassan, J. (2002). *A house next door to trauma: Learning from Holocaust survivors how to respond to atrocity.* London: Jessica Kingsley Publications.

HelpAge International (1999). How older people lose out in emergencies. *Ageing & Development, 4,* 2.

HelpAge International (2002). *Older People in disasters and humanitarian crises: Guidelines for Best Practice.* London: Author.

Hudson, B. (1992). Ensuring an abuse-free environment: A learning program for nursing home staff. *Journal of Elder Abuse & Neglect, 4,* 25–36.

Keikelame, J., & Ferreira, M. (March, 2000). *Mpathekombi, ya bantu abadala: Elder abuse in black townships on the Cape Flats.* HSRC/UCT Centre for Gerontology.

Kivelä, S.L., Köngäs-Saviaro, P., Kesti, E., Pahkala, K. & Ijäs, M.L. (1992). Abuse in old age: Epidemiological data from Finland. *Journal of Elder Abuse & Neglect, 4,* 1–18.

Kwan, A.Y. (2000). *The gray wave.* Unpublished manuscript.

Lachs, M.S., Williams, E., O'Brien, S., Hurst, L., Pillemer, K., & Charlson, M. (1998). The mortality of elder mistreatment. *Journal of the American Medical Association, 280,* 428–432.

Millar, B. (1996). New focus: Traumaspotting. *Health Services Journal, 106,* 16.

NGO Committee on Ageing. (2000). Report prepared for the Millennium Forum.

Ogg, J., & Bennett, G. (1992). Elder abuse in Britain. *British Medical Journal, 305,* 998–999.

Phifer, J.F. (1990). Psychological distress and somatic symptoms after natural disaster: Differential vulnerability among older adults. *Psychology and Aging, 5,* 412–420.

Phifer, J., & Norris, F. (1989). Psychological symptoms in older adults following natural disaster: Nature, timing, duration, and course. *Journal of Gerontology, 44,* 207–217.

Pillemer, K., & Finkelhor, D. (1988). Prevalence of elder abuse: A random sample survey. *The Gerontologist, 28,* 51–57.

Pillemer, K., & Moore, D.W. (1989). Abuse of patients in nursing homes: Findings from a survey of staff. *The Gerontologist, 29,* 314–320.

Podnieks, E. (1992). National survey on abuse of the elderly in Canada. *Journal of Elder Abuse & Neglect, 4,* 5–58.

Schiamberg, L.B., & Gans, D. (1999). An ecological framework for contextualising risk factors in elder abuse by adult children. *Journal of Elder Abuse & Neglect, 11,* 79–103.

Spencer, C. (1999). *Considering the social and economic costs of abuse in later life. Summary.* Vancouver, BC: Gerontology Research Centre, Simon Fraser University.

Till, C., & Clark, H. (Eds.) (2000). Violence and abuse. *Ageways: Practical issues in ageing and development, 59.*

WHO/INPEA (2002). *Missing voices: Views of older persons on elder abuse.* Geneva: World Health Organization.

Whittaker, T. (1997). Rethinking elder abuse: Towards an age and gender integrated theory of elder abuse. In P. Decalmer & G. Glendenning (Eds.), *The mistreatment of elderly people* (2nd ed., pp. 116–128). Thousand Oaks, CA: Sage Publications, Inc.

Websites

Canadian Network for the Prevention of Elder Abuse	www.mun.ca/elderabuse
HelpAge International	www.helpage.org
International Association of Gerontology	www.sfu.ca/iag
International Network for the Prevention of Elder Abuse	www.inpea.net
National Center on Elder Abuse (US)	www.elderabusecenter.org
National Committee for the Prevention of Elder Abuse	www.preventelderabuse.org
UN Programme on Ageing—The UN Secretariat	www.un.org/esa/socdev/ageing
World Health Organization (Ageing and Life Course)	www.who.int/hpr/ageing

Chapter 7

People with Mental and Physical Disabilities

Kim T. Mueser, Virginia A. Hiday, Lisa A. Goodman, and Denise Valenti-Hein

Culture and economic development influence how disability is perceived, distributed, and responded to. Physical disability resulting from disease, malnutrition, and accidents is more common in developing nations than in more developed nations (United Nations General Assembly, Resolution 37/53, Dec. 3, 1982). Poor prenatal nutrition, obstetric skills, and perinatal care are other sources of disability. Once a disability occurs, the affected child has considerably less chance of surviving due to impoverished living conditions (De Jong, 1987). Poverty and harsh living conditions may result in extreme solutions, including abandonment (Carreire, 1971; Lévy-Bruhl, 1921). This higher prevalence of disabilities in developing nations has negative and, surprisingly, also positive consequences for those who have physical or mental disabilities. On the one hand, because of poverty and lack of health services, persons with physical disabilities in developing nations are less likely than those in more developed nations to have technical aids and accommodations that facilitate their interactions and functioning. On the other hand, perhaps because disabilities are more common in developing countries, and also because in these countries individuals are more integrated into family and mainstream society, persons with both physical and mental disabilities appear to be better accepted in developing nations.

For example, surveys sponsored by the World Health Organization have reported that individuals with severe mental illnesses such as schizophrenia have better outcomes in developing countries, where they are more likely to live with families in their communities (Sartorius et al., 1986). Unfortunately, traditional structures are breaking down in many developing countries. As countries go through the transition to development with mechanization and commercialization of agriculture, migration from farms and small towns to cities, and monetary systems replacing barter systems, extended families and communities disintegrate and are no longer able to provide the traditional supports that have assisted people with mental disabilities in remaining in their communities and achieving the more favorable outcomes. The plight of the mentally disabled in developing countries is further compounded by a lack of skilled health workers and by poverty exacerbated by an uneven global economy.

In developed countries, where families are smaller and disperse during the day, where home and work are separate, where life is faster-paced and more compartmentalized, and where most daily encounters are limited, impersonal, and transitory, people with mental and cognitive disabilities are less likely to have a role in their families' lives and in their communities. For over a century, developed nations tended to place individuals with mental disabilities in large public institutions, but for the past 40 years, deinstitutionalization has led to more people with mental illness and cognitive disabilities living on their own, in group homes, or on the streets, no longer institutionalized but not fully integrated back into their families and communities.

Adding to the increased vulnerability of the population of persons with disabilities and poor outcome in the legal arena is the mythology carried by society at large. Several sources have reviewed commonly held myths regarding people with disabilities (Baladerian, 1991; Smith, Valenti-Hein, & Heller, 1985). Some of these myths, such as the idea that people with disabilities are sheltered from harm, are used to deny that crimes are perpetrated against them. Others, such as the belief that people with disabilities do not understand what is happening to them or are devoid of feelings, are used to minimize the impact of the abuse. Still others, such as the belief that people with disabilities are deceitful and unreliable reporters or have poor memories, serve to deny the victim justice throughout the legal system.

In this chapter we review the nature and scope of conditions and events that threaten death, severe bodily harm, or severe psychological injury in the lives of persons with physical and mental disabilities. Although awareness of the problem of trauma exposure in persons with disabilities is relatively new, an emerging body of research from developed nations indicates that individuals with disabilities are especially vulnerable to trauma exposure and its consequences. Persons with disabilities often depend on others to get their needs met, increasing their likelihood of, and susceptibility to, exploitation and injury. Likewise, individuals with disabilities are exceptionally sensitive to the effects of stress, which can have a deleterious effect on the course of their illnesses and their overall functional capacity.

According to the United Nations, the term *disability* summarizes a great number of different functional limitations: "**... any restriction or lack (resulting from an impairment) of ability to perform an activity in the manner or within the range considered normal for a human being. People may be disabled by physical, mental or sensory impairment, mental conditions, or mental illness**" (World Programme of Action Concerning Disabled Persons adopted by the United Nations General Assembly resolution 37/52 on 3 December 1982; see http://www.un.org/esa/socdev/enable).

In this chapter we use the broad categorization of physical and mental disabilities, recognizing that both include a wide range of impairments—and that notions of what is and what is not normal change with time and place. Because mental disabilities are commonly divided further to distinguish between psychiatric and cognitive disabilities, we distinguish between those who have a serious mental illness (e.g., schizophrenia, bipolar disorder, major depression) and those who have impairments in cognitive functioning (e.g., mental retardation, traumatic brain injury, autism). Nonetheless, physical, psychiatric, and cognitive disabilities may overlap, with many individuals having two or even all three types. The overlap between different types of disability is especially common in persons with developmental disabilities: **i.e., mental or physical disabilities that are severe and chronic, that arise during childhood or adolescence, that tend to continue indefinitely, and that interfere with functions such as self-care, communication, learning, mobility, self-direction, capacity for independent living, and economic self-sufficiency.** Despite the common overlapping of these disabilities, the literature reporting research studies, advocacy programs, and prevention and intervention services tends to deal separately with each of the three types.

There are crucial differences among the disability groups, but in this chapter we concentrate on their similarities rather than their differences. The three groups are similar in sharing a condition that makes them less able than members of the general population to fend for themselves. Their impairments make them easy targets for victimization. The United Nations has recognized the necessity of addressing not only the unique needs of these individuals, such as rehabilitation and technical aids to facilitate mobility, communication, and daily living, but also their societies' shortcomings regarding accommodation and integration. Examples of physical obstacles to participation include raised structures without ramps, light switches that cannot be reached, and telephone lines without telecommunication devices for deaf access. Normative obstacles include notions of perfection and beauty, which devalue persons with disabilities, marginalizing them as "children of a lesser god." Even though adaptations, accommodations (e.g., electrical and mechanical aids), and structured environments are able to facilitate some degree of independence, many people with disabilities continue to be unserved or underserved by these supports, and remain dependent on others for assistance, as well as for opportunities to participate in sociocultural and economic affairs.

We begin with a review of the rates of different common disabilities in the general population. This is followed by a discussion of the nature of severe threats and injury in the lives of persons with disabilities. The discussion is divided into three categories based on the source of harm: societal, institutional, and interpersonal. We then describe current methods for responding to trauma in persons with disabilities. The chapter concludes with recommendations for dealing with trauma in individuals with physical and mental disabilities.

NATURE AND SCOPE OF THE PROBLEM

Rates of Physical and Mental Disabilities

There are many different types of physical and mental disabilities, and their severity ranges from mild to severe and incapacitating. We focus here on those disabilities that have the most profound impact on functioning, including the ability to care for oneself, to work, to establish and maintain social relationships, and to develop and pursue recreational and leisure activities. Estimates of prevalence rates are drawn from community surveys, national registers, and observations of expert investigators (Goldman, 1984; National Information Center for Children and Youth with Disabilities, 1999; Robins & Regier, 1991; United Nations Decade Of Disabled Persons, 1983–1992 (United Nations General Assembly, Resolution 37/53, Dec. 3, 1982). The United Nations estimates that a total of 500 million persons worldwide are disabled by physical, mental, or sensory impairment, and that the number is growing. It further estimates that in most countries one out of ten persons has a disability, but that in some poor, developing countries, the disabled population rises to 20%. It is estimated that the prevalence of epilepsy in some areas of Africa and Asia is as high as 3.7–4.9% (Adamolekun, 1995). Estimates of the prevalence of mental disability among children have varied widely, from 2% in Sudan to 15% in India (De Jong, 1987; Giel et al., 1988).

Studies from developed nations provide estimates of multiple specific disabilities. Among the more common physical disabilities are hearing impairment (.5%), cerebral palsy (.3%), and spinal bifida (.1%). Estimates of the most common cognitive disabilities show mental retardation, epilepsy, and lifetime traumatic brain injury each to be 1% of the population, followed by autism at .05% (National Information Center for Children and Youth with Disabilities, 1999). Most estimates of severe and persistent psychiatric disorders suggest a prevalence rate between 2% and 3%, with the main disorders being schizophrenia (1%) and bipolar disorder, also called manic depression at .5% (Goldman, 1984; Robins & Regier, 1991). Some of the more common psychiatric disorders, which tend to be somewhat less severe, are major depression, anxiety disorders (e.g., obsessive-compulsive disorder, panic disorder, posttraumatic stress disorder), and personality disorders (e.g., borderline personality disorder, schizotypal personality disorder, paranoid personality disorder), although for some individuals these disorders are severe and debilitating. The primary focus of this chapter is on physical and mental disabilities that are either acquired at birth or develop over the course of childhood, adolescence, and early adulthood, including the effects of childhood trauma. However, disability may also be directly due to the effects of societal or international conflict, such as torture and systematic rape, exposure to combat, or the large-scale displacement of individuals, resulting in deprivation and increased vulnerability to violence.

Cultural Issues

Culture has a marked influence on how mental illness is perceived and responded to. Expectations of what is normal functioning, for example, are shaped by cultural views of gender, class, economics, and religion. These then define what is normal for that society, designating other behaviors as "abnormal" or "disabled." Such definitions become particularly evident with migration and cultural pluralism, which prompted the National Institute of Mental Health in the US to establish in 1991 a working group on culture and diagnosis aimed at making culture more central to the process of establishing psychiatric diagnoses.

Cultural pluralism brings with it awareness that behavior dismissed as abnormal in one place may actually be respected and honored in another. For example, the trance-like phenomenon of possession that scientifically oriented cultures may dismiss as irrational may be seen in other cultures as a normative and restorative response to a stressful event. *Espiritismo* in Puerto Rican culture is a system of beliefs involving interactions between the invisible spirit world and the visible world in which spirits can attach themselves to persons (Comas-Díaz, 1981; Morales-Dorta, 1976). Spirits are hierarchically ordered in terms of their moral perfection, and the practice of espiritismo helps individuals who are spiritually ill achieve higher levels of this perfection. Troubled persons are not identified as "sick" nor are they blamed for their difficulties; in some cases, symptoms such as hallucinations may be interpreted favorably as signs that the person is advanced in his or her spiritual development, resulting in prestige (Comas-Díaz, 1981). Thus, certain cultural interpretations of mental illness may promote more acceptance of persons who display characteristic symptoms, as well as avoid the common assumption that these phenomenological experiences are the consequence of a chronic, unremitting condition.

While cultures differ in how mental illness is interpreted and managed, and respect for cultural differences is paramount, it should not be assumed that mental health needs are being adequately addressed within a particular cultural group, especially during sociocultural, economic, and political upheaval. The following illustrates how the provision of mental health intervention was both a feasible and welcome service in one traditional culture.

> *In Siem Reap, Cambodia, following establishment of a community mental health service in 1995, patients traveled long distances from all around the country to seek treatment at the center. The number of patients who attended the center grew dramatically during a short period. Most of the early attendees were those with severe mental illnesses. There were fewer people with trauma-related disorders, although the numbers increased, which suggests that the initial barriers of stigma and suspicion decreased over time. The impact of treatment was dramatic. Individuals responded rapidly to the introduction of standard antipsychotic medications and supportive community follow-up. When visited by a consultant team some months after the initiation of treatment, a psychotic man who had previously been chained to a tree for 8 months was found to be working in the rice fields with his family, apparently restored fully to his usual mental state (Silove, Ekblad, & Mollica, 2000). In areas in Cambodia with high concentrations of returnees from Thai border camps, the consumption of mental health care services was many times higher than in areas that had never known any allopathic mental health care service over and above the services that were delivered by local healers and monks. The reason for the difference was that, although both groups regarded mental disorders as a serious problem, only the returnees from the border camps knew from their previous experience in Thailand that allopathic treatment for mental disorders existed (Somasundaram, Van De Put, Eisenbruch, & De Jong, 1999).*

The plight of the mentally disabled in developing countries is compounded by a variety of factors, such as poverty, differences in help-seeking behavior, and lack of skilled health care workers. In many places, people understand disability as a disease sent by God, or caused by witchcraft

or sorcery, whereas scientific interpretation attributes disabilities to problems such as cerebral damage from diseases such as malaria, meningitis,
or parasitoses involving the brain. People believing in spiritual causes of
disability are likely to seek religious or magical cures, which sometimes
work but can also exacerbate the disability.

> In remote areas of Guinea Bissau it is the tradition for any mentally disabled,
> deformed, albino, or Mongoloid infant to undergo the following ceremony: After
> sending the mother to her family, the baby is left on the floodline of a sea arm. A
> calabash with some food, an egg, and rum are left with the child. If next day the child
> is gone, it is taken as evidence that the child is not a human being but the product of
> some magic-religious act who has been taken away by the water spirit in the form of
> a snake. If the calabash has disappeared, it is taken as evidence that the snake thinks
> the baby is a human who will grow up normally (De Jong, 1987).

Sources of Threat

A variety of threats contribute to the vulnerability of persons with
disabilities to traumatic events. In this section, we consider three broad
categories of threats, including those arising from society, from institutions,
and from interpersonal relationships.

Societal Threats. Any large-scale conflict or social upheaval that
threatens death, physical injury, or psychological harm to members of the
general population is likely to affect those with disabilities even more. In
times of large-scale conflict, such as a war or disaster where the physical
environment is destroyed, those with disabilities may be less able to act to
move themselves out of harm's way. They are less able to flee with other
residents when a town is attacked, less able to negotiate torn-up buildings,
streets, and fields, and less able to collect and carry supplies necessary for
their and others' survival.

> When Russian troops attacked the city of Grozny in Chechnya, in an attempt
> to destroy the opposing forces, individuals with physical and mental disabilities
> suffered the worst. While many other Chechen refugees fled the city, it was the elderly
> and disabled who were left behind, unable to flee. When military commanders gave
> Chechen civilians an ultimatum to get out of their home city by Dec. 11, 1999 or be
> "destroyed," serious concerns arose for how many individuals with disabilities could
> be killed in the conflict due to their inability to flee (Paddock & Kuhn, 1999).

Mental illness and retardation pose additional threats. In contrast to
those without mental disabilities, mentally disordered or retarded individuals may be less able to follow safety and evacuation instructions, less able
to assist in the tasks necessary to the survival of their group or themselves,

less likely to have access to critical resources, and more likely to need the help of others. Because their disabilities and dependence are exacerbated by societal conflict and upheaval, persons with disabilities are more in need at the same time that others may be preoccupied with their own survival and less able to assist. People with disabilities can, therefore, be expected to be more affected by large-scale, societal disruptions such as disaster, war, and migration.

> *Many refugees from the conflict in Yugoslavia who are physically disabled live in economic disparity in refugee compounds on the outskirts of Belgrade. Refugees with physical disabilities have no citizenship rights, no ability to work legally, and no access to adequate health care. There are no special services for refugees with physical disabilities and most see little hope for any economic opportunity (Gall, 1999).*

Even during times without large-scale conflict or social upheaval, persons with disabilities are more likely than others to suffer the consequences of social deprivation (see Chapter 3). Because of their disabilities, they require more specialized adaptations (e.g., Braille, technical and mobility assistance) to be able to work. Many are unable to work fully, and thus are vulnerable to poverty. Unemployment, homelessness, disease, and malnutrition, in turn, are likely to take a heavier toll on these individuals. A birth, accident, or sickness that impairs a child or adult places heavy demands on a family's limited physical and emotional resources. Individuals with disabilities who have family or friends to provide for their basic needs are still often unable to participate fully in community activities unless they are fortunate enough to have technical aids and an environment free of obstacles.

When technical aids are abundant and the physical environment is relatively free of obstacles, disabled persons must nevertheless negotiate obstacles in the social landscape of their communities. People who live with disabilities are especially susceptible to being excluded from participation in society because of the social stigma so often placed on them. Their lives are frequently marked by neglect, scorn, scapegoating, bullying, and violence. Maltreatment due to their stigmatized status has been a problem throughout the history of mankind, as shown by the following examples. In ancient Greece, the *Pharmakos* or scapegoat—who was beaten up, expelled, and sometimes wounded to the death—was often a mentally or physically disabled person. Among some nomadic groups in East Africa, the mentally disabled were not only maltreated but were often sexually exploited or sacrificed. In Haiti, people with bad luck could supposedly change their luck by having intercourse with a mentally disabled person. And in Greece and southwest France, "village fools" were often mentally disabled women who were sexually abused. People with disabilities may be even more socially marginalized by conflict. In extreme cases, persons with disabilities may become the direct targets of violence, as was seen in Hitler's genocide of such individuals.

During the genocide that occurred in Rwanda in 1994, people stormed the only psychiatric hospital in the capital of Kigali and killed all of the patients.

In mental disabilities, psychiatric symptoms such as severe depression, hallucinations, delusions, and cognitive impairments such as disorganization, compromised planning ability, and lack of social judgment can further interfere with the anticipation of dangerous situations and appropriate self-defense. Visible vulnerabilities, isolation, lack of work, difficulties anticipating and avoiding dangerous situations, and the absence of truly protective living environments also make individuals with disabilities easy targets for criminal violence. Numerous studies in developed nations have documented the high prevalence of criminal victimization among those with mental disabilities. For example, one recent study in the US reported violent criminal victimization experienced by persons with a mental illness to be twice as high as in the general population (Hiday, Swartz, Swanson, Borum, & Wagner, 1999), and another study in a large US city reported a history of physical and/or sexual assaults in homeless mentally ill women to be above 90% (Goodman, Dutton, & Harris, 1995).

Institutional Threats. As mentioned above, deinstitutionalization in developed nations has led to a great reduction in the numbers of people with cognitive disabilities and mental illnesses living in large institutions. As these institutions' populations have declined, and as the patient rights movement has achieved legal protections for institutionalized persons with disabilities, problems of overcrowding, inhumane conditions, excessive coercion, and abuse have been drastically reduced. But even with adequate staff, supplies, and facilities, cases of patient abuse by staff still occur.

A teenage male patient who was admitted to a psychiatric hospital was awakened on several nights by a male attendant who was fondling his genitals. Each time, when the patient expressed shock and asked him to stop, the attendant complied, but he returned the next night. The patient stated that he got little sleep during his two-week stay in the hospital because he felt he had to stay awake to protect himself.

In large part, such remaining cases of institutional abuse are due to failures in screening and training of staff and to social powerlessness, family isolation, communication deficits, and weakened defenses of the population in institutions. Unfortunately, many developing nations in transition have not experienced the same reforms in their institutions, so that today many persons with mental retardation and mental illness are held in crowded institutions with inadequate staff, supplies, and medicine. The problems of institutions in these nations are often compounded by inadequate resources available during or following war. Mental Disability Rights International, which investigates conditions in mental hospitals, has found persons with cognitive disabilities and mental illness living in inhumane conditions in remote asylums in virtually every transitional and developing country it has visited. Such institutional confinement violates the *United Nations International Covenant on Civil and Political Rights*, whose Article 7 holds that "no one shall be subjected to torture or cruel, inhuman or degrading treatment" (International Covenant on Civil and Political Rights, United Nations Treaty Series, No. 14668, Vol. 999, p. 171–187, 1977). Furthermore, Mental Disability Rights International finds that most of the people in these mental institutions could live in the community if they were supplied with assisted housing. Thus, even disregarding inhuman conditions, keeping them institutionalized is abusive.

> *As a result of the conflict in the Balkans, many adults and children with physical and mental handicaps have been displaced from their communities and forced to live in institutions. In the Demir Kapjar center, south of Skopje, 340 adults and 120 children are institutionalized for their handicaps. There is one care assistant for every 20 patients: "limbless adults languish motionless on the floor," patients sit in their soiled clothes and children are strapped to beds. Some patients actually have no disabilities; one girl was considered to be handicapped due to a "squint," and another healthy child happened to have been born to parents with disabilities (Randall & Kapija, 1999).*

In many developing countries, there are few institutions for persons with mental and physical disabilities, and they have fewer inpatients compared to facilities in more developed nations. Having few or no institutions can be seen as an advantage, because these societies do not have to deinstitutionalize. Rather, efforts to improve treatment of disabilities in developing nations can be directed at establishing community-based care that maintains and is built upon existing social support structures.

Interpersonal Threats.   Many studies in developed nations have assessed the incidence and prevalence of interpersonal violence to people with disabilities. Estimates of the risk of traumatic exposure vary across studies. However, the vast majority of studies are consistent in finding that individuals with disabilities are more likely to be victimized than persons without disabilities (Carmen, Rieker, & Mills, 1984; Goodman, Rosenberg,

Mueser, & Drake, 1997; Sobsey, 1994). The extent of increased risk depends on several factors, including the specific population, method of collecting information, definition of abuse, and whether single or multiple victimization is considered.

Much research has shown that children with physical disabilities are more likely to be subject to maltreatment, including physical and sexual abuse (White, Benedict, Wulff, & Kelley, 1987). Less research is available concerning the mistreatment of adults with physical disabilities, but studies are generally consistent with the literature from childhood: adults with physical disabilities are more likely to be abused than persons in the general population, with care providers commonly one important source of abuse (e.g., Young, Nosek, Howland, Chanpong, & Rintala, 1997). Some evidence indicates that individuals with a combination of physical and cognitive disability are at highest risk for abuse, followed by persons with a single disability (Mullan & Cole, 1991).

> A woman with spina bifida living in the United States was abused by her husband for six years. He would get angry when she refused to have sex and would yell and grab at her. He would exert control over her by preventing her from leaving rooms or taking her crutches. Once he cut off her clothes while she slept (Young et al., 1997).

Multiple studies in developed nations report higher rates of traumatic experiences among persons with cognitive disabilities than among others in the community (Sobsey, 1994). Studies of cases of physical and sexual abuse reported to treatment and legal agencies indicate that a disproportionately large number have a cognitive disability. One study of agencies serving victims of abuse who also had disabilities found that 67% of the clients had an intellectual disability, 18% had a physical impairment, 14% had a hearing impairment, and 6% had a psychiatric diagnosis; a total of 19% of abused clients had multiple disabilities (Sobsey & Doe, 1991).

> A young woman with cerebral palsy moved from a small town in the US to a transitional residence in a city. Coming from a rural environment where she had limited contact with others made her vulnerable to men who showed an interest in her. Soon after arriving she was invited to parties at private homes that featured alcohol. At one such party she was sexually assaulted. A man fondled her breasts, touched her labia, and manipulated her to touch his groin. After the event she expressed guilt and confusion, and believed the incident was her fault (Watson-Armstrong, O'Rourke, & Schatzlein, 1994).

The relationship of trauma to mental illness is complex and differs in some ways from its relationship with other disabilities. In contrast to cognitive and physical disabilities, interpersonal trauma in childhood often *precedes* the development of psychiatric disorders (Bushnell, Wells, &

Oakely-Browne, 1992; Duncan, Saunders, Kilpatrick, Hanson, & Resnick, 1996; Polusny & Follette, 1995), suggesting that trauma may increase vulnerability to mental illness. Similarly to other disabilities, once a mental illness has developed, persons are more likely to be interpersonally victimized (Goodman et al., 1997). Most documentation of trauma in persons with mental disabilities comes from studies of persons in psychiatric treatment, which have examined patients' experience of physical and sexual abuse. However, general population surveys have also found high rates of psychiatric comorbidity among persons with a lifetime history of posttraumatic stress disorder (Kessler, Sonnega, Bromet, Hughes, & Nelson, 1995), who by definition have experienced a traumatic event. Overall, the research suggests that trauma may contribute to the onset of mental disabilities, and also that mental illness may increase the likelihood of subsequent traumatization.

Routine psychiatric examination often fails to uncover abuse among mentally ill persons in treatment, but standardized interviews that inquire directly about exposure to specific violent or otherwise abusive threats and acts report rates higher than those in the general population. History of child abuse among adult psychiatric patients is very high, ranging from 65% to 81% in studies that probe for multiple types of abuse (physical, sexual, neglect) and that use broader definitions of violence, such as emotional and verbal abuse (Greenfield, Strakowski, Tohen, Batson, & Kolbrener, 1994; Jacobson & Herald, 1990; Rose, Peabody, & Stratigeas, 1991; Ross, Anderson, & Clark, 1994). Adult abuse and victimization are also high among persons with mental disabilities (Hutchings & Dutton, 1993; Jacobson, 1989; Jacobson & Richardson, 1987; Lipschitz et al., 1996), especially among those who are homeless (Davies-Netzley, Hurlburt, & Hough, 1996; Goodman et al., 1995). One study that probed for recent violence in newly hospitalized psychiatric patients found that 62% of both males and females reported physical victimization by their partners and 46% described abuse by other family members (Cascardi, Mueser, DeGiralomo, & Murrin, 1996). The high rates of abuse in persons with a psychiatric disorder has led some to characterize such experiences as "normative" in this population (Goodman, Dutton, & Harris, 1997).

NATURE OF THE RELATIONSHIP BETWEEN VICTIMIZATION AND DISABILITIES

A variety of explanations have been offered for the higher prevalence of interpersonal victimization of persons with disabilities. Some of these are applicable to a particular disability, whereas others are more general. They can be grouped into five general categories: increased dependence upon others, disability-related vulnerability, the effects of disability on poverty, the effects of abuse on disability, and the relationship between disability and substance abuse. A brief description of each explanation is provided below.

Dependence upon Others

Persons with physical and mental disabilities often have an increased dependence on others for getting their basic needs met. This dependence, combined with a desire for acceptance, and with awareness of the social stigma associated with disability, may result in persons with disabilities being victimized by people upon whom they are dependent (e.g., caregivers), or with whom they have close relationships (e.g., spouses) or hope to develop close relationships (Watson-Armstrong et al., 1994). This vulnerability may be related in part to the blurring of boundaries that may occur when individuals with disabilities receive personal care from another (e.g., touching a person's body when helping him or her to bathe). Inherent in the dependency of many persons with disabilities is fear about the loss of needed supports, which can lead to a willingness to endure interpersonal trauma, and even protect close ones who are violent. Similarly, the intense desire for acceptance, personal closeness (including sexual expression), and a sense of integration with the world of people without disabilities can lead an individual with disabilities to accept violent and exploitative relationships out of the belief that it is the best he or she can "do."

> *A young woman in the US with a severe mental illness and mild mental retardation was admitted to a psychiatric hospital with suicidal ideation. This hospitalization was part of a pattern of hospitalizations occurring at approximately the same time each year for over five years. Review of the patient's history indicated that her hospitalizations coincided with the anniversary of her sister's suicide ten years before. Further exploration revealed that the patient's sister had been sexually abused by her father, who subsequently turned his attention to the patient after the sister's death. This sexual abuse had stopped recently, although the patient continued to live at home. In addition to her mental illness, the patient also had posttraumatic stress disorder, for which she was treated (Mueser & Taylor, 1997).*

The Effects of Disability on Poverty

Individuals with disabilities are more likely to live in impoverished areas, both rural or urban. Impoverished urban neighborhoods tend to have high crime rates that increase the risk of victimization for all residents, but particularly those with disabilities. Their visible vulnerabilities, isolation, lack of work, and lack of protected environments make them easy targets for criminal violence (Hiday, Swartz, Swanson, Borum, & Wagner, 1999), especially from individuals who prey on the weak (Levey & Lagos, 1994).

Disability-Related Vulnerability to Abuse

Impairments directly related to psychiatric disorders or cognitive disability may increase the vulnerability of persons to trauma. Psychiatric symptoms such as severe depression, hallucinations, delusions, and cognitive problems such as disorganization, poor abstraction and planning skills, and lack of social judgment can interfere with their ability to anticipate dangerous situations and to defend themselves in such situations (Goodman et al., 1997). For example, a multi-site survey of trauma in 782 persons with severe mental illnesses such as schizophrenia, schizoaffective disorder, bipolar disorder, and major depression indicated that 35% had been physically or sexually assaulted *in the last year alone* (Goodman et al., 2001). In addition, agitated, bizarre, incoherent, antagonistic, or suspicious behaviors can lead to tension and conflict with others, which may result in a person with a disability being victimized because others become violent or coercive to that person, or because the person lashes out physically and others react in the same way (Hiday, 1995).

The Effects of Abuse on Disability

Another explanation for the association between abuse and psychiatric disability is that abuse may worsen the disability. Specifically, posttraumatic stress disorder (PTSD) can exacerbate the impairment and course of disability, especially severe mental illness. When abuse results in PTSD, specific symptoms of PTSD, such as avoidance of trauma-related stimuli, continued distress due to re-experiencing the trauma, and overarousal, may directly affect the course of a severe mental illness, and contribute to retraumatization, substance abuse, and lack of social support (Mueser, Rosenberg, Goodman, & Trumbetta, 2002). It is also plausible that abuse worsens impairment for persons with cognitive disabilities, while the interactions between abuse and severity of physical disability remain largely unknown.

The Impact of Substance Use Problems on Trauma

The relationship between mental illness, substance use problems, and trauma provides yet another explanation for the high vulnerability of persons with severe mental illness to interpersonal victimization. People with severe mental illness in developed nations (e.g., the US, Europe, or Australia) have high rates of comorbid substance abuse (Duke, Pantelis, & Barnes, 1994; Fowler, Carr, Carter, & Lewin, 1998; Kessler et al., 1996; Regier et al., 1990), and substance abuse has been linked to subsequent traumatization (Kilpatrick et al., 1997). Substance abuse may make persons with a disability more likely to frequent dangerous areas and to interact with potentially exploitative people (e.g., drug sellers, persons with addictions), which makes them more likely to become victims of interpersonal violence (Goodman et al., 1995; Hiday et al., 1999). This explanation, similar to the poverty explanation, suggests that some of the increased exposure to trauma in persons with disabilities is due to a "third variable" functionally related to the disability (substance abuse), rather than the disability itself.

EFFECTS OF TRAUMA

Numerous reviews from developed nations document the multitude of negative consequences associated with recent and past occurrence of severe threats and injury, especially physical and sexual victimization for individuals with disabilities (e.g., Finkelhor & Browne, 1985; Goodman et al., 1997; Nosek, 1996; Sobsey, 1994). As in the general population, the consequences of abuse include depression, anxiety, suicide attempts, substance abuse, aggression, poor self-esteem, social isolation, and sexual "acting-out" behavior. Many of the consequences span the different disability groups, and there is a tendency for persons with developmental and physical disabilities who have been abused also to receive psychiatric diagnoses, such as schizophrenia and major depression (e.g., Ryan, 1994). It is unclear whether the apparently strong association between trauma and psychiatric disabilities is due to the increased risk of abuse in persons with psychiatric disorders, the increased risk of psychiatric disorders in abused persons, some combination thereof, or a shared etiology between the two. Among individuals with psychiatric disorders and cognitive disorders, additional consequences of trauma exposure include homelessness, more frequent hospitalizations and emergency room visits, and engagement in behaviors that put them at risk for infectious diseases (e.g., Goodman et al., 2001).

As in the general population, one of the most prominent consequences of violent victimization in persons with disabilities is PTSD. Despite this, the research literature on PTSD in persons with disabilities is quite sparse, with only a handful of published studies, all from developed nations using convenience samples. The limited data suggest that, as expected, individuals with disabilities are at increased risk for developing PTSD. For example,

Ryan (1994) performed evaluations on 310 consecutive admissions to a team consultation service for persons with developmental disabilities, and found that 16.5% met criteria for current PTSD. This rate is approximately double the rate of *lifetime* PTSD in the general population (e.g., Breslau, Davis, Andreski, & Peterson, 1991; Kessler et al., 1995). Several studies of PTSD in persons with severe psychiatric disorders indicate even higher rates. Specifically, across five studies of PTSD in people with severe psychiatric disabilities, the rate of current PTSD ranged from 29% to 43% (Cascardi et al., 1996; Craine, Henson, Colliver, & MacLean, 1988; Mueser et al., 1998; Mueser & Rosenberg, 2001; Switzer et al., 1999).

ASSESSMENT ISSUES

Findings on the high prevalence and devastating effects of abuse in people with disabilities underscore the importance of routine inquiry into past and present exposure to violence as part of regular intake, as well as ongoing assessments. Yet abuse is often not evaluated in persons with disabilities. Even when an incident is reported, many cases are dismissed because of a lack of substantiating evidence, likely due to a poor understanding of interviewing methods for individuals with disabilities (Sobsey & Varnhagen, 1989). Common consequences of abuse, such as PTSD, are also rarely documented. For example, across the five studies mentioned above that found high rates of PTSD in persons with severe mental illness, fewer than 5% of those with PTSD diagnoses had this disorder documented in their medical charts (Cascardi et al., 1996; Craine et al., 1988; Mueser et al., 1998; Mueser & Rosenberg, 2001; Switzer et al., 1999). Given the low detection rates of PTSD in psychiatric populations, it can be assumed that PTSD is similarly under-detected in individuals with developmental and physical disabilities.

One reason for the failure to detect abuse and PTSD in people with disabilities may be the problem of *diagnostic overshadowing*, in which the most prominent diagnosis is made (e.g., major psychiatric, cognitive, or physical disability), while another comorbid diagnosis is ignored (e.g., PTSD). Two other reasons for the under-detection of abuse and its consequences in persons with disabilities, which are briefly discussed below, include questions of the credibility of reports by individuals with disabilities and societal attitudes toward those individuals.

Memory and Report Credibility

Reports of interpersonal violence, and sexual abuse in particular, by people with a disability may be assumed to be the product of cognitive impairment or emotional or psychotic distortions. Problems with memory and susceptibility to suggestion in individuals with developmental disabilities may also lead to their verbal reports of abuse being dismissed. Despite these limitations, research on the nature of memory impairment in persons with developmental disabilities challenges the notion that physical and sexual abuse would be more (or less) likely to be recalled by these individuals than by persons with no disability (e.g., Ellis, Palmer & Reeves, 1998; Rothbart-Seidman, 2001).

Gudjonsson and Gunn (1982) found that suggestibility was a problem primarily when an individual with mild mental retardation was confronted with sophisticated or abstract ideas that had no basis in direct observation. When direct observation of an event was involved, responses were consistent and resistive to suggestions. Newer research with adults with cognitive deficits found that women with mental retardation were highly susceptible to misleading questions regarding a witnessed incident involving genital touch (Rothbart-Seidman, 2001). This research also found, however, that the ability to report accurately when questions were presented in a non-suggestive manner was equivalent to that in women with average intelligence. That abstract forms of language and leading questions influence the degree of suggestibility strongly indicates a need for non-suggestive and developmentally appropriate language in interviewing to ensure that clients are able to communicate all that they know (Valenti-Hein & Schwartz, 1995).

Similar concerns have been raised about the role of affective and psychotic distortions in reports of trauma by persons with severe mental illness. Doubts about the veracity of reports are difficult to refute. However, thus far, the little work that exists to address the reliability of reports of victimization suggests that the reports of persons with severe mental illness are reliable over time, and consistent within measures of PTSD (Goodman et al., 1999; Mueser & Rosenberg, 2001). Although the literature on the relationship between psychiatric symptoms and abuse is quite varied, there is no consistent trend indicating that specific symptoms are strong predictors of abuse reports. The notion that psychiatric symptoms lead to over-reporting of interpersonal violence, while often raised, has little empirical support.

INTERVENTIONS

The broadest efforts to address the problem of trauma in persons with a disability begin at the societal level, chiefly with respect to national and international efforts to safeguard their basic rights. As people with disabilities are often less capable of advocating for themselves, their rights are not likely to be respected, and are often not formally recognized. The most basic of these rights include food, housing, medical care, work, and education. There have been international efforts to heighten awareness and to establish these rights (e.g., the UN Decade of Disabled Persons 1983–1992), as well as national efforts to prohibit discrimination against persons with disabilities (e.g., the *Americans with Disabilities Act* in the U.S.A.; Kaufmann, 1993). At the community and neighborhood levels, a major focus has been to educate the public about the nature of disabilities in order to decrease the stigma that leads to fear and abuse of individuals with disabilities. In many nations, such approaches (i.e., social marketing) are aimed at changing public perceptions of disability through public speaking, exposure to positive role models, and positive coverage in the popular media in order to reduce barriers to social integration, thereby also reducing the trauma associated with social rejection and self-stigmatization. As much abuse of persons with disabilities occurs within the institutions responsible for their care, another level of intervention has involved the appropriate screening and training of staff members, development of oversight and grievance procedures in order to detect and respond rapidly to possible cases of abuse, and creating structures whereby individuals with disabilities can have input into their care. At the family level, policies are aimed at providing families with the support they need to cope with the challenges of caring for or helping a person with a disability. Core features of such support include education about disabilities and how to cope with them, financial aid, and emotional assistance (e.g., family self-help groups). On the individual level, policies aim at teaching basic safety skills to persons with disabilities, and, to a limited extent, treating PTSD and other post-trauma symptoms.

Developing-country initiatives often demonstrate innovative rehabilitation, self-help, and participatory strategies that do not rely on expensive professional health services. Many families among Sudanese refugees living in North Uganda have found that caring for a disabled child is particularly taxing given their living conditions. They have welcomed the idea of a special income-generating project that also gives the disabled family member an added value and an engaging activity (see below). The Goat Project emerged through consultations between a family and the staff of the Transcultural Psychosocial Organisation. After the project began, many more families with disabled children expressed interest in it. Each disabled child was given two goats, which would produce a daily supply of milk and occasional income once they had multiplied. The disabled children surprised many in the community by their responsible handling of the goats.

Steven is 10 years old. He developed normally until he was two years old, when late one night he had a high fever and convulsions, apparently due to cerebral malaria. The family lived far from a health clinic, so no treatment was given. Soon afterwards he began to have convulsions a few times a week and never learned to speak fully. The family realized he was different from their other children and brought him to a traditional healer for a cure. The healer believed that the problem was due to the family not performing a proper burial ritual for an uncle who died in Sudan. Much money was spent to perform this ritual, but the child did not improve. The father left the family for fear of having more disabled children.

Steven's mother sought help from the Transcultural Psychosocial Organisation. The counselor explained that the disability was caused by damage to his brain, probably due to the fever. She explained that there was no cure, but that with perseverance the family could teach the child self-help skills. The mother was eager to educate the child. The father participated, and soon returned to the family. The child was taught to assist in household tasks. He was delighted when given the goats. When the father asked for money instead, the child declared "No, these are my goats." Steven responsibly cares for the goats and is eagerly awaiting the birth of their first offspring. (Source: Transcultural Psychosocial Organisation)

Some organizations in developed nations have begun programs using non-professionals offering specialized services to address abuse in populations of persons with specific disabilities. For example, the Abused Deaf Women's Advocacy Services (ADWAS) in Seattle, Washington in the US has developed a community-based program to respond to and deal with cases of sexual assault and domestic violence (Merkin & Smith, 1995). This comprehensive program includes a 24-hour crisis line, advocacy (including individual, systems, and legal advocacy), safe housing, counseling, education, and outreach.

Currently, there is a paucity of well-articulated treatments for trauma and its effects in individuals with severe mental illness (Mueser & Rosenberg, 2001) or cognitive disabilities (Mansell, Sobsey, & Calder, 1992). Considering the low detection rates of abuse in persons with a disability, this is no surprise.

In developed nations, traditional psychotherapy techniques with a psychoeducational approach focusing on understanding appropriate relationships, assertiveness, and communication have been found useful with cognitively disabled individuals (Szymanski & Tanguay, 1980). By defining a loving and caring relationship, clients can learn which of their experiences are abusive. Assertiveness skills provide the empowerment to say "no." Many individuals with disabilities are socialized into compliance, and thus permission to say "no" can be a powerful tool. Expressive therapy (i.e., art or movement therapy) has also been emerging as a favored treatment technique for people with cognitive disabilities, particularly when there are limitations in language skills. These therapies can empower the individual to communicate her or his story, as can non-medical self-help treatment.

Similarly, with respect to psychiatric populations, Harris (1998) has developed a weekly 9- to 12-month psychosocial group intervention and accompanying treatment manual for physically or sexually victimized women with severe mental illness. The intervention builds on a social skills training model to address difficulties in three domains likely to be affected by physical and sexual victimization: (1) intrapersonal skills, including self-knowledge, self-soothing, self-esteem, and self-trust; (2) interpersonal skills, including self-expression, social perception and labeling, self-protection, self-assertion, and relational mutuality; and (3) global skills, including identity formation, initiative-taking, and problem-solving.

Rosenberg, Mueser, and colleagues (Rosenberg et al., 2001) have recently developed two interventions for persons with severe mental illness that are more narrowly focused on the treatment of PTSD. One intervention is a 12- to 16-week individual treatment program, while the other is a 21-week group intervention. Both programs are based on cognitive-behavioral methods and include psychoeducation, breathing retraining for relaxation, and cognitive restructuring to address negative emotions stemming from abusive experiences.

RECOMMENDATIONS

International and National

In keeping with national culture, aspirations, and resources, measures should generally prioritize prevention of disability, equality of opportunities for disabled persons, and elimination of obstacles in the environment, both physical and cultural. Specific recommendations include:

- Safeguard and reaffirm the right to basic needs such as food, clothing, housing, health, income, and economic and social supports for persons with disabilities.
- Provide or expand disability benefits for workers.
- Pass legislation to make discrimination against people with disabilities illegal.
- Pass legislation to encourage employment of workers with physical and mental disabilities.

Community

- Raise awareness about prejudice and engage the public and disabled persons in finding ways of eliminating it.
- Ensure participation by representatives of disabled persons in community decision-making.
- Educate social and humanitarian workers about traumatic stress and abuse of persons with disabilities and how to deal with it.
- Make support services accessible to people with disabilities.
- Recruit and train volunteers to visit isolated persons with disabilities, families giving care to these individuals, and institutionalized persons.
- Create assisted housing for those without shelter who do not need institutional care.
- Provide access to emergency shelters for victims with disabilities.
- Provide or expand employment services for persons with disabilities.
- Remove environmental barriers that exclude people with physical challenges from opportunities for education, employment, social services, and recreation.
- Develop a proactive, coordinated community approach to investigating and prosecuting cases of abuse of people with disabilities.
- Provide linkages between programs serving victims in different disability groups.

Institutional

- Provide staff with ongoing training and resources to avoid the burnout and frustration that can lead to abuse of clients with disabilities.
- Train staff in institutions and in residential facilities on the nature of abuse and neglect and ways to prevent them.
- Develop a resident's bill of rights that emphasizes the right to live free of abuse and neglect.
- Have management and staff establish a "zero tolerance" policy statement for abuse within each of their institutions.
- Screen staff with background and attitudinal checks to avoid hiring persons with the potential for inflicting abuse, such as those with criminal backgrounds.
- Set staffing requirements and schedules so that staff will be able to give appropriate attention and care to their charges.
- Provide necessary resources to maintain a clean, pleasant, and uncrowded environment.
- Develop a resident council and family council so that the persons served and their families have input into their care and more control over their lives.

Families

- Facilitate convening of self-help groups for family caretakers of persons with disabilities.
- Train workers and service providers to give support and work collaboratively with family caregivers.
- Provide necessary resources to families caring for a member with a disability, including fiscal resources, respite, and skills for managing conflict.
- Engage families in discussions about the nature, consequences, and treatment of abuse in a member with a disability.

Individuals

- Organize self-help groups.
- Link victims with "natural helpers."
- Increase self-esteem by facilitating contact with role models who have disabilities or who are in recovery.
- Establish community programs for the purpose of empowering persons with disabilities, such as assertiveness training.
- Teach safety skills, including self-defense.
- Inform individuals of their rights, including the right to be free of sexual harassment, threats, and physical intimidation.
- Teach appropriate interpersonal skills to help persons with a disability express their feelings (including affection and intimacy), to assert themselves in the face of pressure, and to obtain assistance from others when their rights have been infringed.
- Teach sexual education within the context of socialization to enable persons with disabilities to learn important information about choices and decision-making skills with respect to matters of intimacy and sex.
- Provide individual or group therapy services for traumatized individuals to help them integrate their experiences and reduce their distress, including symptoms of PTSD.

REFERENCES

Adamolekum, B. (1995). The aetiologies of epilepsy in tropical Africa. *Tropical Geographic Medicine, 47(3)*, 115–117.

Baladerian, N.J. (1991). The sexual abuse of people with developmental disabilities. *Sexuality and Disability, 9(4)*, 323–335.

Breslau, N., Davis, G.C., Andreski, P., & Peterson, E. (1991). Traumatic events and post-traumatic stress disorder in an urban population of young adults. *Archives of General Psychiatry, 48*, 216–222.

Bushnell, J.A., Wells, J.E., & Oakely-Browne, M. (1992). Long-term effects of intrafamilial sexual abuse in childhood. *Acta Psychiatrica Scandinavica, 85*, 136–142.

Carmen, E., Rieker, P.P., & Mills, T. (1984). Victims of violence and psychiatric illness. *American Journal of Psychiatry, 141*, 378–383.

Carreire, A. (1971). O infanticídio ritual em Africa. *Boletim Cultural da Guiné Portuguesa, 26*, 101, 149–217 & 26, 102, 321–377.

Cascardi, M., Mueser, K.T., DeGiralomo, J., & Murrin, M. (1996). Physical aggression against psychiatric inpatients by family members and partners: A descriptive study. *Psychiatric Services, 47*, 531–533.

Craine, L.S., Henson, C.E., Colliver, J.A., & MacLean, D.G. (1988). Prevalence of a history of sexual abuse among female psychiatric patients in a state hospital system. *Hospital and Community Psychiatry, 39*, 300–304.

Comas-Diaz, L. (1981). Puerto Rican espiritismo and psychotherapy. *American Journal of Orthopsychiatry, 51*, 636–645.

Davies-Netzley, S., Hurlburt, M.S., & Hough, R. (1996). Childhood abuse as a precursor to homelessness for homeless women in severe mental illness. *Violence and Victims, 11*, 129–142.

De Jong, J.T.V.M. (1987). *A descent into African psychiatry*. Amsterdam: Royal Tropical Institute.

Duke, P.J., Pantelis, C., & Barnes, T.R.E. (1994). South Westminster schizophrenia survey: Alcohol use and its relationship to symptoms, tardive dyskinesia and illness onset. *British Journal of Psychiatry, 164*, 630–636.

Duncan, R.D., Saunders, B.E., Kilpatrick, D.G., Hanson, R.F., & Resnick, H.S. (1996). Childhood physical assault as a risk factor for PTSD, depression, and substance abuse: Findings for a national survey. *American Journal of Orthopsychiatry, 66*, 437–448.

Ellis, N.R., Palmer, R.L., & Reeves, C.L. (1998). Developmental and intellectual differences in frequency processing. *Developmental Psychology, 24*, 38–45.

Finkelhor, D., & Browne, A. (1985). The traumatic impact of childhood sexual abuse: A conceptualization. *American Journal of Orthopsychiatry, 55*, 530–541.

Fowler, I.L., Carr, V.J., Carter, N.T., & Lewin, T.J. (1998). Patterns of current and lifetime substance use in schizophrenia. *Schizophrenia Bulletin, 24*, 443–455.

Gall, C. (1999, June 8). Crisis in the Balkans: Dispossessed Serbs: The refugees of a past war still suffer. *The New York Times*, p. 18.

Giel, R., Harding, T.W., ten Horn, G.H.M.M., Ladrido-Ignacio, L., Murthy, R.S., Siraq, A.O., Suleiman, M.A., & Wig, N.N. (1988). The detection of childhood mental disorders in primary care in some developing countries. In A.S. Henderson & G.D. Burrows (Eds.), *Handbook of social psychiatry* (pp. 233–244). Oxford: Elsevier.

Goldman, H.H. (1984). Epidemiology. In J.A. Talbott (Ed.), *The chronic mental patient: Five years later* (pp. 15–31). Orlando: Grune & Stratton.

Goodman, L.A., Dutton, M.A., & Harris, M. (1995). Physical and sexual assault prevalence among episodically homeless women with serious mental illness. *American Journal of Orthopsychiatry, 65*, 468–478.

Goodman, L.A., Dutton, M.A., & Harris, M. (1997). The relationship between violence dimensions and symptom severity among homeless, mentally ill women. *Journal of Traumatic Stress, 10*, 51–70.

Goodman, L.A., Rosenberg, S.D., Mueser, K.T., & Drake, R.E. (1997). Physical and sexual assault history in women with serious mental illness: Prevalence, correlates, treatment, and future research directions. *Schizophrenia Bulletin, 23*, 685–696.

Goodman, L.A., Salyers, M.P., Mueser, K.T., Rosenberg, S.D., Swartz, M., Essock, S.M., Osher, F.C., & Butterfield, M.I. (2001). Recent victimization in women and men with severe mental illness: Prevalence and correlates. *Journal of Traumatic Stress, 14*, 615–632.

Goodman, L.A., Thompson, K.M., Weinfurt, K., Corl, S., Acker, P., Mueser, K.T., & Rosenberg, S.D. (1999). Reliability of reports of violent victimization and PTSD among men and women with SMI. *Journal of Traumatic Stress, 12*, 587–599.

Greenfield, S.F., Strakowski, S.M., Tohen, M., Batson, S.C., & Kolbrener, M.L. (1994). Childhood abuse in first-episode psychosis. *British Journal of Psychiatry, 164*, 831–834.

Gudjonsson, G.H., & Gunn, J. (1982). The competence and reliability of a witness in a criminal court: A case report. *British Journal of Psychiatry, 141*, 624–627.

Harris, M. (1998). *Trauma recovery and empowerment: A clinician's guide for working with women in groups.* New York: The Free Press.

Hiday, V.A. (1995). The social context of mental illness and violence. *Journal of Health and Social Behavior, 36*, 122–137.

Hiday, V.A., Swartz, M.S., Swanson, J.W., Borum, R., & Wagner, H.R. (1999). Criminal victimization of persons with severe mental illness. *Psychiatric Services, 50*, 62–68.

Hutchings, P.S., & Dutton, M.A. (1993). Sexual assault history in a community mental health center clinical population. *Community Mental Health Journal, 29*, 59–63.

Jacobson, A. (1989). Physical and sexual assault histories among psychiatric outpatients. *American Journal of Psychiatry, 146*, 755–758.

Jacobson, A., & Herald, C. (1990). The relevance of childhood sexual abuse to adult psychiatric inpatient care. *Hospital and Community Psychiatry, 41*, 154–158.

Jacobson, A., & Richardson, B. (1987). Assault experiences of 100 psychiatric inpatients: Evidence of the need for routine inquiry. *American Journal of Psychiatry, 144*, 508–513.

Kaufmann, C. (1993). Reasonable accommodation to mental health disabilities at work: Legal constructs and practical applications. *International Journal of Psychiatry and Law, 21*, 153–174.

Kessler, R.C., Nelson, C.B., McGonagle, K.A., Edlund, M.J., Frank, R.G., & Leaf, P.J. (1996). The epidemiology of co-occurring addictive and mental disorders: implications for prevention and service utilization. *American Journal of Orthopsychiatry, 66*, 17–31.

Kessler, R.C., Sonnega, A., Bromet, E., Hughes, M., & Nelson, C.B. (1995). Posttraumatic stress disorder in the national comorbidity survey. *Archives of General Psychiatry, 52*, 1048–1060.

Kilpatrick, D.G., Acierno, R., Resnick, H.S., Saunders, B.E., & Best, C.L. (1997). A 2-year longitudinal analysis of the relationships between violent assault and substance use in women. *Journal of Consulting and Clinical Psychology, 65*, 834–847.

Levey, J.C., & Lagos, V.K. (1994). Children with disabilities. In L.D. Eron, J.H. Gentry, & P. Schlegel (Eds.), *Reason to hope: A psychosocial perspective on violence and youth* (pp. 197–213). Washington, DC: American Psychological Association.

Lévy-Bruhl, L. (1921). *La Mentalité Primitive.* Paris: Librairie Felix Alcan.

Lipschitz, D.S., Kaplan, M.L., Sorkenn, J.B., Faedda, G.L., Chorney, P., & Asnis, G.M. (1996). Prevalence and characteristics of physical and sexual abuse among psychiatric outpatients. *Psychiatric Services, 47*, 189–191.

Mansell, S., Sobsey, D., & Calder, P. (1992). Sexual abuse treatment for persons with developmental disability. *Professional Psychology: Research and Practice, 23*, 404–409.

Merkin, L., & Smith, M.J. (1995). A community based model providing services for deaf and deaf-blind victims of sexual assault and domestic violence. *Sexuality and Disability, 13*, 97–106.

Morales-Dorta, J. (1976). *Puerto Rican espiritismo: Religion and psychotherapy.* New York: Vantage Press.

Mueser, K.T., Goodman, L.B., Trumbetta, S.L., Rosenberg, S.D., Osher, F.C., Vidaver, R., Auciello, P., & Foy, D.W. (1998). Trauma and posttraumatic stress disorder in severe mental illness. *Journal of Consulting and Clinical Psychology, 66*, 493–499.

Mueser, K.T., & Rosenberg, S.D. (2001). Treatment of PTSD in persons with severe mental illness. In J.P. Wilson, M.J. Friedman, & J.D. Lindy (Eds.), *Treating psychological trauma and PTSD* (pp. 354–382). New York: Guilford.

Mueser, K.T., Rosenberg, S.D., Goodman, L.A., & Trumbetta, S.L. (2002). Trauma, PTSD, and the course of severe mental illness: An interactive model. *Schizophrenia Research, 53,* 153–173.

Mueser, K.T., Salyers, M.P., Rosenberg, S.D., Ford, J.D., Fox, L., & Cardy, P. (2001). A psychometric evaluation of trauma and PTSD: Assessments in persons with severe mental illness. *Psychological Assessment, 13,* 110–117.

Mueser, K.T., & Taylor, K.L. (1997). A cognitive-behavioral approach. In M. Harris & C.L. Landis (Eds.), *Sexual abuse in the lives of women diagnosed with serious mental illness* (pp. 67–90). Amsterdam: Harwood Academic Publishers.

Mullan, P.B., & Cole, S.S. (1991). Health care providers' perceptions of the vulnerability of persons with disabilities: Sociological frameworks and empirical analyses. *Sexuality and Disability, 9,* 221–242.

National Information Center for Children and Youth with Disabilities (1999). Fact Sheets at www.nichcy.org.

Nosek, M.A. (1996). Sexual abuse of women with disabilities. In M.A. Krotoski, M.A. Nosek, & M.A. Turk (Eds.), *Women with physical disabilities* (pp. 153–173). Baltimore: Paul Brookes.

Paddock, R., & Kuhn, A. (1999, December 11). China backs Russia on Chechen war: Conflict: Moscow has threatened an all out attack on separatist republic's capitol today. *Los Angeles Times,* Part A, p. 6.

Polusny, M.A., & Follette, V.M. (1995). Long-term correlates of child sexual abuse: Theory and review of the empirical literature. *Applied and Preventive Psychology, 4,* 143–166.

Randall, C., & Kapija, D. (1999, May 5). Conflict in the Balkans: Army brings aid to Macedonia's unwanted ones. *The Daily Telegraph,* p. 18.

Regier, D.A., Farmer, M.E., Rae, D.S., Locke, B.Z., Keith, S.J., Judd, L.L., & Goodwin, F.K. (1990). Comorbidity of mental disorders with alcohol and other drug abuse: Results from the Epidemiologic Catchment Area (ECA) study. *Journal of the American Medical Association, 264,* 2511–2518.

Robins, L.N., & Regier, D.A. (1991). *Psychiatric disorders in America: The Epidemiologic Catchment Area Study.* New York: The Free Press.

Rose, S.M., Peabody, C.G., & Stratigeas, B. (1991). Undetected abuse among intensive case management clients. *Hospital and Community Psychiatry, 42,* 499–503.

Rosenberg, S.D., Mueser, K.T., Friedman, M.J., Gorman, P.G., Drake, R.E., Vidaver, R.M., Torrey, W.C., & Jankowski, M.K. (2001). Developing effective treatments for posttraumatic disorders: A review and proposal. *Psychiatric Services, 52,* 1453–1461.

Ross, C.A., Anderson, G., & Clark, P. (1994). Childhood abuse and the positive symptoms of schizophrenia. *Hospital and Community Psychiatry, 45,* 489–491.

Rothbart-Seidman, R. (2001). *The memory of female witnesses with mild mental retardation: Implications for reports of sexual abuse.* Dissertation Abstracts International.

Ryan, R. (1994). Posttraumatic stress disorder in persons with developmental disabilities. *Community Mental Health Journal, 30,* 45–54.

Sartorius, N., Jablensky, A., Korten, A., Ernberg, G., Anker, M., Cooper, J.E., & Day, R. (1986). Early manifestations and first-contact incidence of schizophrenia in different cultures. *Psychological Medicine, 16,* 909–928.

Silove, D., Ekblad, S., & Mollica, R. (2000). The rights of the severely mentally ill in post-conflict societies. *The Lancet, 355,* 1548–1549.

Smith, D., Valenti-Hein, D., & Heller, T. (1985). Interpersonal competencies of retarded adults: Implications for social, vocational, and sexual adjustment. In M. Sigman (Ed.), *Children* with dual disabilities: Mental retardation and mental illness (pp. 71–94). New York: Grune & Stratton.

Sobsey, D. (1994). *Violence and abuse in the lives of people with disabilities*. Baltimore: Paul H. Brookes Publishing.

Sobsey, D., & Doe, T. (1991). Patterns of sexual abuse and assault. *Journal of Sexuality and Disability, 9*, 243–259.

Sobsey, D., & Varnhagen, C. (1989). Sexual abuse of people with disabilities. In M. Csapo & L. Gougen (Eds.), *Special education across Canada: Challenges for the 90s* (pp. 199–218). Vancouver, Canada: Centre for Human Development & Research.

Somasundaram, D., Van De Put, W.A.M., Eisenbruch, M. & De Jong, J.T.V.M. (1999). Starting mental health services in Cambodia. *Social Science and Medicine, 48*, 1029–1042.

Switzer, G.E., Dew, M.A., Thompson, K., Goycoolea, J.M., Derricott, T., & Mullins, S.D. (1999). Posttraumatic stress disorder and service utilization among urban mental health center clients. *Journal of Traumatic Stress, 12*, 25–39.

Szymanski, L.S., & Tanguay, P.E. (Eds.). (1980). *Emotional disorders of mentally retarded persons: Assessments, treatment and consultation*. Baltimore: University Park Press.

Valenti-Hein, D.C., & Schwartz, L.D. (1995). *Sexual Abuse Interview for those with Developmental Disabilities*. Santa Barbara: James Stanfield Company, Inc.

Watson-Armstrong, L.A., O'Rourke, B., & Schatzlein, J. (1994.) Sexual abuse and persons with disabilities: A call for awareness. *Applied Rehabilitation Counseling, 25*, 36–42.

White, R., Benedict, M.I., Wulff, L., & Kelley, M. (1987). Physical disabilities as risk factors for child maltreatment: A selected review. *American Journal of Orthopsychiatry, 57*, 93–101.

Young, M.E., Nosek, M.A., Howland, C., Chanpong, G., & Rintala, D.H. (1997). Prevalence of abuse of women with physical disabilities. *Archives of Physical and Medical Rehabilitation, 78*, S34–S38.

Chapter 8

Violence against Women

Mary Ann Dutton, Dean G. Kilpatrick, Merle Friedman, and Vikram Patel

Shamita Das Dasgupta stated, "We have a word for creatures who have no voice, no voice in that they cannot speak a language understandable to us. It is abola. So those who are not allowed to speak, by their husbands or by institutions or because of violence, are abola" (Pence, 1997).

Justice is made when the offender has made whole by being called to account for the damage he has caused, acknowledging his responsibility for it, and changing his behavior so that it is not repeated (Fortune, 1986, p. 236).

Healing begins when there is no more silence about the atrocities done to women—when that silence is filled with the sounds of human connection and the recognition of human dignity across the abyss of suffering and loss.

DEFINITION AND SCOPE

The focus of this chapter is violence against women. Violence violates basic human rights and results in increasing physical, emotional, social, and economic burdens for women and their families around the world. Developments in women's human rights around the globe bring attention to the violence, sexual violation, deprivation, oppression, and murder committed against women everywhere.

Women's human rights issues were first addressed internationally in the *Interamerican Convention on the Nationality of Women*, a treaty created in the Latin American region in 1933 by the Organization of American States (Toro, 1999). Language that prohibits discrimination based on sex is included in The *Universal Declaration of Human Rights* (UDHR) adopted by the General Assembly in 1948. The United Nations General Assembly defined violence against women in the *Declaration on the Elimination of Violence Against Women*, adopted in 1993, as **"any act of gender-based violence that results in, or is likely to result in, physical, sexual, or psychological harm or suffering to women, including threats of such acts, coercion or arbitrary deprivation of liberty, whether occurring in public or private life"** (United Nations, 1994). In the Declaration, violence against women encompasses, but is not limited to, **"physical, sexual and psychological violence occurring in the family, including battering, sexual abuse of female children in the household, dowry related violence, marital rape, female genital mutilation and other traditional practices harmful to women, non-spousal violence and violence related to exploitation; physical, sexual and psychological violence occurring within the general community, including rape, sexual abuse, sexual harassment and intimidation at work, in educational institutions and elsewhere; trafficking in women and forced prostitution; and physical, sexual and psychological violence perpetrated or condoned by the state, wherever it occurs"** (United Nations, 1994).

This section discusses three aspects of violence against women: (1) physical, sexual, and psychological violence and abuse, including homicide; (2) prostitution; and (3) trafficking. Physical and sexual violence against women occurs in industrialized as well as developing countries. Some countries still maintain that men have a legal right, and indeed an obligation, to physically or sexually assault or even kill their female family members—sometimes in circumstances where violations of proscribed behavior are merely suspected. Even where such violence is not legally sanctioned, at least some level of violence against women is culturally sanctioned in many segments of our global community. Patterns or methods of violence may differ across regions. However, violence against women uniformly includes acts of physical violence (e.g., hitting, throwing acid, igniting with kerosene, using a weapon), sexual violence and abuse (e.g., forced or coerced sexual behavior, female genital mutilation), psychological or emotional abuse (e.g., threats, intimidation, isolation, and withholding of food, basic resources, and basic freedoms), and stalking (e.g., repeated unwanted contacts, following the person, harassment, vandalizing personal property). Violence against women is committed by strangers, acquaintances, caregivers, authorities, intimate partners, and other family members. Sexual assault occurs through the use of varying levels of coercion, ranging from the expectations of wives to serve the sexual needs of their husbands (but not the reverse) to physical force.

The United Nations' *Global Report on Crime and Justice* (1999) indicates that violence against women, like most serious crime, is related to economic hardship. Lower social status is related to greater violence. Where women are more liberated, there is less violence. Fewer than one in three female victims of violence report their victimization to the police.

Violence against women has been recognized as a major health and human rights issue, an important cause of morbidity and mortality. Based on a summary by the World Health Organization of large-scale studies in both industrialized and developing countries (Krug, 1999), men have physically or sexually abused at least one in five of the world's female population at some time in their life. Many, including pregnant women and young girls, are subject to severe, sustained, or repeated attacks over many years.

High rates of violence against women by their intimate partners have been documented in many different countries, among married and unmarried couples, and among heterosexual and same-sex couples. For example, the International Center for Research on Women (2000), in a survey conducted with 9,938 households from three strata in India, found that 40% of women reported experiencing at least one form of physical violence in their married life, and 15% reported experiencing forced sex, with 26% reporting physical violence in the previous 12 months.

The National Violence Against Women Survey (Tjaden & Thoennes, 2000), conducted on 8,000 women and 8,000 men, found that 18% of all women said they had been the victim of a completed or attempted rape at some point during their lifetimes. Eight percent of women and 2% of men reported having been stalked at some point in their lives. Women reported experiencing more intimate partner violence (22%) than did men (7%) during their lives. American Indian/Alaskan Native women and men reported more violence victimization than those from other racial groups. Finally, this same report found that violence against women is most often committed by an intimate partner: 64% of women who reported being raped, physically assaulted, or stalked were victimized by partners (compared to 16% of men).

A national mail survey of Japanese women (Yoshioka & Sorenson, 1994) found that 59% reported experiencing some type of physical abuse by an intimate partner. Among those abused, one-third reported attempted strangulation, a particularly lethal form of violence. Finally, 5% of this sample reported having experienced one or more acts by an intimate partner they considered to be sexually abusive. A woman's legitimacy within a Japanese marriage is defined largely by her fertility. This makes women's infertility—and the sexual coercion that may accompany it—particularly relevant as cultural factors underlying physical and sexual violence within the culture.

The First Palestinian National Survey on Violence Against Women (Haj-Yahia, 1999), involving 2,410 married women from the West Bank and the Gaza Strip, found that 52% of the Palestinian women reported they had experienced one or more acts of physical violence at least once during the past year. An additional 27% of these women reported that their husbands had sex with them without their consent, whereas an additional 31% reported that their husbands attempted to do so.

Crimes of violence against women are often not reported to police. Based on findings from the Fifth United Nations Survey of Crime Trends and Criminal Justice Systems reported in the United Nations' *Global Report on Crime and Justice* (United Nations, 1999), less than one in three female victims of violence report their victimization to police. The National Violence Against Women survey in the US (Tjaden & Thoennes, 2000) found that reports were made to police in only 17% of rape cases involving female victims, 27% of physical assault cases involving female victims, and 14% of physical assault cases involving male victims. Reasons physical assault victims gave for not reporting victimization to police were that "police couldn't do anything," "police wouldn't believe them," and "wanted to protect the attacker, relationship, or children." Some evidence suggests that the police view women's claims of having been battered as non-credible, unworthy of police time (Belknap, 1995). Fewer than 1% of perpetrators of physical assault were convicted or were sentenced to jail or prison.

Ironically, the *Global Report* indicated that rape was the crime for which countries most often reported data in the Fifth United Nations Survey. This is surprising, since it is widely believed that rape is one of the most under-reported crimes, and since rape victims themselves tend to report this crime (or their victimization) to police less often than do other crime victims.

According to Amnesty International, on February 1, 2000, the human rights section of the United Nations Mission in Sierra Leone (UNAMSIL) reported that harassment, abduction, and sexual violence were occurring almost daily in the area around Port Loko. Pregnancies resulting from these rapes were so frequent that they "could not be counted."

It is often the case that murders of women involve specific gender-based motives. For example, "honor killings" involve the murder of women who are viewed as dishonoring their families through being accused of an extramarital affair, when they desire to remarry after divorce, or even when they are raped. The Muslim Women's League, a nonprofit

American Muslim organization, states that "honor killings" are erroneously justified by a distorted interpretation of religion, especially of Islam. As late as 2000, the Jordanian Lower House failed to abolish Article 340 of the Penal Code, which provides for lenient sentences when men kill their female relatives in the name of "honor."

Dowry deaths, or "bride burnings," in India involve the killing of women due to insufficient funds or dowry provided by the woman's family to the new husband. An increased emphasis on consumerism has been blamed for an increase in the demand for cash and gifts from a new bride's family—even after the marriage. Dowry deaths are described as a "modern" development in India, situated within the commercialization of marriage transactions in a predominately patriarchal social structure (Vindhya, 2000). Although such killings are punishable by law, courts tend to offer lenient sentences.

In spite of increased resources focused on violence against women, domestic homicide against women in the United States has failed to decline substantially, although the frequency of women killing their male partners has decreased. The overall rates have declined from 1976 to 1998: male victims have declined an average of 4% a year, but female victims only an average of 1% a year (Rennison & Welchans, 2000). Women comprise 62% of the intimate partner homicide victims in the US.

Separation of an intimate relationship heightens the risk of homicide. The *Family Violence in Canada: Statistical Profile 2001* (Trainor & Mihorean, 2001) reported that ex-marital partners were responsible for 28% of all homicides of women (compared to 10% of male homicides). Although the absolute number of homicides against separated women were fewer than for cohabiting women, when calculated as the rate per million couples, the rate of homicide for separated women was greater. It is not uncommon for a domestic homicide perpetrator to defend the murder of his estranged partner by citing that he was distraught over the extramarital affair or relationship separation.

Rape is a tool of hatred used against a group of people—as well as a crime against individual women. However, crimes of violence against women historically were not considered war crimes. Recently, the international human rights community has recognized rape as a war crime and a crime against humanity. Human Rights Watch reported credible accounts of 96 cases of sexual assault by Yugoslav soldiers, Serbian police, or paramilitaries during the period of NATO bombing, although the actual number may be much higher.[1] An historic verdict before an international tribunal at The Hague, which focused entirely on crimes of sexual violence,

---

[1] http://www.hrw.org/reports/2000/fry/index.htm

involved the conviction of three Bosnian Serbs of crimes against humanity for using "rape as an instrument of terror." They received jail terms of up to 28 years. The tribunal ruled that rape does not have to be ordered by superiors to be considered the highest level of atrocity.

> *Kim Yoon Shim was a Korean woman and one of 200,000 women the Japanese armed forces took captive for use as sexual slaves in military brothels—"comfort stations"—during World War II. She writes, "Day and night, the Japanese military raped us repeatedly. . . . My wish is that the Government of Japan admit its wrongs, apologize for its crimes, and punish the offenders . . . record the true facts of sex slavery in its textbooks" (Yoon Shim, 1999, pp. 127–128).*

Prostitution and trafficking are forms of violence targeted mainly against women and children. **Trafficking is defined as the illicit and clandestine movement of persons across national and international borders**, according to the 1994 revised UN Convention on the Suppression of the Traffic in Persons and the Exploitation of the Prostitution of Others, originally adopted in 1949. In addition, other illegal activities are related to trafficking, such as forced domestic labor, false marriages, clandestine employment, and false adoption.

Recruiters, traffickers, and crime syndicates profit from forcing women and girl children into sexually or economically oppressive and exploitative situations. For example, in 1997 they made $7 billion in profits from these activities (USAID Office of Women in Development, 1999)—more profit than from international trade in illicit weapons. The UN estimates that 4 million women, children, and men become victims of international trafficking each year. This has been referred to as a "modern form of slavery." Their destitute families sell some into slavery. "Employment brokers" who promise employment to those in desperate economic situations draw other victims. Trafficking is inextricably linked to poverty. Thus, it is no surprise that trafficking generally flows from poorer regions to wealthier areas, which provide the demand and can afford the payment.

> *One case of trafficking involved a prominent couple in the US who offered a woman a job as a domestic worker through contacts in her small town in Central America. Once in the US, her passport was held by her employers and she was not allowed to leave the house unaccompanied by them. She was required to work long hours, and was physically and sexually assaulted as well. She finally sought help, while meeting the family's children after school, by passing a note to a school bus driver.*

These examples underscore the importance of understanding the context and consequences of violence against women in order to craft more effective strategies for violence prevention. Further, they indicate the need to examine the differential risk of victimization of women by social strata and ethnic groups in all parts of the world. They also point to the importance of targeting repeat victimization in prevention efforts. Special attention needs to be paid when the victimization is compounded by oppression, dominance, and control that occurs even during periods of nonviolence.

IMPACT OF VIOLENCE AGAINST WOMEN

Societal

There are tremendous costs to society—both economic and social—resulting from violence against women. The economic burden to society of violence against women follows, in part, from the community response to such violence and its aftermath. When violence against women occurs, the medical, psychological, and legal sequelae increase demand for public services. These include emergency shelter, law enforcement, criminal and civil courts, prison and detention of offenders, crime prevention and detection, job training and health services for victims, alcohol and drug treatment programs, and foster care. For example, according to the World Health Organization,[2] studies from Zimbabwe, Nicaragua, and the United States indicate that women who have been physically or sexually assaulted use health services more than women with no history of violence, thus increasing the public health care burden. Greater health care costs to society result from injury and chronic health problems, sexually transmitted diseases such as AIDS/HIV, unplanned pregnancies, birth defects resulting from violence-related fetal injury, and premature death (Laurence & Spalter-Roth, 1996). Increased health care and mental health care costs apply also to children who witness violence against women in the home. Children exposed to domestic violence have more behavior problems, including hyperactivity, emotional disorders, aggression, and delinquency (Trainor & Milhorean, 2001). These too result in greater need for services.

The economic burden of violence against women is also evident in the workplace. Workplace-related costs include greater job loss, lost productivity due to disruption in the workplace caused by violence or its aftermath, and decreased worker productivity in the workplace or school of victims and their children. For example, the World Health Organization reported in a *June 2000 Fact Sheet* (No. 239) a study of abused women in Managua, Nicaragua, which found that abused women earned 46% less than women

---

[2] http://www.who.int/violence_injury_prevention/vaw/infopack.htm

who did not suffer abuse, even after controlling for other factors that affect earnings.[3]

Societal costs also include the perpetuation of violence from one generation to the next. Violence against women exposes children in the family to the violence, as well as to its aftermath, and childhood exposure in turn is the most consistent correlate of later adult domestic violence (Simons & Johnson, 1998). Children's exposure to domestic violence increases the risk for later criminal victimization as well, especially for girls (Mitchell & Finkelhor, 2001).

Community/Neighborhood/Family

It is important to consider not only the impact of crime victimization per se in oppressed and underprivileged groups, but also the related or combined impact of other abuses of power. Examples include repeated oppression based on race, culture, gender, sexual preference, or physical disability. "Insidious trauma" (Root, 1992) refers to repetitive and cumulative abuse experiences against less-privileged individuals by those who have power over their access to resources and their well-being. For example, the combined impact of violence, racism, and homophobia increases the challenges faced by lesbian battered women of color. The rape of a homeless and impoverished woman of color is another, too frequent, example. Root (1992) suggests, "Insidious trauma's imprint rests in an acute self-awareness that one's safety is very tentative" (p. 375).

Violence victimization creates an atmosphere of insecurity and threat. Notably, the fear of rape is considered nearly universal in the daily lives of women. Indeed, repeated studies in different countries have shown that the fear of rape among young women is greater than the fear of any other type of crime, due to its likelihood as well as its severity. The fear of rape leads women to adapt their social and lifestyle preferences accordingly. The emotional toil and the lost opportunities that follow from the fear of rape and violence on the streets and in their homes rob women and their families of their basic human rights and opportunities to grow and prosper.

Violence against women impacts all members of the family. For example, domestic homicide impacts families when children are left without a parent or are torn between feuding family members attempting to gain custody (Kaplan, 1998). There remain many instances where perpetrators of serious violence are awarded unsupervised access to their children. In some instances their violence is construed as "out of character," attributed

---

[3] http://www.who.int/inf-fs/en/fact239.html

to the perpetrator's "despair" about the dissolution of the (battering) relationship. In addition, separation of children from grandparents and other extended family members disrupts family relationships.

Individual

Violence against women impacts their well-being in all aspects. The next section focuses on the physical and psychological impact of violence against women.

Physical Impact. Violence against women increases their risk of physical health problems and death. Health status among victims can be affected through at least three possible routes: (1) physical injury resulting directly from the violence, (2) impaired physical health following from the victimization experience, and (3) increased health-risk behaviors.

Women assaulted by intimates are more likely to be injured than women assaulted by strangers (52% vs. 20%) (Bachman & Saltzman, 1995). A recent study (Thompson, Saltzman, & Johnson, 2001) found that being severely injured was $8^1/_2$ times more likely among women with a previous abuse history involving six or more incidents perpetrated by the same partner, 7 times more likely among women who feared that their lives were in danger, 3 times more likely if the violence began before the union, 3 times more likely if the perpetrator was using alcohol at the time of the assault, and more than $2^1/_2$ times more likely if the level of emotional abuse was also high.

A comprehensive review of the health effects of interpersonal violence (Acierno, Resnick, & Kilpatrick, 1997; Kilpatrick, Resnick, & Acierno, 1997; Resnick, Acierno, & Kilpatrick, 1997) showed a relationship between violence and a host of physical health problems and risk factors for health morbidity and mortality. For example, a recent review (Golding, 1999b) found that sexual assault is usually associated with poor general health and limitations in physical functioning, as well as with specific health problems such as chronic pelvic pain, premenstrual disturbance, other gynecologic symptoms, fibromyalgia, headache, other pain syndromes, and gastrointestinal disorders. Depression did not account for the poorer health of these women. Another study (Stein & Barrett-Connor, 2000) found that a history of sexual assault was associated with an increased risk of arthritis and breast cancer. Further, a "dose-response" effect was observed, such that multiple episodes of sexual assault carried a two- to three-fold increased risk of these diseases compared with a single episode.

Risk of HIV/AIDS is a major public health problem associated with crime victimization—especially sexual assault and trafficking. Indeed, the

World Health Organization noted that the primary risk factor for HIV among women is violence (Farley & Kelly, 2000). This has implications for a wide variety of victimized groups, including battered women, rape victims, and prostitutes. The risk of HIV/AIDS associated with trafficking varies within regions of the world. For example, where prostitution is controlled by organized crime, as in Mumbai, India, women are less likely to have information or the means to protect themselves from infection, compared to when sex workers are organized for their own protection, as in Calcutta (USAID Office of Women in Development, 1999).

Another serious consequence of violence is revictimization (Browne & Finklehor, 1986). Adult sexual victimization is more likely among those sexually abused in childhood. Further, many individuals who find themselves revictimized through prostitution have been assaulted sexually and physically in childhood, often by multiple perpetrators and by persons both inside and outside the family (Farley & Kelly, 2000).

Death is the most extreme physical health outcome associated with crime victimization. The leading cause of death worldwide is injury (Krug, 1999), including intentional and self-inflicted injury—two types of injury related to violence against women. Death and injury from suicide attempts is another serious health concern associated with crime victimization—especially sexual assault and domestic violence. In high-income countries, self-inflicted injuries and interpersonal violence are two of the three leading causes of death among people aged 15 to 44 years (Krug, 1999). Self-inflicted injuries are the leading injury-related cause of death in China.

Psychological Impact.   Violent crime victimization produces a wide range of emotions in its wake, many of which are normal human reactions to traumatic experience. Yet, a failure to recognize that the experience, labeling, and expression of emotion can vary widely between cultures (Kitayama & Markus, 1994), as well as between the genders, can lead one group to label another's expression as deviant or dysfunctional.

Violence against women results in a variety of different mental health outcomes. For example, victims of crime in the US have been shown to have higher rates of major depression, suicidal thoughts and attempts, sexual dysfunction, alcohol and drug abuse problems, anxiety disorders, dissociative disorders, and personality disorders than non-victims (Acierno, Kilpatrick, & Resnick, 1999; Boudreaux, Kilpatrick, Resnick, Best, & Saunders, 1998; Kessler, Sonnega, Bromet, Hughes, & Nelson, 1995). A recent review of mental health problems among women with a history of intimate partner violence in the US (Golding, 1999a) reported that victims had a 3–5 times greater likelihood of depression, suicidality, posttraumatic stress disorder [PTSD], and substance abuse than non-victims.

A recent interview study examined cultural influences on PTSD among 475 women, men, and transgendered persons currently and recently prostituted in five countries, including South Africa, Thailand, Turkey, the United States of America, and Zambia (Farley, Baral, Kiremire, & Sezgin, 1998). Across countries, 73% reported physical assault while prostituting, 62% reported having been raped since entering prostitution, and 67% percent met criteria for a diagnosis of PTSD. The study suggested that the harm of prostitution is not culturally specific. Yet, consideration of cultural variation in the expression, configuration, and impairment associated with PTSD and other violence-related mental health symptoms is greatly needed.

Rates of PTSD in the general US population have been documented as higher among women than among men (Breslau, Chilcoat, Kessler, Peterson, & Lucia, 1999). In South Africa, PTSD has also been found to be higher among those who have experienced interpersonal violence (vs. other types of crime) (Seedat & Stein, 2000). Life threat is another important factor contributing to PTSD. Crime victims who experience physical injuries, as well as those who thought they might be killed or seriously injured during the crime, are much more likely to develop PTSD than crime victims without injuries or life threat (Freedy, Resnick, Kilpatrick, Dansky, & Tidwell, 1994; Kilpatrick et al., 1989; Resnick, Kilpatrick, Dansky, Saunders, & Best, 1993).

Many of those with PTSD do not recover spontaneously without appropriate treatment. Some crime victims have been found to have persistent PTSD for years (Freedy et al., 1994; Hanson, Kilpatrick, Falsetti, & Resnick, 1995). Finally, a prior history of trauma has been repeatedly shown to increase the negative effect of a subsequent traumatic event (McFarlane, 2000).

The relationship between exposure to traumatic events and mental health impact is a complex one. Studies have shown that the psychological abuse component of intimate partner violence—especially dominance and control—is as important as physical violence in terms of its link to posttraumatic stress symptoms (Follingstad, Rutledge, Berg, Hause, & Polek, 1990). These findings support the notion that understanding the context in which women experience violence is important for understanding its psychological impact and the environments in which women recover best.

It is important to consider a wide range of consequences related to the individual effects of violence against women. There are economic consequences when women cannot work because of injuries or being forbidden to leave the house. Social isolation can result when women are embarrassed or feel shame in revealing that they have been abused. Their ongoing perception of risk alters the way victimized women live their lives.

Relationships with children change, as women fear for a daughter's or son's future in a world filled with violence. Trust in others is often seriously damaged. The psychological effects of violence against women manifest themselves in defined psychological diagnoses, as well as in the day-to-day fabric of their lives.

PREVENTION AND INTERVENTION FOR VIOLENCE AGAINST WOMEN

This section will follow the inverted pyramid structure that illustrates levels of intervention from top to bottom, as societal/global, community-based, and individual/family interventions. To date there has been a relatively greater emphasis on community-based and legal solutions to the problem of violence against women in the world community, while empirically-supported and clinical solutions are less well-developed. The following are examined as societal/global efforts: legislation and UN declarations, international criminal courts and tribunals, and criminal justice systems. Community-based interventions include restorative justice efforts, community audits and fatality reviews, interventions by non-profit or non-governmental organizations, community-based education, and professional training and education. Individual and family efforts refer to information, support, and services delivered to individuals and families.

Societal/Global Interventions

Legislation and UN Declarations. The 1985 United Nations' *Declaration of Basic Principles of Justice for Victims of Crime and Abuse of Power* is a major international policy effort for improving response to crime victims, including violent crimes against women. The Declaration, the culmination of a long-standing concern of for victims of crime, has encouraged Member States to make changes in their criminal justice systems that would improve the treatment of crime victims. The UN Declaration outlines principles of justice for victims of crime that fall into four basic categories: (1) providing access to justice and fair treatment, (2) restitution, (3) compensation, and (4) assistance.

In 1996, the UN Commission of Crime Prevention and Criminal Justice adopted a resolution calling for the development of two manuals designed to assist in the implementation of the UN Declaration. The first manual was *Guide for Policymakers on the Implementation of the UN Declaration of Basic*

Principles of Justice for Victims of Crime and Abuse of Power (1999).[4] This guide
is organized to address briefly each of the 21 items in the UN Declaration.
It provides background information, discusses why the recommendation
was made, and gives examples of how Member States have successfully
implemented recommendations. The second manual, *Handbook on Justice
for Victims* (1999),[5] outlines basic steps for developing comprehensive victim assistance services for victims internationally. It too is comprehensive
in scope. Experts from almost 40 nations contributed to its development,
and the manuals clearly are mindful of cultural, economic, and other differences across Member States.

The *Platform for Action*[6] was adopted at the 1995 4th UN Conference on
Women, held in Beijing. Although it addresses far more than crimes against
women, a major focus is on human rights accorded to women, including
freedom from rape, assault, and other forms of violence.

The *Violence Against Women Act*,[7] passed in the US legislature in 1994
and reauthorized in 2000 for 5 years at $3.33 billion, is one example of legis-
lation focused on crimes against women. The legislation is broad and provides for strengthening law enforcement, victim services, services to limit
the effects of violence on children, strengthening education and training
on violence against women, and aid to battered immigrant women. Crime
victims' rights legislation provides for additional rights to crime victims,
such as 1) the right to be present during criminal proceedings, 2) the right
to be notified of the perpetrator's release from incarceration, 3) the right to
be heard, and 4) compensation for medical expenses and other costs from
the Crime Victim Fund.

Crime Victim Assistance—including assistance for victims of violence
against women—is sometimes organized at the international level. An
International Victim Compensation Program Directory[8] was developed based
on a survey of 174 countries. It has not yet been demonstrated whether
officially granting victims more rights has had a major impact on the way
they are treated by, or on their satisfaction with, the criminal justice system. Importantly, victims' rights are not always honored. One United States
study (Kilpatrick, Beatty, & Howley, 1998) ranked states on the basis of the
strength of legal protection they provided to crime victims, and conducted
interviews with crime victims from two strong-protection and two weak-
protection states. Victims of intimate partner assault were consistently less

[4] http://www.uncjin.org/Standards/policy.pdf
[5] http://www.uncjin.org/Standards/9857854.pdf
[6] http://usinfo.state.gov/topical/global/women/plat.htm
[7] http://www.ojp.usdoj.gov/vawo/laws/vawo2000/
[8] http://www.ojp.usdoj.gov/ovc/intdir/intdir.htm

likely to be satisfied with the criminal justice system than were those assaulted by a non-partner. However, this difference was most evident in weak-protection states.

In 2000, the US Congress passed the *Victims of Trafficking and Violence Protection Act*, the first comprehensive US legislation to combat trafficking. The new law provides for (1) protection for trafficking victims through establishing domestic and international policies, (2) prosecution of and enforcement against traffickers by establishing new crime categories, increasing penalties, making mandatory restitution, and other measures, and (3) prevention of trafficking (e.g., through economic opportunity).

Hague Convention. The *Hague Convention on Civil Aspects of International Child Abduction*, signed by 45 countries, assists in the recovery of children taken across national borders, often by one parent fleeing the other. The abduction or kidnapping of children is a frequent threat by an abusive partner who has the means to take a child to a different country where he may have dual citizenship or where other family members may aide in keeping the child from the mother. Indeed, domestic violence has been shown to be a major factor in a substantial number of parental abductions in the US (Plass, Finkelhor, & Hotaling, 1997). The *Hague Convention* assists parents in obtaining lawful custody of an abducted child. The success rates vary based on the extent to which the courts of each country implement the treaty, but the rate among countries who have signed the treaty, on average, exceeds the very low rate for countries that have not signed it.

Tribunals/International Criminal Court. The criminal tribunals and the new international criminal court offer the important mechanism of criminal prosecution for dealing with crimes committed during wartime. At its fifty-second session, the General Assembly convened the UN Diplomatic Conference of Plenipotentiaries on the Establishment of an International Criminal Court, subsequently held in Rome, Italy, "to finalize and adopt a convention on the establishment of an international criminal court." Discussions of an international criminal court had been ongoing since the Nuremberg trials, but spurred by the horrific events in the former Yugoslavia and Rwanda, the need for a permanent mechanism to prosecute such cases was recognized. The court was established July 1, 2002 and is located in The Hague. Kofi Annan, United Nations Secretary-General, stated in an address to the International Bar Association on June 12, 1997,[9]

---

[9] UN Press Release Press Release SG/SM/6257

In the prospect of an international criminal court lies the promise of universal justice. That is the simple and soaring hope of this vision. We are close to its realization. We will do our part to see it through till the end. We ask you . . . to do yours in our struggle to ensure that no ruler, no State, no junta and no army anywhere can abuse human rights with impunity. Only then will the innocents of distant wars and conflicts know that they, too, may sleep under the cover of justice; that they, too, have rights, and that those who violate those rights will be punished.

Article 5 of the *Statute of the International Tribune*, adopted in 1993 and amended in 2000, states that the International Criminal Court has the power to prosecute persons responsible for crimes—including murder, enslavement, deportation, imprisonment, torture, and rape—when they are committed in armed conflict, whether international or internal in character, and when they are directed against any civilian population. Thus, a future international criminal court has the opportunity to prosecute the crimes of violence targeted against women—especially rape—that occur during wars and other armed conflicts, and by so doing continue to bring awareness to violence against women as one of the major atrocities perpetrated in our global community.

Under recent Belgian legislation, introduced in 1993 and modified in 1999, the possibility of bringing war criminals to account was extended both in terms of citizenship and time. Using established legal concepts of universal jurisdiction, Belgian legislators have set aside limitations of time, citizenship, and diplomatic status; foreign heads of state can now be held accountable for their crimes, whenever they were committed.

Criminal Justice System.   The criminal justice system is a government-based infrastructure that exists in every nation and that is thought to have the capacity to make victims' crime-related outcomes better or worse, depending on how victims are treated. Many crimes—especially crimes against women—do not come to the attention of the authorities. However, when they do, the criminal justice system serves a gatekeeping function by referring to, and in some cases, paying for, a variety of non-legal interventions discussed below.

Specialized units have been used to address the specific needs of domestic violence and/or sexual assault cases. Women's Special Police Stations or Delegacias de Mulheres (DEAM) were developed in Brazil in 1985 and staffed by policewomen and social workers, offering both psychological counseling and legal aid (Aboim, 1997). In 1997, approximately 100 DEAMs existed. Specialized law enforcement and prosecution units have been developed in the US following the enactment of the *Violence Against Women Act* in 1994. These units provide specialized training to police officers and prosecutors of these crimes. They often work closely with victim advocates to assist victims of domestic violence and other types of crimes. Specialized prosecution units often approach crimes of violence against women more seriously than prosecutors without this specialized training. One illustration is the use of "evidence-based" prosecution methods, akin to those used in homicide cases, which rely less on victim cooperation and more on the taking of evidence at the scene of the crime. Successful prosecutions have been shown to be higher in specialized prosecution units.

The justice system also provides for civil remedies for victims of violence. Civil protection orders, referred to as "interdicts" in South Africa, constitute an order by a court for a person alleged to have engaged in violent behavior to restrain from engaging in violence or abuse and to stay away from the victim. In some countries, these orders can be obtained without representation by a lawyer, making them relatively accessible to a large number of people. Additional provisions are often included in these orders. In the case of civil protection orders issued to victims of family violence, these remedies can include an order to pay financial support to the victim and/or her children; to vacate the joint residence; to refrain from contacting the victim by phone, mail, through third parties, or other means; to turn in a gun to authorities; or to attend counseling. Specific arrangements concerning temporary custody and visitation of children can also be ordered. Violating a protection order is defined as a criminal offense in many jurisdictions, even if the act on which the violation is based (e.g., contacting the victim) is itself not a criminal violation. For example, the passage in 1993 of the *Prevention of Family Violence Act* in South Africa requires police to arrest the abuser if he continues his abuse, even though there is no specific law against domestic violence (Levi, 1997b).

Fewer than one in five victims of physical assault in a US national survey (Tjaden & Thoennes, 2000), however, reported using civil protection orders, and when they did, the orders were often violated by the perpetrator. Interestingly, a temporary order (typically lasting 14 days) was as effective as a permanent order (typically lasting 1 year) in terms of deterrence of abuse, including physical violence, threats, or property damage (Harrell & Smith, 1996). Training of law enforcement officers, judges, and other court personnel is needed to maximize the effectiveness of civil protection orders, especially in terms of education concerning the dynamics of family violence and the types of remedies that are most helpful to victims and their children.

A domestic violence victim in the US obtained a protective order against her abusive husband. However, the police waited several days before serving him with the order. During this time, the victim made a final desperate call to the police, saying that her

husband had threatened to come to her house and kill her. Although the police rushed
to the scene, she lay dead on the stairs when they arrived, next to his dead body, both
of them riddled with bullet holes.

Although remedies may be available to protect women from violence, they are of no value unless they are properly implemented and monitored. Violations must be addressed swiftly. Educating judges and other justice system personnel is critically important for improving the criminal justice response to crime victimization. One study of 109 judges in the district courts, high courts, and Supreme Court of India (Sakshi, 1996, 1998 [2nd printing]) concluded that deeply held attitudes and beliefs about women or gender bias in the legal system demanded attention. The study identified the need to educate judges to understand gender inequality in situations of violence and how that influences their personal perceptions of men and women. The authors concluded that the nature of justice to which victims of violence have access depends on such education and training.

Indeed, the response of the justice system to victims of sexual assault and domestic violence is often inadequate across the range of functions: "conviction rates for partner violence and rape by known acquaintances are minuscule; mandatory arrest, protection orders, and diversion programs inadequately deter rebattering; few losses are compensated; and the adversarial justice process is retraumatizing, exacerbating survivor self-blame" (Koss, 2000, p. 1332).

Most cases involving rape or domestic violence do not proceed to prosecution. For example, one study of dowry deaths in India found the overall conviction rate to be 11% across the four sections of the criminal code under which dowry deaths are most commonly registered (Vindhya, 2000). Furthermore, the process of criminal prosecution can revictimize the victim by repeated demands to tell the story of what happened, the necessity of testifying about the events in a public courtroom and in front of the perpetrator, and being subject to cross-examination that may be demeaning and accusatory. Victim advocates who are part of the prosecutor's office—when available—offer support to the victim during this difficult process. However, the fear of retaliation by the perpetrator or other family members, a sense of futility that criminal justice sanctions will actually help the victim, and concerns that conviction may threaten her economic security and ability to raise her children, are reasons that these crimes of violence against women are reported so infrequently.

Court watches, or criminal justice system monitoring projects, involve advocates explicitly observing the actions of judges and lawyers within the court system. One example is the International Centre for Human Rights and Democratic Development, which organized a coalition of women's groups in Rwanda to advocate for prosecution, to monitor prosecution proceedings, and to support women involved in gender-based violent crimes (Brunet & Helal, 1998).

Batterer and sex-offender treatment programs are often part of a coordinated community response involving the justice system and mental health or other educational professionals. Although their efficacy is still being established—especially for culturally diverse groups of perpetrators—the results of a large-scale multi-site study of 800 batterers from four treatment programs across the US found that overall, nearly two-thirds of male batterers did not reassault their partners during the first year after being ordered to treatment. However, nearly half (42%-47%) had reassaulted their initial or new partners after 30 months, and most of the assaults took place within the first 6-month period (Gondolf, 2000).

Community-Focused Interventions

"A hundred years ago among the Tlingit people living in what is now southeast Alaska, there was a belief that one should not beat one's wife. If ever a husband deviated from this norm and beat his wife, his clan was required to pay her clan in material goods. The whole community came together for a potlatch to exchange the goods. The whole community knew why they were there. Wife-beating was expensive; wife-beating was shameful. There was very little wife-beating among the Tlingit people a hundred years ago" (Fortune, 1986, p. 236).

Restorative Justice. An indigenous system of restorative justice and conflict resolution involves all parties acknowledging the emotional and material loss to a victim. Offenders and their families are held responsible for a victim's injuries, pay restitution, and apologize not only to the victim but also to her/his family and to the community. These practices are common in Africa and Asia. It has been argued that modern criminal justice systems, in Nigeria for example, do not provide the same effective response to crime victims as older, indigenous systems of restorative justice and conflict resolution (Elechi, 1999). Research on restorative justice processes for victims in the villages of Vanimo, Papua New Guinea noted the capacity of victims for adaptation and highlighted the continued resilience of custom in resolving grievances. Western criminal justice views crime as primarily an offense against the state, with the crime victim serving as a secondary focus. In contrast, restorative justice views the crime victim as the primary victim and the state as a secondary victim (Umbreit, 1994).

Western countries have begun to adopt restorative justice programs from developing countries. The major focus of restorative justice is to hold offenders accountable by making them repay victims for their actions

(Kilpatrick & Koss, 2001; Zehr, 1990). A common type of restorative justice in the US is a victim-offender reconciliation program. Such programs provide victims with the chance to face their offender. The victim explains how the crime has affected her life. The offender works out an agreement with the victim as to how he or she will pay back the victim for her crime-related losses. Trained professionals mediate this reconciliation process. Satisfaction with these methods comes from having a chance to learn from the perpetrator why the crime was committed, receiving restitution, and hearing the perpetrator apologize.

Using four separate victim-offender mediation programs in the United States, Umbreit (Umbreit, 1994) compared victims and offenders in three conditions: 1) a mediation condition, 2) a comparison condition in which subjects were referred but did not participate, and 3) a comparison condition in which subjects were not referred but were matched on key variables. In this study, most victims and offenders who participated in mediation expressed satisfaction; victims expressed less fear of being revictimized by the offender than before the program. These findings suggest that these mediation programs produce promising results that warrant additional research. However, victim-offender mediation programs are not without problems, and the extent to which they are applicable to serious violent crime, especially crimes involving persons in ongoing relationships such as domestic violence, has been seriously questioned (Stubbs, 2002).

It is unclear whether women who are victimized by violent crimes would be more interested in mediation programs than in seeing offenders receiving substantial punishment or getting treatment. There are serious concerns and significant challenges to ensuring that violence is effectively confronted and women are protected (Zellerer, 1999). Further, emphasis on apology (and forgiveness) in some approaches to restorative justice poses an important concern for domestic violence cases. Domestic violence offenders often use apology as a means of manipulation (Stubbs, 2002), enticing their victims into believing they are repentant and have changed. In this sense, a restorative justice process could re-enact the same controlling dynamic commonly found in abusive relationships—this time with the imprimatur of the criminal justice system. Restorative justice must be situated within a more general meaning of justice that does not encourage "social structural violence"—violence done to people through the exercise of power, and hierarchical social arrangements that support this maintenance of power (Gil, 1996; Sullivan & Tifft, 1998).

Services of Non-Profit/Non-Governmental (NGO) Organizations.
There are many non-profit or non-governmental organizations that focus on the prevention of violence against women. International women's

organizations, some of which have been in existence for well over a century, have been central in bringing attention to violence against women to the international consciousness (Harris, 1996). The Instituto Méxicano de Investigación de Familia y Población (Mexican Institute for Research on Family and Population), in collaboration with the Center for Health and Gender Equity, developed a 12-session pilot workshop aimed to develop a cadre of local women who could help victims of violence in the community (Trainor & Mihorean, 2001). The workshop was followed by a six-month community awareness and education campaign, where buttons and posters were distributed in shops, on lampposts, and in local institutions. Lessons learned included the importance of (1) formative research to identify community needs; (2) shared control with community organizers, governmental, and nongovernmental organizations; (3) providing support and training to community leaders; (4) educating all members of the community, including women, men, and children; and (5) building on positive attitudes.

Community organizing is the underlying mechanism used by advocates working against domestic violence in Seely Lake, Montana, US, to build the foundation for community-based efforts to respond more effectively to domestic violence. Rather than bring services into this small rural community from larger cities, organizers worked with local community members to help define their needs and to develop resources for responding to them. For example, local advocates are contacted immediately when local law enforcement officers receive a call involving domestic violence. The program builds on the foundation of a closely-knit local community, whose members are known to each other and for whom the investment is in changing—rather than punishing—offenders. The community organizers helped the community articulate its support for bystander involvement, rather than detachment, in situations involving domestic violence.

Rape crisis centers and battered women's shelters provide services to rape victims, battered women, and their children. IFSHA, an NGO in New Delhi, provides healing of violence and trauma through meditation. Battered women's shelters provide housing, food, clothing, legal advocacy, safety planning, and counseling for domestic violence victims and their children. Rape crisis centers offer legal advocacy and counseling. While both rape crisis centers and battered women's shelters had their origins as grassroots organizations, increased attention in the past decade has led to more federal support for such services in the US and elsewhere.

Family Violence in Canada reports that 63% of shelters provide culturally sensitive services to Aboriginal women. Culturally sensitive services include recognition of traditional healing methods, use of spiritual elders and teachers, access to Aboriginal interpreters and Aboriginal materials, and understanding of Aboriginal cultural beliefs and norms. A network of culturally specific domestic violence services for South Asian women are developing in Canada, India, the United States, and the United Kingdom.[10]

Community Audits and Fatality Reviews. Institutional ethnography is the basis for conducting a "community or safety audit," a systematic investigation of one or more points of institutional action on a particular case or series of cases. An audit can be focused on a single institutional step (e.g., a pre-sentence investigation report), or it can investigate a series of steps in a process (e.g., a call to police, arrest, or arraignment). The audit can be designed specifically for certain tasks: for example, to uncover the system's bias for or against specific groups of people (e.g., Native Americans, migrant workers, those in lower socioeconomic classes). The safety audit is not intended as a performance review of specific individuals.

The *Domestic Violence Safety and Accountability Audit*, developed by Ellen Pence of the Domestic Abuse Intervention Project of Minnesota,[11] has been an important tool for identifying and tracking the process for each component of the criminal justice system in the US in order to identify strengths, gaps, and failures in protecting victims and holding perpetrators accountable. Mending the Sacred Hoop, the Native American arm of Minnesota Program Development, Inc., is currently forming a collaboration to conduct a community-controlled assessment of criminal and civil justice intervention with Native American women who are battered.

Domestic Violence Fatality Reviews are used to identify factors associated with the failure to prevent a domestic homicide. A fatality review team analyzes specific deaths to identify where the community and its institutional systems failed to prevent the death, toward the goal of preventing future fatalities. Domestic violence death reviews refer to a "deliberative process for identification of deaths, both homicide and suicide, caused by domestic violence, for examination of the systemic interventions into known incidents of domestic violence occurring in the family of the deceased prior to the death, for consideration of altered systemic response to avert future domestic violence deaths, or for development of recommendations for coordinated community prevention and intervention initiatives to eradicate domestic violence" (Hart, 1995). See Violence Against Women Online resources for an online summary of US national developments.[12]

---

[10] http://www.umiacs.umd.edu/users/sawweb/sawnet/violence.html
[11] http://www.praxisinternational.org
[12] http://www.vaw.umn.edu/FinalDocuments/fatality.htm

Community-Based Education. School-based prevention programs target children at an early age, typically for violence prevention aimed at reducing date rape and domestic violence among dating couples. For example, Women's Aid in Ireland maintains a student program called Breaking the Silence on Violence, which combines education about violence with art and community work in secondary schools. The program is intended to provide the opportunity for both male and female students to challenge existing and perceived notions about violence against women.

Public education is another common prevention effort used widely across the world. For example, Women's Aid in Ireland uses "forum theatre" to engage the public in preventing violence against women (Levi, 1997a). Forum theatre begins by performing a piece of drama devised by people who share a common experience (i.e., assault) that tells a story and identifies people and organizations that are oppressive, and those that are supportive. The piece is played for a short time and then a facilitator stops to explain that the piece will be played again, and this time anyone in the audience can suggest changes in the story. The characters then improvise based on the direction from the audience. A discussion of the realities of living through a victimization experience—or ongoing violence—and obstacles for responding to it are discussed with the audience.

Professional Training and Education. Educating religious leaders is essential, since the religious community plays a key role in both prevention of and intervention to end violence, especially violence in the family. The Center for Prevention of Sexual and Domestic Violence is an interreligious organization working in the US and Canada that focuses on training clergy on issues of misconduct and responding to abuse victims in their congregations. The Center's Seminary Project is designed to work with seminary faculty and administration to develop, implement, and evaluate a comprehensive curriculum that promotes ethical conduct and relational integrity in all areas of seminary and community life, preparing participating seminary teams to implement the curriculum in their own communities.

Educational efforts are ongoing in most other domains of professional practice. Communities Against Violence Network[13]—is an online international network of anti-violence advocates and experts. The *Global Violence Prevention* (funded through the University of Minnesota) is an interactive web site designed to teach professionals about violence prevention and intervention.[14] The DART Center for Journalism and Trauma, housed at the University of Washington in the US, is a resource center for

[13] http://www.cavnet2.org/
[14] http://www.globalvp.umn.edu/

students, educators, journalists, and news organizations interested in the intersection of journalism and trauma issues, such as domestic violence and rape.

Individual/Family-Focused Intervention

Interventions should be consistent with social or cultural customs. The social, economic, and political context influences the nature, impact, and indeed even the feasibility, of community and institutional responses to crime victimization. Thus, prevention and intervention must be relevant to the victim in her life context. Prevention and intervention are particularly challenging in the context of intimate and domestic victimization. Women who are victimized by intimate partner violence often do not seek help. These and similar findings, along with anecdotal reports, signal the need to identify and offer the types of services that crime victims need in settings where they live and work. Fewer than 2% of women in the household survey of women in India (International Center for Research on Women, 2000) sought help from a women's organization, police, health care setting, mental health center, or local official.

Service-delivery mechanisms located in the communities where crime victims live and work provide important access to information, support, and services. For example, the Coalition to Abolish Slavery & Trafficking, a coalition of non-profit service providers, grassroots advocacy groups, and activities in the US, assists persons from Asia, Latin America, and Central Europe who were trafficked for the purpose of forced labor and slavery-like practices. Services include (1) referral to basic human services through a network of ethnic community service providers, (2) assistance with immigration and other legal issues, (3) training for government agencies, law enforcement, and immigration agencies, (4) media outreach and public education, (5) advocacy for public policy change, and (6) research and documentation.

Some violence victims have special needs, such as physical disabilities. However, these services require additional education and training of service providers. A training guide and resource kit, *Building Bridges Between Domestic Violence & Sexual Assault Agencies, Disability Service Agencies, People with Disabilities, Families and Caregivers*,[15] provides such information.

An innovative early intervention for rape victims shows promising preliminary results (Resnick, Acierno, Holmes, Kilpatrick, & Jager, 1999). This videotaped intervention is designed to be used with rape victims

---

[15] http://www.austin-safeplace.org/training/default.htm

during forensic examinations conducted a few hours after the rape, typically in an emergency department setting. The video presents the forensic medical exam and why it is being conducted, common post-rape mental health problems, and constructive ways to address such problems if they occur. Providing this information seems to help reduce acute distress and the risk of long-term mental health problems such as PTSD. This approach has potential to be modified for delivery in other settings.

Several cognitive-behavioral treatments have been found to be effective for victimization-related mental health problems. A description of these treatment procedures is found in Chapter 4 and elsewhere (Meadows & Foa, 1999). In particular, the efficacy of cognitive behavioral treatment is well-established, and it tends to persist over time after the completion of treatment, with limited side effects. While these interventions have been examined with rape victims, there is less evidence available for domestic violence victims. An advantage of these treatments is that some of them may be delivered by crime victim advocates with no formal mental health training. For example, the Stress Inoculation Training package (Veronen, Kilpatrick, & Resnick, 1979) was conducted by rape crisis counselors who had received special training and supervision.

RECOMMENDATIONS

Societal/Global

- Adopt recommendations for criminal justice system reform from the United Nations' Declaration of Basic Principles of Justice for Victims of Crime and Abuse of Power, including elaborations in the *Handbook on Justice for Victims* and the *Guide for Policymakers*. Categories include access to justice and fair treatment, restitution to victims, compensation for losses, and material, medical, psychological, and social assistance.
- Strengthen economic opportunities for countries, communities, families, and individuals in order to reduce the oppression of poverty and economic dependence, structural forces that compound the impact of individual violence.
- Develop international standards of victim assistance and victim rights.
- Develop networks to provide technical assistance and publicize these.
- Support national and international development of materials for widespread public distribution that provide information about violence, its consequences, and what victims, families, and their communities can do to prevent crime-related mental health problems.

- Strengthen international laws to adequately address trafficking, child abduction, and other offenses involving transport across borders.
- Pass legislative reform to ensure that governments pay for and/or provide mental health intervention for crime victims throughout the criminal justice process and beyond.
- Develop restorative justice approaches for some forms of violence against women, particularly those involving widespread, government-sanctioned violence and other human rights abuses, and crimes whose victims wish to hold their perpetrators accountable through direct confrontation.
- Aim to transform the social structures of our global societies, which foster and maintain violence and abuses of power against women, through efforts to change social values, policies, and institutions as well as individual consciousness.

Community/Neighborhood

- Increase culturally sensitive training for professionals within social institutions—such as government, health care, law enforcement, and the courts—so that these professionals will better understand the context in which violence against women occurs.
- Increase public awareness of all forms of violence against women, in a manner that is free of racial and ethnic bias.
- Develop prevention efforts through policy, legal reform, community intervention, and clinical practice.
- Develop links between the mental health community and crime victims' compensation and victims' assistance programs, as well as criminal and juvenile justice agencies, to ensure that victims of violence against women have access to adequate counseling or mental health treatment at each stage of the justice process, from the time the crime occurs through incarceration, pardon, parole, and appeal.
- Establish multidisciplinary teams, including victim service providers, primary care providers, law enforcement officers, emergency medical responders, mental health professionals, corrections officers, and clergy, to respond to violence against women.
- Train teachers at all levels to identify and provide interventions with children who witness violence in their homes.
- Adapt routine community activities to incorporate targeted prevention efforts with children, dating and newly married couples, pregnant women, and other groups with special needs.
- Support social activism to strengthen the safety net provided by communities, led by former victims of violence.

- Encourage culturally appropriate community rituals that promote healing and that hold perpetrators accountable.
- Teach appropriate and safe strategies for responding to community members who observe the victimization of women in their homes, in their places of worship, and on the street.

Individual/Family

- Provide economic and educational opportunities for women to reduce their dependence on family members and others who use violence against them and their children.
- Develop interventions for victims, perpetrators, and family members that are sensitive to, and based on, cultural and ethnic differences.
- Develop interventions and counseling services for victims with multiple mental health problems. Special attention should be given to individuals suffering from repeated victimization and individuals with limited access to financial and social services or health care resources.
- Develop volunteer programs to work with high-risk families to provide support and information, to decrease isolation, and to increase access to resources as a means of violence prevention.
- Conduct research to determine what modifications are necessary for the successful application of existing services for victims and perpetrators in a variety of cultural settings.
- Develop low-cost and culturally-sensitive preventive measures that can be implemented with large numbers of people.

REFERENCES

Aboim, M.L. (1997). Brazil: Domestic violence and the women's movement. In L. Marin, H. Zia, & E. Soler (Eds.), *Ending domestic violence: Report from the global frontlines* (pp. 7–13). San Francisco: The Family Violence Prevention Fund.

Acierno, R., Resnick, H.S., & Kilpatrick, D.G. (1997). Health impact of interpersonal violence: I. Prevalence rates, case identification, and risk factors for sexual assault, physical assault, and domestic violence in men and women. *Behavioral Medicine, 23,* 53–64.

Acierno, R.E., Kilpatrick, D.G., & Resnick, H.S. (1999). Posttraumatic stress disorder: Prevalence, risk factors and comorbidity relative to criminal victimization. In P.A. Saigh & D. Bremner (Eds.), *Posttraumatic stress disorder: A comprehensive approach to research and treatment.* New York: Allyn & Bacon.

Bachman, R., & Saltzman, L.E. (1995). *Violence against women: Estimates from the redesigned survey* (NCJ 154348). Washington, D.C.: Bureau of Justice Statistics, US Department of Justice.

Belknap, J. (1995). Law enforcement officers' attitudes about the appropriate responses to woman battering. *International Review of Victimology, 4*, 47–62.

Boudreaux, E., Kilpatrick, D.G., Resnick, H.S., Best, C.L., & Saunders, B.E. (1998). Criminal victimization, posttraumatic stress disorder, and comorbid psychopathology among a community sample of women. *Journal of Traumatic Stress, 11*, 665–678.

Breslau, N., Chilcoat, H.D., Kessler, R.C., Peterson, E.L., & Lucia, V.C. (1999). Vulnerability to assaultive violence: Further specification of the sex difference in post-traumatic stress disorder. *Psychological Medicine, 29*, 813–821.

Browne, A., & Finklehor, D. (1986). Impact of child sexual abuse: A review of the research. *Psychological Bulletin, 99*, 66–77.

Brunet, A., & Helal, I.S. (1998). Monitoring the prosecution of gender-related crimes in Rwanda: A brief field report. *Peace & Conflict: Journal of Peace Psychology, 4*, 393–397.

Elechi, O.O. (1999). Victims under restorative justice systems: The afikpo (Ehugbo) Nigeria model. *International Review of Victimology, 6*, 359–375.

Farley, M., Baral, I., Kiremire, M., & Sezgin, U. (1998). Prostitution in five countries: Violence and post-traumatic stress disorder. *Feminism and Psychology, 8*(4), 405–426.

Farley, M., & Kelly, V. (2000). Prostitution: A critical review of the medical and social sciences literature. *Women and Criminal Justice, 11*(4), 29–64.

Follingstad, D.R., Rutledge, L.L., Berg, B.J., Hause, E.S., & Polek, D.S. (1990). The role of emotional abuse in physically abusive relationships. *Journal of Family Violence, 5*, 107–120.

Fortune, M.M. (1986). Justice-making in the aftermath of woman-battering. In D.J. Sonkin (Ed.), *Domestic violence on trial: Psychological and legal dimensions of family violence* (pp. 237–248). New York: Springer Publishing Company.

Freedy, J.R., Resnick, H.S., Kilpatrick, D.G., Dansky, B.S., & Tidwell, R.P. (1994). The psychological adjustment of recent crime victims in the criminal justice system. *Journal of Interpersonal Violence, 9*, 450–468.

Gil, D.G. (1996). Preventing violence in a structurally violent society: Mission impossible. *American Psychologist, 66*, 77–84.

Golding, J.M. (1999a). Intimate partner violence as a risk factor for mental disorders: A meta-analysis. *Journal of Family Violence, 14*, 99–132.

Golding, J.M. (1999b). Sexual-assault history and long-term physical health problems: Evidence from clinical and population epidemiology. *Current Directions in Psychological Science, 8*, 191–194.

Gondolf, E.W. (2000). A 30-month follow-up of court-referred batterers in four cities. *International Journal of Offender Therapy and Comparative Criminology, 44*, 111–128.

Haj-Yahia, M.M. (1999). Wife abuse and its psychological consequences as revealed by the first Palestinian National Survey on Violence Against Women. *Journal of Family Psychology, 13*, 642–662.

Hanson, R. Kilpatrick, D.G., Falsetti, S.A, & Resnick, H.S. (1995). Violent crime and mental health. In J.R. Freedy & S.E. Hobfoll (Eds.), *Traumatic stress: From theory to practice* (pp. 129-161). New York: Plenum Press.

Harrell, A., & Smith, B.E. (1996). Effects of restraining orders on domestic violence victims. In E.S. Buzawa & C.G. Buzawa (Eds.), *Do arrests and restraining orders work?* (pp. 214–242). Thousand Oaks, CA: Sage Publications.

Harris, R.W. (1996). Traumatized women: Dealing with violence against women. In Y. Danieli, N.S. Rodley, & L. Weisaeth (Eds.), *International responses to traumatic stress: Humanitarian, human rights, justice, peace and development contributions, collaborative actions and future initiatives* (pp. 367–382). Amityville, NY: Baywood Publishing Co., Inc.

Hart, B. (1995, February). *Domestic violence death review.* Legal Committee, National Council of Juvenile and Family Court Judges.

International Center for Research on Women (2000). *Domestic violence in India: A summary report of a multi-site household survey.* Washington, D.C.: USAID/India.

Kaplan, T. (1998). Marital conflict by proxy after father kills mother: The family therapist as an expert witness in court. *Family Process, 37,* 479–494.

Kessler, R.C., Sonnega, A., Bromet, E., Hughes, M., & Nelson, C.B. (1995). Posttraumatic stress disorder in the National Comorbidity Survey. *Archives of General Psychiatry, 52,* 1048–1060.

Kilpatrick, D.G., Beatty, D., & Howley, S.S. (1998). *The rights of crime victims—Does legal protection make a difference?* US Government Printing Office.

Kilpatrick, D.G., & Koss, M.P. (2001). Homicide and physical assault. In E. Gerrity, T.M. Keane, & F. Tuma (Eds.), *Mental health consequences of torture.* (pp. 195–209). New York: Plenum.

Kilpatrick, D.G., Resnick, H.S., & Acierno, R. (1997). Health impact of interpersonal violence. III: Policy implications. *Behavioral Medicine, 23,* 79–94.

Kilpatrick, D.G., Saunders, B.E., Amick-McMullan, A., Best, C.L., Veronen, L.J., & Resnick, H.S. (1989). Victim and crime factors associated with the development of crime-related post-traumatic stress disorder. *Behavior Therapy, 20,* 199–214.

Kitayama, S., & Markus, H.R. (1994). *Emotion and culture.* Washington, D.C.: American Psychological Association.

Koss, M.P. (2000). Blame, shame, and community: Justice responses to violence against women. *American Psychologist, 55*(11), 1332–1343.

Krug, E. (1999). *Injury: A leading cause of the global burden of disease.* Geneva, Switzerland: Violence and Injury Prevention, Department for Disability/Injury Prevention and Rehabilitation, Social Change and Mental Health Cluster, World Health Organization.

Laurence, L., & Spalter-Roth, R. (1996). *Measuring the costs of domestic violence against women and the cost-effectiveness of interventions: An initial assessment and proposals for further research.* Washington, DC: Institute for Women's Policy Research.

Levi, R.S. (1997a). Ireland: We must say it again. In L. Marin, H. Zia, & E. Soler (Eds.), *Ending domestic violence: Report from the global frontlines* (pp. 38–43). San Francisco: The Family Violence Prevention Fund.

Levi, R.S. (1997b). South Africa: Peace starts at home. In L. Marin, H. Zia, & E. Soler (Eds.), *Ending domestic violence: Report from the global frontlines* (pp. 50–55). San Francisco: The Family Violence Prevention Fund.

McFarlane, A.C. (2000). Posttraumatic stress disorder: A model of the longitudinal course and the role of the risk factors. *Journal of Clinical Psychiatry, 61,* 15–23.

Meadows, E.A., & Foa, E.B. (1999). Cognitive-behavioral treatment of traumatized adults. In P.A. Saigh & J.D. Bremner (Eds.), *Posttraumatic stress disorder: A comprehensive textbook.* Needham Heights, MA: Allyn and Bacon.

Mitchell, K.J., & Finkelhor, D. (2001). Risk of crime victimization among youth exposed to domestic violence. *Journal of Interpersonal Violence, 16,* 944–964.

Pence, E. (1997). *Safety for battered women in a textually mediated legal system.* Doctoral dissertation, University of Toronto.

Plass, P.S., Finkelhor, D., & Hotaling, G.T. (1997). Risk factors for family abduction: Demographic and family interaction characteristics. *Journal of Family Violence, 12,* 333–348.

Rennison, C.M., & Welchans, S. (2000). *Intimate partner violence.* Washington, D.C.: US Department of Justice, Office of Justice Programs.

Resnick, H., Acierno, R., Holmes, M., Kilpatrick, D.G., & Jager, N. (1999). Prevention of post-rape psychopathology: Preliminary findings of a controlled acute rape treatment study. *Journal of Anxiety Disorders, 13*, 359–370.

Resnick, H.S., Acierno, R., & Kilpatrick, D.G. (1997). Health impact of interpersonal violence: II. Medical and mental health outcomes. *Behavioral Medicine, 23*, 65–78.

Resnick, H.S., Kilpatrick, D.G., Dansky, B.S., Saunders, B.E., & Best, C.L. (1993). Prevalence of civilian trauma and PTSD in a representative national sample of women. *Journal of Consulting and Clinical Psychology, 61*, 984–991.

Root, M. (1992). Women of color and traumatic stress in "domestic captivity": Gender and race as disempowering statuses. In A.J. Marsella, M.J. Friedman, E.T. Gerrity, & R.M. Scurfield (Eds.), *Ethnocultural aspects of posttraumatic stress disorder: Issues, research, and clinical applications*. Washington, D.C.: American Psychological Association.

Sakshi. (1996, 1998 (2nd printing)). *Gender and judges: A judicial point of view*. New Delhi: Sakshi.

Seedat, S., & Stein, D.J. (2000). Trauma and post-traumatic stress disorder in women: A review. *International Clinical Psychopharmacology, 15*, S25–S33.

Simons, R.L., & Johnson, C. (1998). An examination of competing explanations for the intergenerational transmission of domestic violence. In Y. Danieli (Ed.), *International handbook of multigenerational legacies of trauma*. New York: Plenum Press.

Stein, M.B., & Barrett-Connor, E. (2000). Sexual assault and physical health: Findings from a population-based study of older adults. *Psychosomatic Medicine, 62*, 838–843.

Stubbs, J. (2002). Domestic violence and women's safety: Feminist challenges to restorative justice. In H. Strang & J. Braithwaite (Eds.), *Restorative justice and family violence: New ideas and learning from the past*. Cambridge: Cambridge University Press.

Sullivan, D., & Tifft, L. (1998). The transformative and economic dimensions of restorative justice. *Humanity & Society, 22*, 38–54.

Thompson, M.P., Saltzman, L.E., & Johnson, H. (2001). Risk factors for physical injury among women assaulted by current or former spouses. *Violence Against Women, 7*, 886–899.

Tjaden, P., & Thoennes, N. (2000). *Extent, nature, and consequence of intimate partner violence* (NCJ 181867). Washington, D.C.: National Institute of Justice and the Centers for Disease Control and Prevention.

Toro, M.S. (1999). Recognizing and realizing women's human rights. Part I: Sexual politics and human rights. In Y. Danieli, E. Stamatopoulou, & C.J. Dias (Eds.), *The Universal Declaration of Human Rights: Fifty years and beyond* (pp. 115–120). Amityville, NY: Baywood Publishing Company, Inc.

Trainor, C., & Mihorean, K. (Eds.). (2001). *Family violence in Canada: A statistical profile 2001*. Minister of Industry, Ottawa, Canada. (Catalogue No. 85-224-XIE).

Umbreit, M. (1994). *Victim meets offender: The impact of restorative justice and mediation*. Monery, NY: Criminal Justice Press.

United Nations (1994). *Declaration on the Elimination of Violence against Women*. New York.

United Nations (1999). *Global Report on Crime and Justice*. New York: Oxford University Press.

USAID Office of Women in Development (1999, February). Women as chattel: The emerging Global market in trafficking. *Gender Matters Quarterly, 1*.

Veronen, L.J., Kilpatrick, D.G., & Resnick, P.A. (1979). Treatment of fear and anxiety in rape victims: Implications for the criminal justice system. In W.H. Parsonage (Ed.), *Perspectives on victimology* (pp. 148–159). Beverly Hills, CA: Sage, 1979.

Vindhya, U. (2000). "Dowry deaths" in Andhra Pradesh, India: Response of the criminal justice system. *Violence Against Women, 6*, 1085–1108.

Yoon Shim, K. (1999). Lessening the suffering after wartime sexual slavery. In Y. Danieli, E. Stamatopoulou, & C.J. Dias (Eds.), *The Universal Declaration of Human Rights: Fifty Years and Beyond* (pp. 127–128). Amityville, NY: Baywood Publishing Company, Inc.

Yoshioka, M., & Sorenson, S.B. (1994). Physical, sexual, and emotional abuse by male intimates: Experiences of women in Japan. *Violence and Victims, 9,* 63–77.

Zehr, H. (1990). *Changing lenses: A new focus for crime and justice.* Scottsdale, PA: Herald.

Zellerer, E. (1999). Restorative justice in indigenous communities: Critical issues in confronting violence against women. *International Review of Victimology, 6,* 345–358.

Chapter 9

Survivors of Mass Violence and Torture

Stuart Turner, Sahika Yuksel, and Derrick Silove

The chapter focuses on adult survivors of torture and mass violence living within their own communities—as distinct from refugees who have moved to other countries or internally displaced people (IDP) who are living in another part of the same country (see Chapter 11). With psychosocial aid in mind, we emphasize the psychological meaning of events, in addition to legal definitions, and on the ways that communities, families, and individuals may respond to those events. A woman who has been raped has survived an act of violent domination, whether it was a soldier or a stranger who was responsible, and there will be many similarities in the meaning of these events and in their effects. The differences may be less in the act of violation itself than in the opportunity to seek aid (how easy is it to report a rape by a soldier or a paramilitary, and to whom should it be reported?) and in the meaning conveyed by the act (e.g., is it an attack on a woman, or an attack on women of a specific ethnic group?).

Torture encourages the development of what Barudy (1989) has described as a "repressive ecology"—a state of generalized insecurity, terror, lack of confidence, and rupture of social relations. Various forms of violence may be seen as having similar repressive purposes. For example, ethnic violence or ethnic cleansing is one way of influencing a community, and selective torture of individuals is another. For this reason, a broad definition of torture is to be preferred. Terms such as "low-grade warfare" or "mass violence" are used to refer to these broader attacks on communities, and they emphasize the social rather than the individual dimension. Informed by this understanding, torture (which may be seen as an extreme form of repressive violence) needs to be placed in a social as well as an individual context.

Torture has been defined in various ways. Importantly, its application and meaning have varied in different times. In Roman and medieval times, for example, it was incorporated into a judicial process. A confession was regarded as the "Queen of Proofs." The focus of the legal process, therefore, was directed at obtaining confessions in people suspected on other grounds as guilty. Torture was then seen as a valid means of obtaining a confession. The strength of suspicion was considered by a court, which then had the power to order torture. Methods of torture were sometimes categorized in degrees according to the strength of this suspicion. The use of the phrase "third degree" is a remnant from this use of torture. This was the most severe of the degrees of torture that a court could authorize. Unfortunately for those involved, a confession obtained under torture and then retracted would often be considered a reason for suspicion, and the court could then authorize further torture! In modern times, torture has a different meaning/goal (repression) and a different method of practice (i.e., covert activity). The definition in the United Nations Convention against Torture (1984) clarifies this point.

> **For the purposes of this Convention, the term "torture" means any act by which severe pain or suffering, whether physical or mental, is intentionally inflicted on a person for such purposes as obtaining from him or a third person information or a confession, punishing him for an act he or a third person has committed or is suspected of having committed, or intimidating or coercing him or a third person, or for any reason based on discrimination of any kind, when such pain or suffering is inflicted by or at the instigation of or with the consent or acquiescence of a public official or other person acting in an official capacity. It does not include pain or suffering arising from, inherent in or incidental to lawful sanctions (Article 1.1, *Convention against Torture and Other Cruel, Inhuman or Degrading Treatment or Punishment*, Resolution 39/46 adopted by the General Assembly on 10 December 1984, entering into force on 26 June 1987).**

This definition points to its use in, for example, obtaining information (coercively), punishment, and intimidation. These are repressive actions—whatever the context.

In terms of its psychological/contextual meaning, this emphasizes that torture involves:

- severe pain or suffering
- a public official or other person acting in an official capacity
- a purpose essentially to do with achieving psychological (repressive or coercive) change

- in individuals (e.g., intimidation or confession)
- in communities (discrimination).

Torture is intentional and systematic. It takes place covertly, in a world where rules are arbitrary and where control over even the simplest personal decision may be lost. Officials who use torture typically deny its use both to their own (protected) communities and to outsiders.

From a social perspective, the context in which torture occurs is as important to understand as the experience itself. Where torture occurs, it is important that those at risk (either because of their actions or by virtue of belonging to a particular group) are fully aware of this aspect. In other words, the fear of torture can have a marked effect even when torture itself has not been used on that individual. Similarly, other official actions can enhance this effect. The use of soldiers (or paramilitary troops and non-state militias) to round up groups of people, the enforced displacement of communities (including ethnic cleansing), a policy of detentions for particular communities—all take on a larger meaning, where there is, in addition, the use of torture. These broader activities go beyond the UN definition of torture but provide a related backdrop of fear and intimidation that has been described as low-grade warfare.

Torture may be undertaken for a variety of reasons, often in defense of current manifestations of power, wealth, or culture, and is frequently directed against powers seen as superior or as a covert threat to communal cohesion and tradition. Once undertaken, it frequently knows no bounds. Torture and related fear-provoking measures may be construed as a means of repression by challenging directly the relationships of trust people share with one another (Turner, 1995). If one person is arrested and faces torture, it will be natural to wonder what he or she might say about those with whom he or she lives and works. If he or she is actively engaged in op-position to an official (or sometimes unofficial) authority, then those who are also involved will experience fear themselves. The more the detainee knows, the more fear will be felt—so others in the community may begin to feel that it is safer to withhold information, safer not to oppose, and safer not to trust. Thus torture, whether it is actually applied or merely a risk, often holds people apart and represses communities by disrupting people's ability to trust. Although this is the common response, in a pro-portion of people it leads to even stronger opposition. It therefore produces a social radicalization—many being held in a state of unhappy repression and some being strengthened in active opposition.

These pressures on people may persist over long periods—even whole lifetimes. The effects can therefore be fundamental and persistent. In some parts of the world, adult survivors of torture and low-grade warfare describe discrimination and violence going back as far as they can recall. Elsewhere, people who have previously lived under conditions of freedom may, as regimes change, be subjected to violence and torture. It is likely that there are significant differences in the way people react to these two conditions.

NATURE AND SCOPE OF THE PROBLEM

Torture continues to be a serious problem in the world today. The eradication of the practice of torture in the world was one of the major challenges taken up by the United Nations only a few years after its establishment. The *Convention against Torture and Other Cruel, Inhuman or Degrading Treatment or Punishment* was adopted by the General Assembly in December 1984 and entered into force in June 1987. In a report to the 55th session of the General Assembly, the Secretary-General reported on the status of this convention (July, 2000). By July 1st 2000, the Convention had been acceded to or ratified by 119 states. Nine additional states had signed the Convention.

In establishing this convention, the UN set up a monitoring body as well, the Committee against Torture (Fact Sheet 17; http://www.unhchr.ch/html/menu6/2/fs17.htm), whose main function is to ensure that the convention is observed and implemented. The committee came into being in January 1988 and met for the first time in April of that year. It has a range of powers in relation to States that have recognized the competence of the committee to receive and investigate communications from other states (Article 21 of the *Convention against Torture and Other Cruel, Inhuman or Degrading Treatment or Punishment*) or from individuals (Article 22 of the same Convention). At the time of the report to the General Assembly in July 2000, 41 States had made this declaration in relation to both these Articles.

It is difficult to obtain good epidemiological evidence about the prevalence of these practices. Those detained and tortured may be released, or they may "disappear." Typically, torture exists in conditions of conflict, and material from either side is thus subject to distortion as a part of a pattern of disinformation. Human rights groups are usually given only limited access to survivors and can thus report on only a sample of those who might be affected.

Amnesty International (1999) has documented alarming findings in its annual report: that people "disappeared" (or remained "disappeared" from previous years) in 37 countries; that people were reportedly tortured or ill-treated by security forces, police, or other state authorities in 125 countries, and that confirmed or possible prisoners of conscience were held in 78 countries. There are statistics on refugees and others of concern to the United Nations High Commissioner for Refugees; although an indirect measure, these statistics probably reflect changes in patterns of mass violence and torture across the world—in this case showing an increase of 3.7% from the end of 1998 to the end of 1999, an absolute rise to a total of 22,257,340 (http://www.unhcr.ch).

Also, systematic assault on one community by another may include ethnic cleansing, enforced displacement, false imprisonment, disappearances, (attempted) assassinations, closure of schools and other normal services, prolonged use of curfews, use of anti-personnel landmines, systematic violence, rape, or genocide. The widespread use of rape has been reported from a number of conflict areas. This violation often has severe physical and psychological consequences for its victims (whether men or women) that are typically compounded by the many barriers to disclosing such an attack. These barriers may include fears of being cast out by the community, or of being rejected by a partner, as well as the inner experience of profound shame. Survivors of rape may also report a direct challenge to beliefs of safety arising from the fact that the perpetrator may have been a former neighbor or even a friend from another ethnic group.

Landmines have been another recent topic of attention (*UN Convention on the Prohibition of the Use, Stockpiling, Production and Transfer of Anti-Personnel Mines and on their Destruction,* 1997). There are millions of scattered and unrecorded landmines in more than 50 countries. These not only lay waste large tracts of land, but they also often target poor civilian communities forced to return to unsafe farmland or allow their children to play in dangerous areas. The United Nations Mine Action Service (UN-MAS) is the UN focal point for coordinating the mine-related activities of 11 different UN departments and agencies. Although the effort is still relatively small compared with the scale of need, there is increasing mine-clearing activity and a greater commitment to preventing this problem from building up again.

One group of people who are likely to know what is happening in a country are the health professionals. Survivors of torture often have health problems—both physical and psychological. Practitioners will be in contact with at least a subset of survivors. Unfortunately, health professionals known to be willing to work with victim groups are often targeted for persecution. There is anecdotal evidence that some may be aided by being recognized within an international network or grouping, and there is scope to explore this area further and possibly to systematize these mechanisms. The International Rehabilitation Council for Torture Victims (IRCT) is one example of a group that has been active in reaching out and offering international support to health professionals working under difficult circumstances. There are examples of rehabilitation centers receiving strong support from peer organizations in safer countries, both directly and through letter-writing campaigns. Action from health professionals in other countries may be one deterrent to persecution of health professionals. At the very least, it is made more difficult.

Conversely, health professionals may themselves be part of the process of torture (British Medical Association, 1992). There are principles of medical ethics for health personnel, particularly physicians, in the protection of prisoners and detainees against torture and other cruel, inhuman, or degrading treatment or punishment (General Assembly Resolution 37/194 of December 18, 1982). These principles state that "Health personnel, particularly physicians, charged with the medical care of prisoners and detainees, have a duty to provide them with protection of their physical and mental health and treatment of disease of the same quality and standard as is afforded to those who are not imprisoned or detained." ... and ... "It is a gross contravention of medical ethics, as well as an offence under applicable international instruments, for health personnel, particularly physicians, to engage, actively or passively, in acts which constitute participation in, complicity in, incitement to or attempts to commit torture or other cruel, inhuman or degrading treatment or punishment." (UNHCR Fact Sheet Number 4, *Methods of Combating Torture*; http://www.unhchr.ch/html/menu6/2/fs4.htm). Nonetheless, in reality it can be extremely difficult to adhere to such principles where the health professional is also a target for violence. This is a complex issue, but one that could only be helped by further protective mechanisms for those who wish to defend these principles of ethical practice. This would require international cooperation and scrutiny.

REACTIONS TO TORTURE

A review of reactions to torture must refer first to the investigations that followed the outrage of the Holocaust in the last century, which provide a wealth of material (for further discussion, see Kahana & Kahana, 2001). Eitinger (1964) was a pioneer in the investigation of the emotional sequelae of detention in concentration camps. He identified two primary aspects of the experience, one being an immediate trauma, and the second a tearing-up of a whole social world, leaving many survivors without any "form of anchorage in the world" (p. 188). Matussek (1975) brings much of this material together in an excellent text. There are various approaches to categorization in his book. A crucial conclusion he draws is that there is a broad spectrum of somatic and psychological complaints occurring long after the date of liberation. One analysis points to a distinction between two psychological syndromes (p. 50). The first is characterized as "psychophysiological," comprising symptoms such as poor concentration and memory, tiredness, depression, anxiety dreams, and sleep disturbances, symptoms seen in a co-morbid pattern of posttraumatic stress disorder [PTSD] and major depressive disorder [MDD] (American Psychiatric Association [APA], 1994). The other comprises a separate cluster of symptoms ("psychic syndrome") relating to mistrust, isolation, and alienation, resembling the concept of enduring personality change after catastrophic experience as defined in the current diagnostic criteria of the World Health Organization (WHO, 1993). Matussek (1975) did not avoid discussions of complex issues, such as attempts to understand and forgive; feelings of belonging and alienation, and ideology and faith. These are often overlooked in modern accounts, but are as important now as they were then.

Following a severe, malicious, and often prolonged experience such as torture in the modern world, undertaken within a political context, most people experience distress, but the majority probably do not develop a severe psychiatric disorder. Research into the prevalence of torture is hard to undertake in non-refugee groups, so prevalence studies in people who remain in the community in which they were tortured are very limited. There are also important differences between these various settings in (for example) the types of events experienced and social support systems available. It can be said with confidence, however, that mental health problems are common and that they should be expected in planning a service response. Silove (1999) has proposed that torture and related abuses may challenge five core adaptive systems subserving the psychological functions of "safety," "attachment," "justice," "identity-role," and "existential-meaning." Most individuals and collectives have intrinsic mechanisms for repairing damage to these systems. Indeed, a study of normative reactions to threats such as torture might shed further light on those who develop long-term morbid reactions (Silove, 1999).

Over the last decade, the debate about the physical and psychological effects of torture, especially in the realm of psychiatric disorders, has moved away from discussion of a (largely discredited) concept of a specific torture syndrome to the relative importance of more general psychiatric reactions in torture survivors. This is still surprisingly controversial. The two diagnoses most commonly associated with torture are PTSD and MDD, which commonly co-exist (e.g., Van Velsen, Gorst-Unsworth, & Turner, 1996). Differences in aspects of stress responses following torture have also been identified in research studies. These may relate to the specific nature of the trauma experience rather than to culture (although there may be an interaction effect, with certain forms of torture being more common in some cultures than in others). For example, torture that included sexual assault (e.g., rape) has been statistically associated with avoidance responses (Ramsay, Gorst-Unsworth, & Turner; 1993; Van Velsen et al., 1996). This probably relates to the emotions of humiliation and shame in men and women subjected to sexual assault. In both clinical and legal settings, it is important that there is full recognition that there may be late disclosure of torture—especially where this has involved sexual assault.

The view that survivors of torture face a significantly increased risk of PTSD and MDD is not universally accepted. One of the most strident critics of the application of a PTSD diagnosis to torture (Summerfield, 1999) argues that PTSD is a "reframing of the understandable suffering of a war as a technical problem to which short-term technical solutions like counselling are applicable" (abstract, p. 1449). This argument confounds cause and effect. It is true that but for torture or for war exposure, many would not develop a psychiatric injury. Therefore a primary task has to be to explore the degree to which change can be achieved at a sociopolitical level, which stands to assist the whole community. However, it would be wrong and even cruel to deny aid to those who have undergone this experience and are suffering. In other words, once there has been an injury, whether it is a loss of limb or a psychological wound, if there are available and affordable interventions that will aid recovery, it would be unethical to deny the injured party access to them.

Recently, Silove, Ekblad, and Mollica (2000) have highlighted the way that disagreement in the field seems to stem mainly from this "either-or" fallacy. On the one hand, some have argued that whole populations are traumatized. Critics call this a medicalization of a normative response to severe human rights abuse. Silove et al. suggest that both extremes are mistaken, and they point to the need to identify separate (and sometimes overlapping) subpopulations with distinctive needs. The majority will be able to adapt once peace and order are restored and, for these, the emphasis is best placed on finding peace and rebuilding a social community to support recovery. Others may have severe psychological reactions, and an even smaller subset will have disabling psychiatric illnesses. There should be no conceptual conflict in principle between community development programs and specific therapeutic programs, although decisions about resource allocation will have to be made. Both approaches are important and should be seen as operating in different ways, targeting different subgroups.

The focus on PTSD (e.g., Allodi, 1991), and of establishing treatment programs around this condition, is very helpful to the degree that we now have greater knowledge of the phenomenology, neurobiology, prognosis, and treatment of conditions such as PTSD and MDD, but a broader perspective may be more useful. For a complex traumatic stressor experience such as torture, although PTSD and MDD represent useful diagnostic entities, they do not go far enough in explaining the wide range of symptomatology seen in some torture survivors (Gorst-Unsworth, Van Velsen, & Turner, 1993). PTSD should certainly not be seen as a universal reaction. Similarly, the absence of PTSD does not discredit a history of torture—for the reason that many survivors do not develop PTSD. In 1990, four common elements of torture reactions in refugees were proposed (Turner & Gorst-Unsworth, 1990). These were (a) PTSD symptoms (incomplete emotional processing of shocking events); (b) depressive reactions secondary to loss and other adverse life events; (c) somatoform symptoms; and (d) changes in personal value systems—for example, changed personal, religious, or political thinking, or changes in core beliefs in a just or meaningful world. In other words, it was suggested that PTSD is important but insufficient to explain the range of possible reactions to torture.

One of the most important of these consequences of torture is an alteration in personal beliefs. For example, religious or political values may change, as well as the ability to relate normally to others. These changes may be positive as well as negative. In some people, there may even be changes in personality following torture and related forms of gross human rights abuses (Beltran & Silove, 1999). In diagnostic terms, the ICD-10 diagnosis of enduring personality change after catastrophic experience is a helpful addition to the classification system (WHO, 1993) in describing the impact of some severe negative changes. It captures well some of the problems of isolation, emptiness, and mistrust which may follow torture or a prolonged experience as a hostage. It is an example of a complex trauma reaction. This is a condition that may occur following extreme and/or prolonged stress (e.g., concentration camp experiences, torture, and hostage situations). It may coexist with PTSD and is a chronic and sometimes irreversible sequel to a complex traumatic experience. It is characterized by permanent, usually irreversible, changes, including:

- a hostile or mistrustful attitude towards the world
- social withdrawal
- feelings of emptiness or hopelessness
- a chronic feeling of being "on edge," as if constantly threatened
- estrangement.

Scientific study of enduring personality change is difficult, since it must usually involve retrospective confirmation that there has been a genuine personality change. However, it is helpful conceptually to move beyond the circumscribed clinical syndromes. Torture is a personal experience. It involves a relationship between victim and torturer within a political, cultural, and social context. The individuality of the response equally needs to be acknowledged. For most, this will not be within a diagnostic framework; yet there is a need to recognize complex trauma reactions for those with long-term disabling responses. It is important to find the right balance, acknowledging that these conditions (especially PTSD and depression) are commonly found and that they may be treatable, while at the same time recognizing the complex and human nature of the experience and of the response.

Mr. A. is a 32-year-old shopkeeper. He is married and has three children—all at home. He belonged to a minority ethnic group in his country—one that had experienced persecution over decades. As a child, he recalled seeing soldiers coming into the village in which he was born, rounding everyone up and beating up the village leaders. He had been an activist for democracy, which had led him to attend occasional demonstrations and distribute political material. He had not been involved in violent opposition of any type. As a shopkeeper, he had given supplies to one of the opposition groups and (under duress) to the army.

He presented for help to an NGO service agency in his home town and explained that the "security forces" had arrested him two months earlier. He had apparently been beaten badly and described at least one occasion when he had been knocked unconscious as the soldiers hit him with the butts of their rifles. They had held him down and had beat the soles of his feet with sticks (falaka), causing extreme pain. However, for him, the worst time was when he had witnessed and heard the torture of others, including children. This had left what seemed to be an indelible imprint on his mind. He had nightmares about it. In his mind, the soldiers were sometimes seen as attacking his own children. He could not bear this, and on a few occasions he had been physically sick at the thought.

He found that, after release, he could not talk about his experience to his wife or family. He retreated into an inner world. He found he could not trust other people. He knew that he wanted to continue his struggle, but he felt paralyzed. He felt himself a failure for giving up. Emotionally, he withdrew and became numb. He stopped socializing; it was a struggle to work. Whenever he saw soldiers he experienced fear, and when he left his shop, he was on the lookout for security forces. There were times when he was very tearful. He found it hard to concentrate, and he was always fatigued. His relationship with his wife changed. Their sexual life virtually ended, and they felt increasingly distant from each other.

He belonged to a faith that opposed suicide. In his heart, he could see no point in living, but his beliefs, although they were also challenged, protected him for the time being against taking active steps.

Mr. A. met diagnostic criteria for both PTSD and MDD (APA, 1994). He had persistent pain in both feet following the beatings. He had also changed radically from the person he used to be; effectively, he had "given up," and regarded the world as empty and without purpose, a place in which no one would ever really understand him again.

(This vignette is not based on an individual case history—it is designed to illustrate some of the common issues in a general way.)

There has also been an active debate about the cultural diversity of responses to torture (e.g., De Silva, 1993). Recently, reports confirming the importance of PTSD and MDD in a range of cultural groups (e.g., Cambodian and Bosnian refugees) have suggested important commonalities (Mollica, McInnes, Poole, & Tor, 1998; Mollica et al., 1999). There are important limitations, however, to the epidemiological evidence. Large-scale surveys generally rely on self-report measures, and small-scale surveys using interview measures are often confounded by selection bias (e.g., help-seeking behavior) or problems of sample size. So, although these studies are helpful in confirming the presence of broadly similar responses in different cultures, care is needed in interpreting prevalence rates of any psychiatric diagnosis. For example, Smith Fawzi et al. (1997), having considered new data on the validity of thresholds for the Harvard Trauma Questionnaire, concluded that "future community based studies conducted among refugee populations should include a validation sub-study in order to ascertain the most appropriate cut-off score for each individual context." In a recent large-scale investigation of Kosovan Albanian refugees in the United Kingdom, this approach was adopted, and the validation process substantially reduced the estimated prevalence of psychiatric disorders in the larger sample (Turner, Bowie, Dunn, Shapo, & Yule, in press). However, in this newly arrived group (in which maximal distress was therefore likely), about 50% still had a diagnosis of PTSD. Fewer had a diagnosis of MDD.

Phan and Silove (1997) explored this theme in detail and highlighted the contributions that both emic (informed by ethnographic concepts of the centrality of culture in shaping the psyche and its expressions) and etic (which focuses on the universal elements in the manifestation of psychic distress) approaches can offer. This debate has extended into discussions about treatment. For example, those working with Indochinese refugees have repeatedly pointed to differences in the acceptability of dealing with trauma directly and early in the treatment process. For this group, the process of addressing trauma tends to be slower, and this has to be fully respected.

As previously mentioned, the research base lacks good epidemiological evidence about torture and its effects, with samples inevitably being subject to important selection processes. Within countries that practice torture, it is difficult to access representative samples of survivors, and it is likely to be unsafe for researchers as well as for those being studied. Indeed, the opportunity to undertake ethical research is an important freedom that may need to be defended. The asylum process imposes a different, but equally important, set of selection filters on any sample. Thus, there may be good epidemiological sampling of an asylum or refugee population, but the population itself is subject to selection forces and may not be representative of survivors of torture in the countries of origin.

There are relatively few investigations of torture or "official" violence in non-refugee samples. In a study looking at the effects of torture in a non-refugee group, the importance of expectation and preparation for torture were emphasized. Activists who were tortured had worse experiences than those who had not been politically active; however, the activists were less severely affected by their experiences (Basoglu et al., 1996; Basoglu et al., 1997).

INTERVENTION STRATEGIES

Overall Goals of Any Intervention

It is helpful to conceptualize the response to low-grade warfare and torture at a number of different levels. Moving from a societal (international and political) to a more intensive (individual and therapeutic) structure of response, the following framework is helpful:

- Organized prevention strategies (addressing root causes)
- Reconciliation and redress (healing and prevention of transgenerational transmission)
- Meeting primary needs of survivors (a context for recovery)
- Community strategies (empowerment and healing)
- Service organization under conditions of low-grade warfare and torture
- Gender, culture, and access to services
- Group and family treatment approaches
- Individual treatment approaches

There is a focus on individual treatment approaches in this chapter, but this is primarily due to the nature of the scientific evidence to date. There is a pressing need for more formal evaluation of strategies adopted in different parts of the world. A general account of work with refugees may be found in Van Der Veer (1992).

Policy Interventions

Organized Prevention Strategies. Nation states, through the United Nations, have agreed on a core set of global standards and development aims that are directly and indirectly relevant to torture prevention, together with mechanisms for reaching and maintaining them worldwide. These mechanisms include the formulation of Conventions and their subsequent ratification and the establishment of Committees and Special Rapporteurs. (The United Nations Commission on Human Rights, in resolution 1985/33, appointed a special rapporteur to examine questions relevant to torture, to seek and receive credible and reliable information on such questions, and to respond to that information without delay). Also important is the convening of major conferences and programs of action, and partnerships with institutions and civil-society organizations worldwide.

Civil society or non-governmental organizations [NGOs] are crucial actors in the formulation and implementation of UN standards and goals, including torture prevention. For example, during one of the many global conferences for development in the 1990s, Sadik (1994) remarked that "non-governmental voices are heard, both in monitoring government support of the Programme of Action (on Population and Development) and in helping to implement it. NGOs keep governments honest, and we should not let up on that." Collective action is also needed to stem the sale and use of small arms, weapon systems, and landmines. Of direct relevance to the prevention of torture is the United Nations Committee against Torture, already mentioned, as well as the Special Rapporteur. To assist the many victims of torture, the General Assembly set up the United Nations Voluntary Fund for Victims of Torture pursuant to General Assembly resolution 36/151 of 16 December 1981. This was not an implicit acceptance of torture but was intended to be a means of providing and channeling assistance (including humanitarian, legal, and financial aid) to people who had been tortured and to their families. The Fund supports the provision of medical treatment, physiotherapy, psychiatric and psychological care, and social and economic assistance, as well as supporting training of medical professionals in the techniques needed to treat victims of torture. (UNHCR Fact Sheet Number 4, Methods of Combating Torture; http://www.unhchr.ch/html/menu6/2/fs4.htm).

In spite of these programs, torture continues to be a serious problem. In the introduction to its 1998 Annual Report, Amnesty International (1998) points out examples of situations in which the United Nations Declaration of Human Rights [UDHR] is plainly not being fulfilled. The Amnesty International report also emphasized the importance of the UDHR for all peoples. Thus, the first level of intervention, in the face of mass violence and torture, is to appeal to the perpetrators whenever possible through the United Nations, select Governments, or civil-society organizations. Also, bearing witness to its occurrence by individuals, national, or international bodies may draw enough attention for the perpetrators to desist.

Torture and mass violence are among the commonest preventable causes of psychological disorder in the world today. Any intervention that stands to make it harder to carry out these abuses of human rights will also reduce the burden of human misery and of mental illness. Health practitioners have special access to information about torture and therefore have special obligations. They also need support.

Reconciliation and Redress. A second line of intervention at a national/policy level is the application of psychological experience and practice toward national reconciliation. A recent example of this is the Truth and Reconciliation Commission in the Republic of South Africa (Friedman, 2000; Stein, 1998). Although individual survivors may find it hard to articulate their needs, often through fear or persisting overwhelming distress, and although there are no perfect models of this process, a number of common strands have emerged. Survivors typically wish to be given information about what happened to them, their families, and their communities. This is the first step. Even if punishments against them are reduced or waived in some cases, there is still a widespread desire to see that those responsible publicly acknowledge their actions, apologize, and display contrition. These demands can be seen as hard to reconcile with other political requirements in "national reconstruction," but if ignored, the psychological burdens may simply become entrenched and affect future generations in a cycle of violence and retribution (e.g., Danieli, 1998).

It is also important that survivors are included in the development of restitution and redress strategies (Stamatopoulou, 1996; Redress, 2001). At the discussions on the Draft Statute for the International Criminal Court (ICC) in Rome in 1998, only one tentative article dealt with the principles of justice for victims (Redress, 1998). This is another area in which bitterness may fuel further conflict.

Meeting Primary Needs. The United Nations *Declaration of Human Rights* (UDHR) includes (among others) the rights to "life, liberty and the security of the person," the right to work, and the rights to "food, clothing, housing and medical care." These constitute primary needs and, in many countries where the UDHR has been ratified, they have formally been adopted as rights. These basic human rights are not necessarily more important than people's psychological needs but, if they remain unmet, they are likely to make psychological recovery more difficult. For example, it may be very difficult to focus on emotional issues when one is profoundly hungry.

Similarly, if survivors of torture are forced to seek refuge elsewhere, then the manner in which the receiving country responds is also important to recovery. Steel, Silove, Bird, McGorry, & Mohan (1999) showed that both pre-migration and post-migration experiences were associated with post-traumatic stress symptoms in a group of Tamil asylum-seekers in Australia. There is evidence that those asylum-seekers who travel to a high-income country and who live: a) in prolonged uncertainty (over their status), b) separated from spouse and children, c) with limited accommodation, and d) limited daytime activity have more depressive symptoms than those who have family union and social support (Van Velsen et al., 1996). Gorst-Unsworth and Goldenberg (1998) demonstrated, in refugees, that poor social support was a stronger predictor of depressive morbidity than trauma factors.

Community Strategies (Empowerment and Healing)

There is a limited evidence base concerning the community response to survivors of torture and mass violence. More information would be helpful, although it will likely be hard to obtain. It is very likely that community support is helpful, although for some groups there may be specific barriers to this type of aid.

Some community strategies have indeed been successful. Human rights groups can help to support the vulnerable by publicizing acts of torture and mass violence (internally and internationally). Aid regimes can be linked to community development plans. NGOs working to provide education and training to women and young people may have a particularly important role, where such work is permitted. Indeed, training (developing the capacity for service delivery) is often an important strategy in helping to develop potential counselors and therapists able to work in oppressed communities.

The position of survivors is complex, in that not only have they had to face torture, but they also belong to a group that is subject to other forms of discrimination, to economic and social pressures, and to deprivation of basic human rights. There is often more scope for interventions with refugees—simply because they have left the place in which the torture took place, and therefore both they and those involved in offering relief can operate with greater safety. Nonetheless, many have found the support of their own communities to be of enormous help.

On the other hand, there can be barriers to community support. One of the most obvious examples is the isolation often imposed on women who have been raped.

Ms. C is a woman who was detained by state security forces overnight and then left on the road some distance from her home. She was in a dazed state. Initially she was reluctant to say very much about what had happened. She merely described being beaten by soldiers, and seemed rather vague about it all.

Two years later, she disclosed (for the first time) to a member of a visiting NGO that she had been raped. Her husband did not know, and she said that if he were ever told, it would be the end of her marriage. She believed that members of her community would also regard her as bringing "bad luck" if they ever learned of her rape. They would not want to talk to her. She had bottled it all inside herself. She felt ashamed. So she had kept it all to herself.

(This vignette is not based on an individual case history—it is designed to illustrate some of the common issues in a general way.)

Service Organizations Under Conditions of Low-Grade Warfare and Torture. Torture survivors may be afraid to access general health services, and those who do often report rejection, so it is important that services be targeted especially for this population. Coordination of health services is also needed. Yet, in conditions of low-grade warfare and torture, it is a challenge to establish effective links among medical and psychotherapeutic services for survivors. Despite this, it is surprising to see how many (often NGOs) have successfully done so (Welsh, 1996). Services are required not only for emotional scars but also for severe physical injuries, and for other concerns in the aftermath of rape (access to HIV testing and treatment; access to post-intercourse contraception and to termination-of-pregnancy services). Assuring safety for survivors and staff is a practical imperative.

Moreover, there are often economic pressures that dictate the resources available to work with survivors within the country of persecution. Usually this work is of low priority politically (being officially denied as a problem), and therefore takes a lower place than does the provision of other mental health services. So even if the state is wealthy, there is usually little political enthusiasm to provide good treatment facilities for this group.

International bodies (such as the World Health Organization, the Red Cross and Crescent Societies, and UNICEF) are in a position to offer guidelines and monitoring for basic treatment facilities. These guidelines should be informed by the scientific literature in the field of traumatic stress reactions. One outcome of the joint ISTSS/UN project of which this book is a component might be the formation of expert reference panels to advise in the development and review of guidelines as the evidence base changes. It may be that attempting to achieve a consensus will make for a better framework for local collaboration. Failure to achieve effective inter-agency cooperation is a major barrier to progress.

This begs a difficult question—and that is the degree to which services can be protected. Even if guidelines were in place, would it be possible to work safely in settings in which human rights are violated (and if the staff were safe, would survivors feel able to trust them—or would they see them as associated with the authorities?). There is no easy answer. There is a pressing need for more research to help inform policy and service provision. This should be concerned not only with the narrow evaluation of treatment but also with different models of service delivery.

International bodies may be in a better position to support practitioners operating in dangerous places than national groups. In some countries (e.g., Chile), the medical association was active in supporting isolated practitioners, but this is often not the case. Doctors and other health professionals in the establishment may share its views or be otherwise unavailable to help support these practitioners. However, probably one of the strongest supports for those who have come forth to work with survivors of torture would be international recognition (examples in Welsh, 1996). If torturers knew that their actions would be widely reported and investigated, they might desist. International publicity is a possible deterrent that might be sufficient to protect some practitioners.

> Dr. B was asked to assess someone who gave a history of torture and had the characteristic psychological signs of PTSD. The victim described how men who appeared to belong to the intelligence services perpetrated the torture. Dr. B decided to let a colleague in another country know about the situation as a form of protection. He provided his colleague with limited information about the case and his role in it. He asked his colleague to make some of this information public should anything happen to him. He hoped that this might deter the security services from acting against him. He also decided to join a recently formed network of health professionals working in this field.
>
> (This vignette is not based on an individual case history—it is designed to illustrate some of the common issues in a general way.)

There are international monitoring frameworks that some countries allow. Of course, just as with the International Criminal Court, those most in need are also the most likely to reject such an approach. Nonetheless, these are an important additional support not only in the prevention of torture but also potentially in the support of practitioners.

Gender, Culture, and Access to Services. Gender issues related to torture are too large a subject to cover adequately in the space available. However, this is an area of high importance internationally and especially in the United Nations, and access to health and social care services must be addressed. While it can be hard for any survivor of torture or mass violence to seek help, there are important barriers often faced by women in their dealings with many health and aid systems (Magruder, Mollica, & Friedman, 2001). Especially following certain forms of assault, like sexual violence as a mechanism of torture, it can be difficult to seek help. Rape is not only an assault on women associated with strong, specific, avoidance reactions (Koss & Kilpatrick, 2001; Ramsay et al., 1993; Van Velsen et al., 1996); it is also a crime in which the perpetrator is almost always male. On this basis, it is unreasonable to expect the survivor of rape to disclose this to a man. Of course, men are subjected to rape and sexual humiliation as well. This is especially true in the context of torture, but rape also appears to be a significant problem in penal institutions in general (Coxell & King, 2000). The difficulties in disclosure apply to both male and female victims (Turner, 2000). This is one instance of a general issue: that services need to provide choice as far as possible, respecting the preferences of the service-user whether these are on grounds of gender or on some other criteria.

It is important to acknowledge the importance of cultural as well as gender issues in relation to services for survivors of sexual assault. Disclosure of sexual assault within the community can lead to survivors being ostracized and can lead to marital breakdown. Another barrier, therefore, may be the proximity of the aid worker to her (or his) community, which raises issues to do with trust in services. It is essential to have mechanisms of feedback and to act on these so that services can continue to improve accessibility to all.

It is also important to consider carefully the significance of cultural diversity in relation to selecting individual treatments. While there are those who argue for cultural primacy and those who advocate the importance of more universal approaches, we believe strongly that a flexible implementation model, which reflects local cultural issues, as well as the limited evidence base, is likely to be the most useful way forward.

Group and Family Treatment Approaches

Group treatments have not been widely used with torture survivors. In safe countries, there are problems in bringing together survivors from different conflicts. In countries of oppression, group mobilization of victims is likely to be a source of interest to security forces, perhaps increasing the danger to victims and counselors if carried out overtly, and difficult to organize on a large scale covertly. It is also likely that there will be fundamental problems of trust in many cases. This is unlikely to be a fruitful avenue in many settings—at least until a change in regime.

On the other hand, a cultural perspective might lead to the most culturally appropriate approaches to families and individuals. In some settings, the natural unit for intervention may be the individual, and in others it may be a family or some other unit. These cultural variations must be taken into account when planning a response.

The possible benefits of group approaches have not been evaluated in any systematic way, although Fischman and Ross (1990) have developed a model for time-limited group therapy for refugees with a history of torture. Schlapobersky (1990) has also proposed a model related to this issue.

Individual Treatment Approaches

These approaches are likely to have different levels of applicability from one country to another in accordance with treatment traditions and resource availability. However, it is still important to be aware of the up-to-date evidence. Unfortunately, there is limited evidence of treatment efficacy in work with survivors of torture. Moreover, given the great diversity of symptoms and the complex reactions to this type of trauma, it is important to be cautious in drawing too many parallels with treatments of other forms of trauma.

Having said that, there is still every reason to believe that interventions that are effective in other settings for depression or for PTSD (see Chapter 4) will be effective in survivors of torture (e.g., Foa, Davidson, & Frances, 1999; Sherman, 1998; Van Etten & Taylor, 1998). The evidence base points to the appropriate use of medication (especially SSRI antidepressants) and specific psychological interventions for depression and for PTSD. Differences may be in emphasis rather than the type of treatment. For example, working within a cognitive-behavioral (CBT) paradigm, Basoglu (1992) has stressed the importance of not overwhelming the survivor of torture by covering too much material in one session, as this may interfere with emotional processing. In general, it is likely that extra caution is required in using approaches in which survivors are confronted with memories of past events following complex traumas such as torture.

One problem that may arise, even where resources are available, concerns getting treatment to survivors of torture. Part of the difficulty may be natural avoidance behavior. In a civilian setting in Norway, Weisaeth (1989) undertook a longitudinal study of 246 employees exposed to an industrial disaster involving a fire. He found that those closest to the fire required significantly more invitation to participate than those who were more peripheral. Moreover, if those who had been initially most reluctant to enter the study had been lost, at seven months the total response rate would have been 83%. The last 17% (those most reluctant to enter the study) included 42% of the total number of people with PTSD and the majority (64%) of those with severe PTSD. The implication for service planning is that not only do survivors need to feel able to trust the service (politically), but that those with the worst conditions are less likely to present. It is particularly important that services are as accessible as possible and that further attention is given to these barriers to treatment. However, it is typically difficult (and may be dangerous) to reach out to survivors of torture in their own communities.

Experts recommend a greater-than-usual emphasis on the phased approach to treatment. Herman (1992), for example, identified three phases: an initial phase of establishing safety and trust; a specific treatment phase with the active intervention; and a reintegration phase.

In any therapeutic intervention with survivors of torture and mass violence, the first and the third of these phases is of particular significance. Although conceptually distinct, these phases are often clinically intermingled. Issues of safety and trust, for example, may re-emerge during the specific intervention phase. However, for the purpose of discussion, it will be assumed that these phases are sequential.

The development of trust and a therapeutic alliance are essential components in the *initial phase*. The therapist should be encouraging, patient, and empathic, but also permit time for the survivor to express strong feelings if he or she wishes. Adequate attention must be given to primary needs, to considerations of safety, and to the boundaries of the therapeutic relationship (Turner, McFarlane, & Van Der Kolk, 1996). A survivor of torture needs to be able to trust his or her therapist, even if both are still in the country of torture, and this may require certain kinds of reassurance by the therapist: for example, an expression of commitment to human rights or even, perhaps, clarification of his or her political or religious outlook.

If it is possible, care needs to be given, therefore, to the gender, ethnicity, or other attribute of therapists that may mark them as belonging to one group or other within a setting of conflict. For example, in working with refugees from the former Yugoslavia, it is essential to consider the ethnic background of a therapist or interpreter in relation to that of the patient. Therapy may not be possible or may require more attention to the relationship, given certain matches/combinations of patient/therapist ethnicity.

In the *specific treatment phase*, in addition to the typical treatment approaches, there has been interest in an approach entitled "Testimony," first used for torture survivors in Chile. It sets out to achieve a written record of the survivor's experiences, a record that is the survivor's to possess and to use as he or she wishes. Sessions are tape-recorded and transcribed. These transcripts are the material of future sessions and are revised and developed by the survivor until, at closure, there is a comprehensive narrative. The survivor is an active participant in therapy – the therapist's role being one of clarification and encouragement. By developing a complete picture from fragmented sequences, survivors can learn to "identify, understand, and integrate the meaning of their political commitment and their suffering" (Cienfuegos & Monelli, 1983).

Recently, there has been a renewal of interest in this technique following the report of a pilot study of its application in a group of Bosnian refugees in the USA. In an average of six sessions of treatment, in this small uncontrolled study, there was evidence of significant symptom reduction and improvement in functioning (Weine, Kulenovic, Pavkovic, & Gibbons, 1998).

Psychological reactions such as guilt (associated with excessive responsibility) felt after divulging information against comrades or family can be reframed as understandable, perhaps even inevitable, in the face of extreme pain and powerlessness. Testimony takes account of the sociopolitical context, and, in that way, is an acceptable approach for many survivors, perhaps in conjunction with techniques likely to be effective in the treatment of PTSD. Where shame or guilt is the dominant emotional reaction, a cognitive approach, exploring carefully the meaning of the experience, may also be appropriate.

Reported approaches to torture appear to share common ingredients. For example, the therapeutic approach reported by the Rehabilitation and Research Centre for Torture Victims (RCT) in Copenhagen (Somnier & Genefke, 1986) begins with cognitive restructuring of the traumatic experience, apparently designed to help survivors increase insight into their experiences. The second phase is more emotive, as the patient recalls traumatic events and is permitted to express repressed emotions such as aggression and fear. As recall continues, the patient comes to realize that his or her conduct was not unique, but was instead a predictable response to an overwhelming trauma. The third phase is to re-establish reality by breaking various vicious cycles such as guilt, anxiety, or low self-esteem, integrating his or her experiences into practical everyday activities, and permitting the move away from the victim role.

Psychodynamic models highlight that the reactions of the therapist are important. These may be potentially anti-therapeutic, sometimes associated with intense emotional reactions on the part of the therapist ranging from denial to over-identification, or fear of failure (Comas-Diaz & Padillo, 1990). If therapy takes place within a country of torture, fear (on the part of the therapist as well as the survivor) may inhibit the development of trust and the confrontation of reality. The therapist may experience overwhelming hatred towards the torturer, or may feel helpless and paralyzed. For some survivors, the reality is that only limited gains are possible. However, even these are worthwhile. If there are twelve problems, three or four of which might be relieved, it is still worthwhile to attempt such relief. These concerns suggest the importance of good supervision for those involved in this field.

In the *reintegration phase*, there are the usual matters concerning the reestablishment of relationships, family bonds, work, and other activities. These may affect any survivor of catastrophe. Following the deliberate use of torture, however, there are additional critical issues involving a return to previous political, religious, or other activities. There may be realistic issues of risk for people living in a repressive regime or in the context of civil war. This is likely to be a difficult phase of treatment. There are decisions to be made that are important matters of personal choice but that may affect the therapeutic process.

For people who have faced torture because they chose an activist approach, there may be the dilemma of deciding whether to return to their natural group, with its associated risk for further torture, or to abandon the struggle, which would effectively cut them off from their social supports. Moreover, after release from detention, there may be questions raised about how much information they gave, which, combined with feelings of worry or even a sense of guilt induced by their torturers, may be another alienating factor. Once again, torture may be seen as having profound effects on trust and therefore on relationships.

For people who were tortured for other reasons, there are sometimes severe problems in trying to reconstruct a working model of the world. If they have been tortured without apparent reason, what might they face in future? This is not so much reintegration as it is *rebuilding* a set of beliefs about others and the world they live in.

Finally, torture does not take place in isolation. Typically, family members are also at risk. The survivor of torture may face other losses and changes in close relationships. These too may require a long process of adaptation. There are probably more options for the survivor remaining in the country of persecution than in asylum (because in a country of asylum it is often harder to maintain normal family/other relationships or a political role). However, a decision to stay and to remain active may reactivate safety issues for the survivor and his or her family.

RECOMMENDATIONS

UN/International Level

- Emphasize prevention and support for implementation of basic human rights (e.g., UDHR) in all member states, using whatever influence is possible.

- Consider victims' needs in all developments in international law.
- Consider the needs of health practitioners in developments in international law, both the need to provide treatment and the need to bear witness, without fear of reprisal.
- Improve public awareness of torture wherever it occurs, and wherever its victims find asylum.
- Encourage collaboration among regional agencies.

National Level

- Encourage all nations to follow UN guidelines and outlaw torture.
- Include efforts to respond to the needs of victims; failure to do this is likely to increase the risk of transgenerational transmission and the perpetuation of a cycle of violence.

Context for Service Delivery

- Provide, as far as it is possible, a supportive social and political context in which recovery and empowerment of repressed communities can take place.
- Recognize the importance of training (capacity-building) for sensitive and informed service delivery.
- Ensure that particular attention is given to the needs of women, children, and other groups facing special difficulties, stigma, or discrimination in the access of services.
- Ensure that when survivors of torture reach safe countries, they are actively helped within a supportive, social, and political framework designed to deal quickly with their fears and with any family separation.

Health Service/NGO

- Provide a system for independent medical assessments of survivors of torture.
- Develop rehabilitation centers, with international support.
- Encourage international accreditation and scrutiny of the treatment work in order to raise standards and support workers.
- Use an evidence-based approach to developing treatment services following torture.
- Ensure that sound knowledge of the local culture is taken into account in the development of accessible and appropriate services.

- Support, as appropriate, rigorous and culturally sensitive research to guide the development of treatment.

Individual Practitioners

- Ensure that people have rights to access health care and to exercise choices about the care they receive.
- Ensure that services are designed to acknowledge and respect cultural diversity as well as differences in gender and religion.
- Recognize and reduce barriers to treatment, e.g. by involving service users in planning decisions.
- Provide a phased approach to the organization of treatment.
- Recognize that survivors may disclose a sexual assault later in treatment.
- Recognize that the therapist may have strong emotional reactions during the treatment and that good supervision is needed to identify and deal with these.
- Ensure that there is a program that addresses the needs of therapists.
- Provide (and evaluate) a means of supporting practitioners working in dangerous settings.

REFERENCES

Allodi, F.A. (1991). Assessment and treatment of torture victims: A critical review. *The Journal of Nervous and Mental Disease, 179*, 4–11.

American Psychiatric Association (1994). *Diagnostic and statistical manual of mental disorders* (4th ed.). Washington, DC: Author.

Amnesty International (1998). *Annual report*. London: Amnesty International Publications.

Amnesty International (1999). *Annual report*. London: Amnesty International Publications.

Barudy, J. (1989). A programme of mental health for political refugees: Dealing with the invisible pain of political exile. *Social Science Medicine, 28*, 715–727.

Basoglu, M. (Ed.). (1992). *Torture and its consequences*. Cambridge: Cambridge University Press.

Basoglu, M., Paker, M., Ozmen, E., Tasdemir, O., Sahin, D., Ceyhanli, A., Incesu, C., & Sarimurat, N. (1996). Appraisal of self, social environment, and state authority as a possible mediator of posttraumatic stress disorder in tortured political activists. *Journal of Abnormal Psychology, 105*, 232–236.

Basoglu, M., Mineka, S., Paker, M., Aker, T., Livanou, M., & Gok, S. (1997). Psychological preparedness for trauma as a protective factor in survivors of torture. *Psychological Medicine, 27*, 1421–1433.

Beltran, R., & Silove, D.M. (1999). Expert opinions about the ICD-10 category of enduring personality change after catastrophic experience. *Comprehensive Psychiatry, 40*, 396–403.

British Medical Association (1992). *Medicine betrayed: The participation of doctors in human rights abuses*. London: Zed Books.

Cienfuegos, A.J., & Monelli, C. (1983). The testimony of political repression as a therapeutic instrument. *American Journal of Orthopsychiatry, 53*, 43–51.

Comas-Diaz, L., & Padillo, A.M. (1990). Countertransference in working with victims of political repression. *American Journal of Orthopsychiatry, 60*, 125–134.

Coxell, A., & King, M.B. (2000). Behind locked doors: Sexual assault of men in custodial environments. In G.C. Mezey, & M.B. King (Eds.), *Male victims of sexual assault* (pp. 79–95). Oxford, England: Oxford University Press.

Danieli, Y. (1998). *International handbook of multigenerational legacies of trauma.* New York: Plenum Press, 1998.

De Silva, P. (1993). Post-traumatic stress disorder: Cross-cultural aspects. *International Review of Psychiatry, 5*, 217–229.

Eitinger, L. (1964). *Concentration camp survivors in Norway and Israel.* London: Allen & Unwin.

Fischman, Y., & Ross, J. (1990). Group treatment of exiled survivors of torture. *American Journal of Orthopsychiatry, 60*, 135–142.

Foa, E.B., Davidson, J.R.T., & Frances, A.J. (1999). Treatment of posttraumatic stress disorder (Expert consensus guideline series). *Journal of Clinical Psychiatry* (vol. 60, Supplement 10).

Friedman, M. (2000). The truth and reconciliation commission in South Africa as an attempt to heal a traumatized society. In A.Y. Shalev, R. Yehuda, & A.C. McFarlane (Eds.), *International handbook of human response to trauma* (pp. 399–411). New York: Kluwer Academic/Plenum Publishers.

Gorst-Unsworth, C., & Goldenberg, E. (1998). Psychological sequelae of torture and organised violence suffered by refugees from Iraq: Trauma related factors compared with social factors in exile. *British Journal of Psychiatry, 172*, 90–94.

Gorst-Unsworth, C., Van Velsen, C., & Turner, S. (1993). Prospective pilot study of survivors of torture and organized violence: Examining the existential dilemma. *Journal of Nervous and Mental Disease, 181*, 263–264.

Herman, J.L. (1992). *Trauma and recovery.* New York: Basic Books.

Kahana, B., & Kahana, E. (2001). Holocaust trauma and sequelae. In E. Gerrity, T.M. Keane, & F. Tuma (Eds.), *The mental health consequences of trauma* (pp. 143–157). New York: Kluwer Academic/Plenum Publishers.

Koss, M.P., & Kilpatrick, D.G. (2001). Rape and sexual assault. In E. Gerrity, T.M. Keane, & F. Tuma (Eds.), *The mental health consequences of trauma* (pp. 177–193). New York: Kluwer Academic/Plenum Publishers.

Magruder, K.M., Mollica, R., & Friedman, M. (2001). Mental health services research: Implications for survivors of torture. In E. Gerrity, T.M. Keane, & F. Tuma (Eds.), *The mental health consequences of trauma* (pp. 291–307). New York: Kluwer Academic/Plenum Publishers.

Matussek, P. (1975). *Internment in concentration camps and its consequences.* Berlin: Springer-Verlag.

Mollica, R.F., McInnes, K., Poole, C., & Tor, S. (1998). Dose-effect relationships of trauma to symptoms of depression and post-traumatic stress disorder among Cambodian survivors of mass violence. *British Journal of Psychiatry, 173*, 482–488.

Mollica, R.F., McInnes, K., Sarajlic, N., Lavelle, J., Sarajlic, I., & Massagli, M.P. (1999). Disability associated with psychiatric comorbidity and health status in Bosnian refugees living in Croatia. *Journal of the American Medical Association, 282*, 433–439.

Phan, T., & Silove, D.M. (1997). The influence of culture on psychiatric assessment: The Vietnamese refugee. *Psychiatric Services, 48*, 86–90.

Ramsay, R., Gorst-Unsworth, C., & Turner, S. (1993). Psychiatric morbidity in survivors of organised state violence including torture. *British Journal of Psychiatry, 162*, 55–59.

Redress (1998). *Promoting the right to reparation for survivors of torture; what role for a permanent International Criminal Court?* London: Redress (6 Queen Square, London WC1N 3AR, UK).

Redress (2001). *Torture survivors' perceptions of reparation.* London: Redress (6 Queen Square, London WC1N 3AR, UK).

Sadik, N. (1994, September). *Closing speech at the International Conference on Population and Development.* Cairo, Egypt.

Schlapobersky, J., (1990). Torture as the perversion of a healing relationship. In J. Gruschow & K. Hannibal (Eds.), *Health services for the treatment of torture and trauma survivors* (pp. 51–71). Washington DC: American Association for the Advancement of Science.

Sherman, J.L. (1998). Effects of psychotherapeutic treatments for PTSD: A meta-analysis of controlled clinical trials. *Journal of Traumatic Stress, 11,* 413–435.

Silove, D. (1999). The psychosocial effects of torture, mass human rights violations, and refugee trauma: Towards an integrated conceptual framework. *The Journal of Nervous and Mental Disease, 187,* 200–207.

Silove, D., Ekblad, S., & Mollica, R. (2000). The rights of the severely mentally ill in post-conflict societies. *The Lancet, 355,* 1548–1549.

Smith Fawzi, M.C., Murphy, E., Pham, T., Lin, L., Poole, C., & Mollica, R.F. (1997).The validity of screening for post-traumatic stress disorder and major depression among Vietnamese former political prisoners. *Acta Psychiatrica Scandinavica, 95,* 87–93.

Somnier, F.E., & Genefke, I.K. (1986). Psychotherapy for victims of torture. *British Journal of Psychiatry, 149,* 323–9.

Stamatopoulou, E. (1996). Violations of human rights – United Nations action from the victims perspective. In Y. Danieli, N.S. Rodley, & L. Weisaeth (Eds.), *International responses to traumatic stress.* New York: Baywood.

Steel, Z., Silove, D.M., Bird, K., McGorry, P.D., & Mohan, P. (1999). Pathways from war trauma to posttraumatic stress symptoms among Tamil asylum seekers, refugees, and immigrants. *Journal of Traumatic Stress, 12,* 421–435.

Stein, D.J. (1998). Psychiatric aspects of the Truth and Reconciliation Commission of South Africa. *British Journal of Psychiatry, 173,* 455–457.

Summerfield, D.A. (1999). A critique of seven assumptions behind psychological trauma programmes in war-affected areas. *Social Science and Medicine, 48,* 1449–1462.

Turner, S.W., & Gorst-Unsworth, C. (1990). Psychological sequelae of torture – A descriptive model. *British Journal of Psychiatry, 157,* 475–480.

Turner, S.W. (1995). Torture, refuge and trust. In E.V. Daniel, & J.C. Knudsen (Eds.), *Mistrusting refugees* (pp. 56–72). California: California.

Turner, S.W., McFarlane, A.C., & Van Der Kolk, B.A. (1996). The therapeutic environment and new explorations in the treatment of posttraumatic stress disorder. In B.A. Van Der Kolk, A.C. McFarlane, & L. Weisaeth (Eds.), *Traumatic stress: The effects of overwhelming experience on mind, body, and society* (pp. 537–558). New York: Guilford Press.

Turner, S.W. (2000). Surviving sexual assault and sexual torture. In G.C. Mezey, & M.B. King (Eds.), *Male victims of sexual assault* (pp. 97–111). Oxford, England: Oxford University Press.

Turner, S.W., Bowie, C., Dunn, G., Shapo, L., & Yule, W. (in press). Mental health of Kosovan Albanian Refugees in the UK. *British Journal of Psychiatry.*

Van Der Veer, G. (1992). *Counselling and therapy with refugees: Psychological problems of victims of war, torture and repression.* Chichester: Wiley.

Van Etten, M.L., & Taylor, S. (1998). Comparative efficacy of treatments for post-traumatic stress disorder: A meta-analysis. *Clinical Psychology and Psychotherapy, 5,* 126–144.

Van Velsen, C., Gorst-Unsworth, C., & Turner, S.W. (1996). Survivors of torture and organized violence: Demography and diagnosis. *Journal of Traumatic Stress, 9,* 181–193.

Weine, S.M., Kulenovic, A.D., Pavkovic, I., & Gibbons, R. (1998). Testimony psychotherapy in Bosnian refugees: A pilot study. *American Journal of Psychiatry, 155,* 1720–1726.

Welsh, J. (1996). Violations of human rights: Traumatic stress and the role of NGOs. In Y. Danieli, N.S. Rodley, & L. Weisaeth (Eds.), *International responses to traumatic stress*. New York: Baywood.

Weisaeth, L. (1989). Importance of high response rates in traumatic stress research. *Acta Psychiatrica Scandinavica Supplementum, 355*, 131–137.

World Health Organization (1993). *The ICD-10 classification of mental and behavioural disorders: Diagnostic criteria for research*. Geneva: WHO.

Part III

War and Disasters

COORDINATING HUMANITARIAN ASSISTANCE WITH OCHA: ISSUES OF PSYCHOLOGICAL TRAUMA

Last year alone, nearly 256 million people were affected by natural disasters. Almost the same number of people worldwide are affected by complex emergencies—war, civil strife, terrorism, or genocide. Twenty-two million are displaced. One billion live below the poverty line. The number rises again, if we add the totals in the developed world.

Traumatic stress spares no one. The United Nations Office for the Coordination of Humanitarian Affairs (OCHA) has experienced its own share of trauma and traumatic stress: Its staff has been front-line witnesses to disaster and genocide, and some have lost their lives doing their jobs. OCHA staff who served in Rwanda during or immediately after the genocide, for instance, suffered atrocious and traumatic experiences.

What we now face, at the beginning of the 21st century, is a continuing rise in the demand for humanitarian assistance, not just as result of natural disasters, but also because of an upswing in the number of countries affected by conflict. The nature of conflict itself has changed in recent years. Protracted violence is, more often than not, now aimed at innocent civilians and children, in flagrant disregard for international humanitarian conventions and principles. As a result, on almost a daily basis, we in the humanitarian community encounter the evident impact and insidious effects of trauma on both the populations we assist and among on our own peacekeeping and humanitarian personnel.

In addressing urgent and vital needs—whether they be the protection of civilians, the guaranteeing of humanitarian access to captive populations, supplying food, water, and shelter, or simply trying to negotiate a minimum adherence to humanitarian principles by warring parties—traumatic stress on the affected population as well as on our own humanitarian personnel may be largely overlooked. Yet sustainable recovery—as well as basic human dignity—requires that we attend to mental and physical well-being. Accordingly, the UN system increasingly seeks to mainstream mental health issues into operational assistance strategies— such as traumatic stress awareness counseling in pre-deployment training, as well as training of trainers.

It has become increasingly evident to OCHA that it needed to strengthen its capacity to address the effects of trauma on its staff. Consequently OCHA now utilizes a Geneva-based Center to train, brief, and debrief staff deployed to and arriving from dangerous missions. The psychologists retained in support of UN operations understand OCHA's working conditions and the high-risk field conditions in which it operates. On a regular basis, workshops are conducted through Emergency Field Coordination Training teams. Up to 50–60 staff at a time are rigorously trained on how to recognize and cope with traumatic stress, how to help others and themselves, and how to differentiate between symptoms of stress management and trauma. Much has been achieved recently, yet much more remains to be done.

Trauma Interventions in War and Peace: Prevention, Practice, and Policy sheds light on this significant issue and its pervasiveness. More importantly, because traumatic events can take so many forms, the book quite rightly examines the multi- dimensional character of trauma. In humanitarian crises, trauma spares no strata of population. We see its effects on older persons, on children, on displaced persons, and on former combatants unable to reintegrate into society; we see it drive the emergence of criminalized economies in which the victims of crime, violence, and torture suffer in despair for years, or maybe decades. It is the effects on children, however, that go mostly unnoticed, with implications for their future roles as responsible citizens and the decision-makers of tomorrow.

Trauma Interventions in War and Peace will support the evolving awareness in the humanitarian community of the rampant effects of traumatic stress. We encourage broad awareness of this book and the issues therein. We commend the authors for undertaking this valuable contribution to the field.

MARK BOWDEN
Director, Policy Development and Studies
Office for the Coordination of Humanitarian Affairs
United Nations

OCHA's mission is to mobilize and coordinate the collective efforts of the international community, in particular those of the UN system, to meet in a coherent and timely manner the needs of those exposed to human suffering and material destruction in disasters and emergencies. This involves reducing vulnerability, promoting solutions to root causes, and facilitating the smooth transition from relief to rehabilitation and development.

Chapter 10

Children in Armed Conflict

William Yule, Rune Stuvland, Florence K. Baingana, and Patrick Smith

UNICEF recently estimated that over 80% of the victims of today's warfare are women and children. Civilian populations are deliberately targeted; "ethnic cleansing" and massacres are almost commonplace; populations are held hostage and under siege; even international economic sanctions are used as weapons in the struggles. The Northern Uganda Psychosocial Needs Assessment (NUPSNA) found that the core problem is conflict and insecurity, leading to abductions of young adults and children, displacement of populations both internally and across borders, social breakdown, lack of basic services such as health and education, and failure to meet basic needs. These in turn may lead to a number of psychosocial consequences including anger, violence, depression, anxiety, early and unprotected sexual activity, teenage pregnancy, alcoholism, promiscuity, prostitution, drug abuse, family breakdown, and so on.

Whether it be in Vietnam, Cambodia, Rwanda, or Bosnia, modern wars result in many families with young children fleeing for safety. "Ethnic cleansing" in Yugoslavia dislocated thousands of people. Simply to escape the fighting and risk of reprisal, people uproot and seek safety in other countries. The result is an estimated 19 million or more people who are refugees (within the formal meaning of the term as defined by the 1951 UN Convention), with a further 27 million people living in refugee-like situations, and 25 million being internally displaced but not having crossed any international border (United Nations, 1996; Rutter, 1994). At least half of all refugees and displaced people are children.

It is not difficult to imagine the experiences children may have had in fleeing from their homes under threat, witnessing fighting and destruction, seeing violent acts directed at their loved ones, leaving their friends and possessions behind, marching or being transported in crowded vehicles, spending months in transit camps, and eventually finding temporary respite in a country at peace, while the authorities decide whether the family can be granted permission to remain legally and indefinitely. Children are sometimes separated from their parents and arrive "unaccompanied" in foreign lands. Even if they remain with their parents, parents may not be able to provide adequate care and psychological support due to their economic circumstances and their own trauma.

Children are sometimes willing or unwilling combatants. As such, they may be forced to or may participate in committing murder and other atrocities. In Uganda, abducted children were often forced to murder their colleagues who tried to escape or were too weak to travel. They did this by battering the victim until he/she died. Some were forced to participate in murdering close relatives or neighbors so that they would fear to return. Thus they were effectively ostracized from the community and became bound to the rebels. Some of the girls were married off and/or raped and produced children with the rebels. These children are now referred to as the "fatherless ones."

The experiences that many refugee children have faced are contrary to what most people consider to be the basic needs of every child, which are discussed in the *Declaration of Amsterdam—The Declaration and Recommendations on the Rights of Children in Armed Conflict* (Aldrich & Van Baarda, 1994). These include the need for continuity of care by a loved one; the need for shelter and food; the need for safety and security; the need for good schooling. The *United Nations Convention on the Rights of the Child* (1987) has been endorsed by all but two countries in the world—Somalia and the United States of America. In relation to children and war, some of the most relevant articles about children's rights are:

Article 9—the right not to be separated from parents

Article 11—measures to be taken to combat the illicit transfer and non-return of children abroad

Article 19—right to the protection of the child from all forms of physical or mental violence, injury or abuse, and neglect or negligent treatment

Article 24—right of access to health care

Article 28—right to education

Article 33—right to protection from the illicit use of narcotic drugs and psychotropic substances

Article 34—protection from sexual exploitation and sexual abuse

Article 35—right to the prevention of abduction, sale, and trafficking in
  children

Article 38—apply rules of international humanitarian law applicable to states
  in armed conflicts which are relevant to the child. This article also refers
  to ensuring that persons who have not attained the age of 15 years do not
  take direct part in hostilities. It further states that "States parties shall take
  all feasible measures to ensure protection and care of children affected by
  armed conflict."

Article 39—in full states that States parties shall take all appropriate measures
  to promote physical and psychological recovery and social reintegration
  of a child victim of any form of neglect, exploitation, or abuse; torture or
  any other form of cruel, inhuman or degrading treatment or punishment;
  or armed conflict. Such recovery and reintegration shall take place in an
  environment which fosters the health, self-respect and dignity of the child.

This Convention also established psychosocial care as a right of every
child, as well as a duty of providers of assistance to children in situations
of abuse, exploitation, and conflict.

The 1996 report of the UN Secretary-General on the Impact of Armed Conflict
on Children (The Machel Report) firmly concluded that psychological recovery and
social reintegration must be a central feature of all humanitarian assistance programmes. The report, based in large part on the conclusions of regional consultations
in Africa, Asia, Latin America and Europe, further states that programmes aimed
at relieving psychological suffering must take into account the social and cultural
context of the children and their families (UNICEF, 1998, p. 4).

This chapter will consider the rights and needs of children, and how
these can best be protected and met in times of armed conflict. It is written
within the framework and principles of the *UN Convention on the Rights of
the Child.*

Children are not just small adults. They are developing beings and
are dependent on adults for their well-being. Children at different stages
of psychological development have different needs, and so a developmental perspective is vital in considering the needs of children exposed to
armed conflict. For example, very young children may not understand
that a nearby exploding shell could have killed them—they may have an
imperfect concept of the finality of death. But that does not necessarily protect them from being terrified by the sound of the explosion, or by seeing
someone blown to pieces.

The effects of war on children can be far-reaching. Not only can children be directly affected by what they witness, but they can also be affected
by its impact on their parents and caretakers. Any of these effects can
distort the child's psychological development, with possibly far-reaching

consequences. Children can develop a wide range of psychological reactions and other reactions to war experiences. This chapter will summarize the evidence on the effects of war on children. In writing it, we are aware that, despite an emerging consensus among agencies involved in helping children affected by war, there are some dissenting voices (Bracken & Petty, 1998). We will attempt to articulate these reservations fairly.

NATURE AND SCOPE OF THE PROBLEM

War is a multifaceted set of traumatic events. Families may be split up; children may be the direct and indirect targets of shelling, sniper fire and fighting in general. Children may be physically wounded, malnourished, unable to attend school, and they may experience disruptions of proper health care. They may be internally displaced. In modern warfare, there may be near-total breakdown of the previous social infrastructure, leaving families and children uncertain of the short- and long-term future. The breakdown in social infrastructure can mean that neither formal nor informal means of delivering services in education, health, and social welfare function. All attempts at rebuilding such services should be carefully planned so that emergency services provided by UNOs and NGOs can be sustained within the framework of the permanent delivery systems.

Children and adolescents will react differently to various war experiences depending on their developmental stages. In particular, when planning how best to respond to the needs of children affected by war, it is necessary to consider separately the needs of pre-school children, primary-school-age children, and teenagers. The issue of child soldiers and the effect of active participation in war on children's development is also of major concern, as highlighted in the Machel report (United Nations, 1996). It will be discussed in a special section below.

While this section of the report focuses on the needs of children, these have to be considered within the needs of the family and the wider community. All humanitarian organizations are in agreement that it is vital to restore some semblance of normality and predictability to children's lives following war. This is best achieved by re-establishing schooling and other normal activities, and by supporting the family in order that they can, in turn, support the child. In addition, there is a need to identify children who have been especially badly affected and arrange support and intervention for them, according to the traditions of the community.

In September 1998, the UNICEF Programme workshop articulated principles on psychosocial care and protection. "The diverse and often violent experiences of armed conflict have profound effects on child development and well-being. The word 'psychosocial' simply underlines the dynamic relationship between psychological and social effects, each continually influencing the other. 'Psychological effects' are those which affect emotions, behavior, thoughts, memory, learning ability, perceptions and understanding. 'Social effects' refer to altered relationships due to death, separation, estrangement and other losses, family and community breakdown, damage to social values and customary practices and the destruction of social facilities and services. Social effects also extend to the economic dimensions, as many individuals and families become destitute through the material and economic devastation of war, thus losing their social status and place in their familiar social network" (UNICEF, 1998, p. 6). That working party also noted the ambiguities associated with the word "trauma," which at times relates to the traumatic event and at times to an hypothesized psychological reaction to that event which in turn compromises psychological development. We concur with the earlier working party's view that "trauma" should be used to refer to "... an event far beyond usual human experience that overwhelms the senses and ability to cope with the event at that time" (UNICEF, 1998, p. 6).

The best way to protect children's rights is not to resort to armed conflict in the first place. However, when civilized ways of settling disputes have broken down, those involved in trying to mitigate the effects of armed conflict on children should do so within the broad framework of an understanding of the *UN Convention on the Rights of the Child*. These rights apply to all children at all times, not merely during times of stability and peace. Children must be provided with access to health, education, and nutrition, along with the family care and protection that ensure their right to childhood. The children retain the right to be brought up within their own cultures and to practice such religions as they choose. If the parents are separated or killed, then the child requires not only care, but also the formation of emotional ties. When the child is unaccompanied and displaced, every effort needs to be made to reunite him or her with the extended family. Cross-national fostering or adoption must be seen as a last resort, for it may serve to weaken the child's cultural identity.

Accepting this framework has many practical implications. While the need for safety, security, shelter, food and clothing is paramount in the initial stages of any armed conflict, UNOs and NGOs have to ensure that their humanitarian programs incorporate an active psychosocial element that goes well beyond the traditional "supplies" approach. The key UN players—UNICEF (United Nations Fund for Children), WHO (World Health Organization), UNHCR (United Nations High Commissioner for Refugees), UNHCHR (United Nations High Commissioner for Human Rights), WFP (World Food Programme), OCHA (United Nations Office for the Coordination of Humanitarian Affairs), the Office of the Special Representative of the Secretary-General for Children and Armed Conflict, and UNESCO—collaborate with each other, with local governments, and with key non-governmental organizations (NGOs) to ensure good-quality health care delivery and education. Given the numbers of children with exceptional needs in war situations, mental health care needs to be community-based. This challenges the traditional individually-oriented therapy that has been the norm in many developed countries during peacetime.

Complex emergencies have a multifaceted impact on children's well-being, including effects on psychological, physical, and social development, on education, on health, on nutrition, and on parental support and guidance, as well as on dynamics within the community. It is therefore imperative that these different facets be addressed when designing interventions for children affected by complex emergencies. Interventions will be most useful when they take into account the parents' psychological state, the dynamics of family and community, the availability and appropriateness of formal education, the availability of health care services, what leisure activities the child has access to, and so on.

This implies the need for a multi-sectoral approach to designing psychosocial interventions for children affected by conflict. Health, probation, child welfare, and education sectors all have vital roles to play. Many NGOs can undertake community-based work that addresses the needs of the children, parents, and community at large so that there is a continuum of care for the child from the school, health center, and within the community.

THE EFFECTS OF WAR-RELATED TRAUMA

Stress Reactions in Children

All or nearly all children exposed to war stressors will show some kind of initial short term emotional reaction (Richman, 1993). This was shown following rioting in Belfast, where children showed increased anxiety, sleep problems, school refusal, loss of appetite, and other somatic symptoms (Fraser, 1974). In Israel, following a fatal bomb attack, children showed fright and panic (Ayalon, 1983). The question for child mental health workers is to what extent these normal reactions disappear without outside help (i.e., outside the family) and to what extent there are severe and/or longer-lasting reactions that do require outside help.

As noted earlier, children respond somewhat differently than adults to major stressors. As a result of trauma and disaster in peacetime, a range of stress reactions have been reported that may also be applicable to wartime stressors (Pynoos, 1994; Yule, 1999).

Most children are troubled by repetitive, intrusive thoughts about the incidents or events. Such thoughts can occur at any time, but particularly when the children are otherwise quiet, as when they are trying to drop off to sleep. At other times, the thoughts and vivid recollections are triggered by reminders in their environment. Vivid flashbacks are not uncommon. Sleep disturbances are very common, particularly in the first few weeks. Fears of the dark and bad dreams, nightmares, and waking through the night are widespread. Separation difficulties are frequent, even among teenagers. For the first few days, children may not want to let their parents out of their sight, and may even revert to sleeping in the parental bed. Many children become much more irritable and angry than previously, with both parents and peers.

Although child survivors often experience a pressure to talk about their experiences, paradoxically, they also find it very difficult to talk with their parents and peers. Often they do not want to upset the adults, and so parents may not be aware of the full extent of their children's suffering. Peers may hold back from asking what happened in case they upset the child further; the survivor often feels this as a rejection.

Children also report a number of cognitive changes. Many experience difficulties in concentration, especially in school work. Others report memory problems, both in mastering new material and in remembering old skills such as reading music. They become very alert to danger in their environment, being adversely affected by reports of other stressors.

Survivors have learned that life is very fragile. This can lead to a loss of faith in the future or a sense of foreshortened future. Their priorities change. Some feel they should live each day to the full and not plan far ahead. Others realize they have been over-concerned with materialistic or petty matters and resolve to rethink their values. Their "assumptive world" has been challenged (Janoff-Bulman, 1985).

Not surprisingly, many develop fears associated with specific aspects of their experiences. They avoid situations they associate with the traumatic event. Many experience "survivor guilt"—about surviving when others died; about what they themselves did to survive; and they may think they should have done more to help others.

Adolescent survivors report significant rates of depression symptoms, some becoming clinically depressed, having suicidal thoughts and taking overdoses in the year after a disaster. A significant number become very anxious after accidents, although the appearance of panic attacks is less frequent and may be delayed. When children have been bereaved, they may need bereavement counseling.

In summary, children and adolescents surviving a life-threatening disaster show a wide range of symptoms which tend to cluster around signs of re-experiencing the traumatic event, trying to avoid dealing with the emotions that this gives rise to, and a range of signs of increased physiological arousal. There may be considerable co-morbidity with depression, generalized anxiety or pathological grief reactions.

In the past decade, there have been many studies of the reactions of children to war as well. Given that such studies are often mounted quickly and conducted under difficult circumstances, their methodologies are not always ideal. Different methods of sampling and different ways of assessing reactions are used, but despite this, a consensus is emerging. Studies from the Middle East, central and southern Africa, Southeast Asia, and Central America reveal consistently high levels of posttraumatic stress reactions across a range of cultures and types of exposure. Some of these studies are described below.

From the peacetime literature, there is a general consensus that the distressing triad of symptoms—upsetting re-experiencing of the event; avoidance of things associated with the event; and increased physiological arousal—are found clearly in some children from the age of 8 years upwards. Younger children show more varied stress reactions, but there are fewer empirical studies of younger age groups. This trio of symptom clusters, when strong enough and continuing long enough, has been identified as posttraumatic stress disorder [PTSD] and has been defined in the two major classificatory systems of mental disorders—namely DSM-IV (American Psychiatric Association [APA], 1994) and ICD-10 (World Health Organization [WHO], 1992).

Single-incident traumatic experiences produce a wide range of reactions that can include PTSD, anxiety, fears, depression and bereavement reactions. Where traumatic events are repeated in peacetime civilian settings—often in cases of physical and sexual abuse—the resulting psychopathology can have far-reaching consequences for mental health. In general, there is evidence that the greater the exposure to a traumatic event, the greater the likelihood that an individual will develop PTSD. Some events—particularly those that involve the child witnessing death and destruction, and which carry a threat to their own integrity—place children at higher risk than others.

As many as 50% of children may develop PTSD after a life-threatening experience, such as surviving a ship sinking (Yule et al., 2000). Seven years after that particular incident, 17% of the then-young adults still met criteria for a diagnosis of PTSD, and many more met criteria for depression and anxiety. Among the messages to be taken from this work is that while a large minority develop PTSD, and a substantial minority continue to suffer from it for many years, there is a majority of children who are more resilient. Considerable effort is under way to identify mechanisms of risk and resilience so that better preventive and intervention strategies can be developed.

The Psychological Effects of War Experiences on Children

If these are the levels of distress that follow a single-episode trauma in peacetime, what can be expected in modern-day war, where the traumatic events are severe, bloody, life-threatening, repeated, and chronic? Many of the children's reactions to adversity are "normal" (i.e., expectable), but that does not mean that normal suffering should not be relieved. The current consensus recognizes that overall levels of psychological distress are raised in children exposed to community violence or war. Although a minority of children are affected, the ones that *are* affected react in predictable ways (Cairns, 1996).

Different studies using different measures and criteria to look at child survivors of a variety of conflicts from many cultures all agree that the rates of distress are raised in children exposed to warfare. Cairns and Wilson (1993) found 10% of children in Northern Ireland were rated by their teachers as reaching "caseness" (that is, they met criteria for a psychiatric diagnosis) compared with 5–7% in societies at peace. In South Africa, Liddell, Kemp, and Moema (1993) reported that 50% of children had suffered psychologically. In Israel, Milgram and Milgram (1976) found that anxiety levels in children increased markedly in 75% of children following the Yom Kippur War. In Lebanon, Saigh (1989) found that around one third of children aged 9 to 13 years developed PTSD. Kinzie, Sack, Angell, Manson, & Rath (1986) found that 50% of adolescent refugees from Cambodia met criteria for PTSD 5 years after reaching the USA. In Rwanda, Gupta, Dyregrov, Gjestad, and Mukanoheli (1996) found that up to 79% of children who survived the genocide were at high-risk of developing PTSD. Fifty percent of refugee children from Nicaragua met criteria for PTSD (Eth & Pynoos, 1985).

In a recent study of the mental health of Kosovar child refugees in Britain, Yule et al. (2001) found that on standardized clinical interviews, 67% of the children met strict DSM-IV criteria for posttraumatic stress disorder. Thus, serious mental health consequences may result from exposure to war both within the country of origin and in any country that offers asylum. The resulting mental health needs should be assessed and met.

Depression. Depression in child and adolescent survivors of war has been far less studied. Mild to moderate depressive symptoms were very common in Kinzie's study of Cambodian refugees, with 21 of 40 meeting a diagnosis of depression (Kinzie et al., 1986). Mghir, Freed, Raskin, and Katon (1995) found similar levels among Afghan refugees. However, Eth and Pynoos (1985) found that only 3 of 30 Central American refugee children were seriously depressed. It may be that the uprooting and associated losses in resettled refugees increase the risk of depression.

For children who remain in the war zone, symptoms of depression are again very common. The small literature we have suggests that during war, the level of depressive symptoms rises, but may subside within a few years of peace (Smith, 1998).

Grief Reactions.   Given that children are directly exposed to war, that they may witness loved ones being killed, and that their fathers and other male relatives may have been killed or lost in action, it is surprising how few studies have looked at bereavement reactions among children affected by war. Kalantari, Yule, and Gardner (1990) reported that among Iranian pre-schoolers, those whose fathers had been killed and accorded the status of "martyr" fared better than those whose fathers were missing in action but not confirmed dead. These latter children showed higher levels of behavioral difficulties.

Following the bombing of a shelter in Iraq in which 750 people were killed, Dyregrov, Gjestad, and Raundalen (2002) found significant and lasting signs of grief among the surviving children. Nader, Pynoos, Fairbanks, Al-Ajeel, and Al-Asfour (1993) found that all but two of their sample of 51 Kuwaiti children reported at least one of nine symptoms of grief, with the average being four.

Risk and Protective Factors.   Peacetime studies are beginning to clarify which children are at greatest risk of developing distressing reactions following traumatic events. As seen above, with the large numbers of children affected by war, it would be helpful to those charged with helping them to be able to promote those factors which protect children and to identify those children at greatest risk.

Given that children during wartime are exposed to many traumatizing events over prolonged periods, it is perhaps inappropriate to generalize from peacetime studies to war. However, a number of recent studies have confirmed that among the most distressing experiences are the violent death of a parent; witnessing killing, especially of close family members; separation and displacement; terror attacks; bombardment and shelling; torture; exposure to bodies and body parts; direct life threat. Studies have repeatedly shown that the greater the number of incidents to which a child is exposed, the higher the level of distress that is displayed.

Studies of children a few years after war and studies of refugees settled abroad suggest that the extent of exposure is less strongly related to current symptoms, and that experiences during resettlement, feelings of loss, and current circumstances are stronger predictors of problems.

Several studies find that girls report more distress, anxiety, and depression than boys following a traumatic stressor, even when level of exposure is controlled. This finding parallels findings from other studies in child psychiatry, and it is still not clear to what extent the difference is biologically or culturally mediated.

As with studies in peacetime, there are few studies that adopt sensitive developmental strategies. Most studies rely on questionnaires for first-stage screening, and so children under 7–8 years who cannot read are rarely studied. Beyond this age, there are few age trends reported.

In peacetime, family support is a protective factor against the effects of traumatic experiences. In the UK in World War II, Freud and Burlingham (1943) concluded that the quality of care experienced by evacuated children was a more important factor than the actual exposure to air raids and other unrelated events. In studies in Lebanon and South Africa, it has been found that the mother's mental health was the main determinant of children's reactions to war/political violence. However, the measures of the children's mental health were made by those same mothers and so were not independent. Both Mghir et al. (1995), in a study of a small group of Afghan refugees, and Smith, Perrin, Yule, Hacam, and Stuvland (2002), in a large study of 300 mother-and-child pairs in Bosnia, found that the mental health of the mothers did indeed explain variations in child mental health even when the latter was independently assessed, but direct exposure to the traumatic event was the most important single predictor.

There are few longitudinal studies of children in peacetime, and even fewer of those affected by war. Dyregrov and Raundalen (1992) followed 94 Iraqi children for two years after the shelter bombing and found that their PTSD symptoms declined only slightly. Kinzie, Sack, Angell, and Clarke (1989) followed 27 of 40 Cambodian refugees 3 years after their first assessment and found that nearly half still had PTSD, while 41% still had depression.

Summary

This overview of recent studies shows all too starkly that war does badly affect children's mental health. Whatever the technical arguments about how symptoms are assessed and whether these are normal or pathological reactions, the findings clearly show that a substantial minority—often a majority—of children report high levels of distress that often meet criteria for diagnosis of serious disorders such as PTSD, depression, and anxiety disorders. Many children are bereaved during war, and this has been insufficiently studied. Large numbers of children are internally displaced or flee to other countries seeking refuge, and they seem at high-risk of developing depressive disorders.

Thus, methods of assessing war-exposed children at high-risk are needed, as well as interventions to help mitigate war's effects in the short term and treat the more severely affected in the longer term. It has been shown that while some symptoms decline over time (in peace), many children remain distressed for many years. Both in the country of origin and in any country that offers refuge, there is a need to provide help for these children.

INTERVENTION STRATEGIES

Community-Based Services

As noted above, all services for children affected by war must be delivered within the existing social and community structures. It is a vital and necessary part of any needs assessment to undertake a proper evaluation of the existing (or previous) services for children—health, education, and social services. Given the experience of UN agencies in recent decades, it would be helpful to have an agreed-upon set of procedures and standards that UNOs and NGOs could follow when undertaking a needs assessment. Without an understanding of previous services and what remains following the war, emergency programs may become isolated from governmental provisions and not be sustainable, no matter how good they are initially.

When communities are involved in warfare, teachers may be called on to fight, may flee along with other civilians, or may be killed—sometimes even deliberately targeted by one of the factions. Thus, the community may lose not only vital school buildings and equipment, but also experienced teachers. Those who remain may themselves be suffering from the effects of the war. It follows from this that in helping to normalize children's lives by providing schooling, those acting as teachers must themselves be properly supported.

Experience from various conflict situations has generally led humanitarian organizations to develop community-based, accessible, and non-stigmatizing services. In practice, where schooling is concerned, this means cooperating with the local authorities to support teachers in their work. Specifically, developing local capacity to meet the needs of children affected by war means training the teachers—in delivering the curriculum as well as having appropriate classroom management skills to meet the changed behavior of the pupils. Training also needs to include recognition of the behavioral and emotional needs of the children. In turn, this implies that teachers should be given some basic training in talking with children about emotionally difficult matters, in providing some basic first-aid to help the children cope with stress reactions, and in knowing how to refer the children (and to whom) for further help if it is needed.

Thus, a pyramidal approach to service delivery is often developed. At the community level, teachers have a pivotal role, as most children will be in school. However, community nurses and physicians also have vital roles to play in helping identify children in need and in organizing services to meet those needs. The use of explanatory leaflets, newspaper articles, and radio and television programs to educate parents about how their children may react, and where to seek help and advice are also strongly recommended.

Where, as often happens, local services are severely strained or have broken down, then both UNOs and NGOs have an important role in providing national or international technical advice and support. This often takes the form of personnel trained in one of the disciplines relevant to child and adolescent mental health services, and with some knowledge and experience of how to help children affected by war. In these situations, it is important to emphasize the training aspect, since emergency services will be time-limited, and skills that accrue to local personnel can be used during the reconstruction phase.

As implied, even where teachers and other community-based personnel can help many children, there will still be a need to develop more specialist services. In recent conflicts, as well as in response to major civilian disasters such as earthquakes, there are now a number of well-developed programs for working with groups of children whose needs cannot be fully met by the first level personnel. Again, there is a great need to provide proper training for those people who will be implementing such group approaches. In addition, there is the whole question of who is to provide the training for the trainers, as well as the issue of ongoing quality control for the services set up. Ideally, these roles should be undertaken by fully qualified local personnel, but they are not always available. Again, there is a need for better, evidence-based packages to be developed by international centers and disseminated by both traditional and distance-learning techniques.

At this level of services, one must not forget the importance of supporting normal community activities for children and adolescents, such as organized sports, youth clubs, and so on. Many NGOs help set up such activities, and their staff can be given relevant counseling skills to listen sensitively to the children, since children often choose to unburden themselves to youth workers rather than teachers or parents. The library-based activities in Croatia constitute one example of good practice in such community activities, and the radio station phone-ins for children in Mostar in Bosnia are another way of helping children share their experiences.

> *During the bombardment and siege, Tajma Kurt, a UNICEF field officer and also a radio producer, helped the children of Mostar to produce their own weekly radio program. A key element, in addition to interviewing pop stars who were passing through on goodwill missions, was children interviewing each other about their war experiences, their reactions to these, and what helped them to cope. Most importantly, each interview ended with the interviewee looking to the future and sharing his or her plans.*
>
> *The program was immensely popular and helped children share their experiences, and the approach shared many of the narrative methods used in counseling. This innovative use of community radio is now advocated by the UN Secretary-General's Special Representative for Children and Armed Conflict (1999-A/54/430 #59) as the "Voices of the Children" project.*

Some families and children will also need to be seen individually, and the precise way such services are organized will depend on local custom. Some programs have been criticized for putting too many resources into building centers rather than into training personnel, and clearly a balance is needed. Children and families do need to be seen in circumstances where their right to privacy is maintained. They need to have confidence in staff and know that their confidentiality will be respected.

In general, when child and adolescent mental health services are being re-established, current views on good practice should be followed. Not only should the interventions be evidence-based, but care should also be given to considering the location of the services. As noted earlier, the bulk of services should be community-based and easily accessible. Specialist services should be dedicated to working with children, adolescents, and their families and should not be located alongside adult psychiatric clinics or hospitals.

Again, resources need to be made available to improve and increase the number of local personnel who can deliver high-quality services to children. This implies that training should be based within the normal educational and professional training system. There should be greater resources and collaboration among agencies to develop appropriate curricula and distance-learning packages so that specific, relevant skills in addition to theoretical foundations can be transmitted.

There is a great need for different UNOs to cooperate in setting up such services. UNICEF, UNHCR, WHO, and UNESCO are the obvious lead players. As stated earlier, mental health services for children should be built into inter-agency collaborations of education, health, and social services agencies. Community and financial support for families will be important, especially where fathers have been killed or are missing. Changes in educational approaches can greatly assist children in getting personal support. The nurturing aspect of education can often be overlooked in the understandable desire to re-establish academic standards following war.

One of the principles behind these suggestions is that with the re-establishment of normal, community-based services, many children will be helped to recover and readjust more quickly. It is important that programs build on children's strengths and resilience. While the minority requiring specialist help will increase during war, they should still receive help in ways that do not disadvantage or stigmatize them.

Identification of Children in Need

Given that wars affect whole communities, needs assessments should be done at a community level. This would include an assessment of the state of existing social structures (families, schools, general health, and mental health resources) as well as an appraisal of the existing services that community offers to promote the recovery and well-being of affected children.

In most recent experiences, schools have been the focus of the community-based delivery of supportive services. Most workers agree that in order to get a semblance of normality back into the children's lives and the lives of their families, schooling should be restarted as soon as possible, even if only on a part-time basis. This being so, schools are the natural place in which to organize psychosocial help, and some aspects of that help can then be offered to all children.

However, experience also shows that some children are more distressed than others and will require additional help. In many communities, receiving counseling or other mental health services can be seen as stigmatizing, so any help offered needs to be not only community-based and non-stigmatizing, but also accessible and, above all, effective. There is a strong impression that some NGOs rush in to offer badly planned or inappropriate help which has not been evaluated.

Whatever the case, there is a perceived need for individual assessment. Economics mean that this has to involve at least a two-stage process: it is cost-effective first to screen all children using an appropriate brief battery of instruments of proven validity, and second to provide small groups or possibly (according to needs and resources) some individual work, for high-risk children.

Assessment (including screening) raises practical and ethical issues. Scales need to be appropriate to the language and culture of the children. If they are being adapted from other cultures, there is a strong onus on the project leader to gather evidence on the validity of the measures in that particular culture. Asking about war experiences may upset some children, so screeners need training in how best to respond to the children so affected. The nature of the questions and their purpose should be explained to local government officials as well as parents, and to children themselves, so that informed consent and assent can be obtained. It is vital to preserve the confidentiality of the information, and the means of doing this must be explained to the satisfaction of the parents. Where information is to be shared with other agencies—as in tracing families, or as forming part of health or education records—this needs to be specifically pointed out. Diagnoses cannot be made on the basis of screening questionnaires alone, and so everyone connected with the screening should refrain from using diagnostic labels in describing any of the children's problems. Assessment can sometimes be justified in order to ascertain need and influence governments to make resources available, but in general, assessment without the possibility for intervention is unethical. In gathering the data, it should always be made clear to what extent the responsible officers will be using the results to publish scientific studies. It is only by improving ways of assessing need and evaluating interventions that the plight of children affected by war will be improved. Not to evaluate these interventions is itself unethical, but it is even more unethical not to obtain informed consent to participate. The same practical and ethical considerations apply to the individual interviewing of children—be it by mental health workers, journalists, or anyone else. Repeated telling may lead to retraumatization and upset (United Nations, 1996).

Many of the problems identified above could be lessened by a strong international and interdisciplinary commitment to developing appropriate screening tools that could be made quickly available in emergencies. The preceding section on the phenomenology of distress is widely accepted among child mental health specialists and education specialists experienced in working with war-affected children. The domains of distress are fairly well identified, but insufficient resources have been put into developing cross-culturally appropriate screening batteries.

In addition, people have their own preferences for particular instruments. It would be useful to have a core battery of instruments that tap into the accepted domains, with individuals having the option of adding measures relevant and specific to the specific war circumstances. This way, over time, different studies would yield results based on comparable instruments and the knowledge base would rapidly improve.

We recommend a broad-based approach to screening children that includes a minimum of well-validated instruments that they, their parents, and/or teachers can complete. It is advisable always to obtain some of the information directly from the child, as studies have shown that parents and teachers grossly underestimate the effects of a traumatic event on the child (e.g., Handford et al., 1986; Korol, Green, & Gleser, 1999). Wherever possible, information from the child should be supplemented with information from parents and teachers. Different approaches need to be developed for assessing younger and pre-school children.

We recommend that the following domains be systematically assessed:

1. The war experiences of the child
2. Stress reactions
3. Other anxiety reactions
4. Depression
5. Bereavement

To this might be added:

6. Parent's mental health
7. Family functioning
8. Child's coping strategies

These latter three are probably more relevant to a second stage in evaluating the needs of children in their family context rather than screening the total population of school children.

In addition, concern has been expressed that simple screening instruments may over-estimate level of symptoms and functioning. It is known from studies in civilian groups that the type of battery recommended above does identify people at high-risk of having disabling problems. Children who score highly (indicating distress) soon after a traumatic event tend to score highly one to seven years later as well. They also have a high level of positive disorders when assessed clinically. This likely holds true in wartime as well.

Even so, now that basic screening technology is fairly well developed, there is an urgent need to develop additional instruments that will indicate levels of difficulty in functioning in everyday life. For example, the Foundation for the Study of Children and War is field-testing an instrument that aims to assess the impact of trauma on children's functioning in the classroom—their concentration, standard of work, and the like—which has greater ecological validity and meaning for their teachers than some of the screening instruments now available. Similar scales should be developed to assess the impact on everyday functioning in the family and community.

Special Circumstances and Special Groups

Child Soldiers.   Children have served armies, either voluntarily or under coercion, in supportive roles in many conflicts. The Machel Report (United Nations, 1996) cites evidence that nearly a quarter of a million child soldiers saw armed conflict in 25 different conflict zones in the late 1980s. Most of these were teenagers, but many were under the age of 10 years. "Involving children as soldiers has been made easier by the proliferation of inexpensive light weapons" (para 27). Thus, child soldiers are no longer only cooks, porters, and messengers; they also become seasoned killers.

Children are recruited in many ways, especially from the poorest, least-privileged sectors. Whether they are street children in Ethiopia, members of whole school classes in Myanmar, or children caught up in the conflicts in El Salvador, Afghanistan, Turkey, Sri Lanka, or Rwanda, both boys and girls are taught to kill. Girls may also be forced to provide sexual services. The whole experience separates them from their families and normal society.

The concern is not only with the exploitation and brutalization of these children but also with the disruption to their education and normal development. The worry is that they will prove difficult to rehabilitate and to reintegrate into society. How does a child who has killed many adults settle back into normal classroom routines? The long-term adjustment of child soldiers has been inadequately studied, but on basic human-rights principles, the practice of recruiting children under 18 should be universally condemned.

> *Twenty child soldiers who had joined the Tamil Tigers in the civil war in Sri Lanka were later interviewed as refugees in Norway. Many joined after they personally had been touched by the violence—often witnessing a friend or family member killed. Revenge, anger, and the belief in fighting for their freedom sustained them initially. After military training, they took part in a variety of actions, including killing and torture. The worst aspect of being a soldier was not so much the hardship as witnessing the death of close friends. One young man recalled, "I planned an attack on an Army camp. The two boys who accompanied me . . . got killed. I am greatly ashamed of what I did. It would have been okay if I had died." Another said, "We had this fear at night, when our movement boys were shot by other movements. It was a psychological torture—as we waited for our turn." Both at the time and later, as they reflected from a greater maturity, many reported feeling marginalized, even ostracized, by their own community. Even so, many remained proud of having been freedom fighters, and did not appear to have been as damaged psychologically as might have been expected. Clearly, children who are forced into committing atrocities will be in a different position. The concern remains that those who are exposed to violence at an early age will have greater problems developing normally (Kanagaratnam, 1996).*

Children with Special Educational Needs.   Children with special educational needs are still not a priority in many countries. Their needs are exacerbated during war, and special consideration needs to be given to meeting those needs. When a previous, segregated system has been destroyed, it is important that the old stigmatizing system is not automatically rebuilt during the emergency or reconstruction phases. Although donors may respond generously to calls to rebuild "orphanages" for mentally handicapped victims of war, re-inventing and rebuilding whole institutions should be avoided. Instead, wherever possible, the education system should be encouraged to move toward meeting individual needs within the community.

Care of Unaccompanied Children.   Children who become separated from their families are at special risk for all sorts of exploitation. Again, there are examples of NGOs and others setting up old-fashioned orphanages to provide shelter for these children without considering more-child-oriented alternatives. Not all countries have a tradition of providing alternative family placements such as foster care, but thought needs to be given as to how best to do this.

Refugees.   Both internally displaced people and asylum seekers often have children and adolescents with them. The families and children often remain in administrative limbo for many years, and the resulting uncertainty about their future has adverse effects on the children's development. There is an onus on the receiving community or country to understand the nature of the experiences the asylum seekers have been through and to develop appropriate ways of meeting their needs (see Chapter 11).

Medical Evacuation.   At the height of war, it is not uncommon for some children to be evacuated to other countries, ostensibly for specialist medical care. The outcomes of such activities needs to be more carefully evaluated, for their impact not only on the child but also on the extended family. Often a parent has to accompany the child and so is unavailable for the other children in the family for months or even years on end. There are concerns in some parts of the international community that, once evacuated, some children do not return and may even disappear. As the Machel report puts it, "In the case of medical evacuations, difficulties often arise when the foster family, thinking the child will have better opportunities in the host country, does not allow the child in their care to return to the original family" (United Nations, 1996, para. 75).

International Adoption.   A specific aspect of child care is the inappropriate harnessing of people's emotional reaction towards pictures of suffering children. Too often in the past, children have been "rescued" by being taken to other countries and fostered or adopted, risking separation from their extended families and losing access to their cultural heritage. Governments need to be more aware of the rights of children in such circumstances and try to channel philanthropic impulses into more-helpful activities. Again, to quote the Machel report, "Ultimately . . . while reports of starving children or overcrowded camps for displaced persons may be dramatic, they do little to support efforts for long-term reconstruction and reconciliation" (United Nations, 1996, para. 28).

Monitoring and Evaluation

Given the enormous resources expended on helping children affected by war, it is important that the effects of all interventions are properly monitored so that efficient and cost-effective, evidence-based programs can be identified and promoted. Monitoring and evaluation are still comparatively in their infancy as far as children affected by war are concerned.

The recommendations made earlier regarding suitable tools for identifying high-risk groups have implications for monitoring. Many of the tools described can be used to assess needs prior to the start of a program starting and then be applied afterwards, both immediately and longer-term, to monitor whether desirable and meaningful change has occurred.

Programs of intervention can and should be monitored at a number of different, complementary levels. As with all child mental health services, there are many stakeholders—including the children, their parents, teachers, and therapists, as well as local officials. Some should be asked to give their opinions, while others can be asked to provide more objective data on children's adjustment. The children themselves can be asked for their views on how they experienced any activity or intervention, with an eye to making improvements. Any training course or seminar for teachers or nurses, for example, should seek feedback on whether the course objectives were attained; on what was seen as good and appropriate, what unhelpful; and on how things could be improved. Assessing client or customer satisfaction is one of many levels of monitoring.

The days are rapidly passing when it was sufficient for donors to learn that their funds had "reached thousands of children" just because 20 teachers would, in a lifetime of teaching, have some effect on many children. Methods of dissemination and ways of reaching large numbers will continue to be important, but the end-point effects are also relevant. Thus, there needs to be monitoring of process in intervention as well as in outcome. Outcome is a multifaceted concept, and evidence needs to be gathered from multiple sources. Some minimum standards should be agreed upon by humanitarian organizations.

Having said that, there are as yet very few published studies of programs of intervention aimed at alleviating the suffering of children affected by war. There are many descriptions of apparently good practice, but few studies with multiple data sources and reliable, validated instruments. This is not very different from the field of child psychology and psychiatry as a whole, but there are opportunities for improving the situation.

Following the earthquakes in Armenia, Goenjian et al. (1997) showed that a structured-group approach to helping children deal with their stress reactions helped reduce distress more quickly among those receiving the intervention, compared with children on a waiting list. Moreover, the treatment specifically helped reduce traumatic stress symptoms but not depression. In the control group, not only did the stress symptoms remain high, but the depression got worse.

In former Yugoslavia, because UNICEF adopted a standard core battery of validated screening measures, it became possible to compare two different approaches to intervention. In West Mostar, teachers wanted children to have art therapy. An acknowledged expert from Croatia trained local teachers, who, in turn, worked with 600 children. Reassessment six months later failed to show any significant reduction in the children's self-reported distress. In contrast, in Novi Sad, Petrovic trained local psychologists in a group-based cognitive behavioral intervention and, working with 100 children, produced significant reductions in symptoms as reported on the same battery. Although this was not a randomized controlled trial, and there were differences in the children's exposures to the war, it illustrates the potential usefulness of programs adopting a core battery that can be applied in different studies, thereby greatly adding to knowledge. Clearly, more studies are needed to better understand the utility of art therapy as a means of reducing the effects of war.

In summary, it is important to evaluate all interventions so that children benefit and resources are not wasted. The technology of good evaluation is improving all the time but is itself costly, and those costs need to be built into the funding of any program.

RECOMMENDATIONS

General Framework and Principles

Our views, based on our diverse experiences of children affected by war, are broadly in agreement with those expressed in the Machel Report (United Nations, 1996). However, we place somewhat greater emphasis on war's psychological effects on children and the need to address these using evidence-based interventions. We agree with the general thrust that all actions have to take place within a relevant community framework.

We strongly recommend that all UNOs and NGOs develop and subscribe to an ethical policy from which stems a code of conduct for assessment, screening, intervention, and research. The rights of the child should be protected at all times. We have argued that the great strides made in the last decade in understanding the effects of war on children and on how best to meet their needs have in large part been made possible by applying rigorous scientific standards to all of the work. This includes assessing the difficulties within their social and cultural context and not solely focusing on isolated reactions. We therefore recommend that there should be more work done through international collaboration on developing even better instruments that can be applied systematically. Such screening and evaluation instruments need to be as simple as possible without doing a disservice to the complexity of the issues being investigated.

We have recognized the need to have practical guidelines to assess existing services and their ability to deal with psychosocial problems presented by children and adolescents. All programs should strive to increase local capacities to provide child and adolescent mental health services through bolstering community structures.

Four articles of the Convention on Children's Rights are fundamental to ensuring that psychosocial services for war-affected children meet the highest standards: Non-discrimination (Article 2), Best interests of the child (Article 3), Right to life (Article 6), and Right of expression (Article 12).

Psychosocial programs should be available to all who require them, irrespective of gender, which faction the child identifies with, and so on. The programs themselves should be based on a thorough understanding of the community's values and culture. Child participation in these programs and in their planning and evaluation is desirable. Programs should have a family and community oriented approach, and should be linked to local services rather than being set up as parallel organizations, to encourage long-term commitment and continuity. We reiterate the Machel Report's concern about "donor pullout," which "can leave populations struggling to survive, particularly if humanitarian assistance has been structured in ways that encourage dependency rather than build family and community strength and integrity" (United Nations, 1996, para. 243).

Finally, we note the need to help the helpers themselves. Whether they be local or international staff, they are exposed directly and vicariously to the traumas of war. They may live in difficult circumstances for many months on end. They need and deserve to be looked after, both physically and psychologically. Good preparation and training, complemented by ongoing support and supervision, are essential to the good functioning of any psychosocial program.

RECOMMENDATIONS

Policy Recommendations

- Base psychosocial programs on a thorough understanding of the community's values and culture.
- Develop suitable training materials for primary health care workers and teachers.
- Develop concise, relevant batteries for needs assessments for use by UNOs and NGOs.
- Improve training for Child and Adolescent Mental Health workers in all countries—especially regarding stress reactions and their treatment.
- Develop strategies to assist in building local capacity to deliver better services.
- Ensure that agency staff is adequately prepared for the impact the work will have on them, and provide proper personal support.
- Give priority to funding interventions that offer the best evidence for efficacy.

Community Program Recommendations

- Reestablish normal sports, leisure, and other recreational activities for children.
- Provide youth leaders with basic counseling skills.
- Use public media to educate the community on the broad effects of war on children.
- Use media to encourage children and adolescents to share their experiences and aspirations.
- Use media to publicize available sources of help.
- Encourage different types of studies to describe examples of good practice that are community-based, and evaluate their effectiveness.
- Develop alternatives to institutional care.
- Encourage "baby-friendly" hospital procedures to support good child health practices in the early months.
- Encourage primary health care workers to support mothers in good nutrition and emotional development practices.
- Develop improved screening batteries.
- Develop better measures to assess needs in pre-school children.

- Ensure that schools are functioning, whatever the physical setup.
- Provide training and support to teachers to help deal with issues raised by children.
- Encourage good family-school liaisons.
- Ensure adequate land-mine-awareness training for all children and families.

Family Recommendations

- Provide education and advice to parents on how their children may have been emotionally affected by the armed conflict.
- Provide material and emotional support to families.
- In particular, support women in supporting their dependents.
- Ensure that proper tracing mechanisms are in place to help reunite families.
- Avoid setting up "total institutions" as opposed to family-style care for unaccompanied or orphaned children.
- Consider international adoption only as a very last resort.
- Support cottage industries to make families economically independent wherever possible.

Individual Child Recommendations

- Undertake interventions with children within the framework of the UN Convention on the Rights of the Child.
- Develop better ways of meeting the needs of child soldiers, especially those who have participated in killing.
- Ensure that the needs of children with special educational needs are better met.
- Make adequate provision for the education and welfare of children physically handicapped by the war (including land-mine damage).
- Encourage self-help groups with access to professional advice.

Evaluation, Development, and Research Recommendations

- Establish the validity of screening measures for different purposes.
- Promote research into better ways of training people to deliver such services.
- Evaluate the effects of medical evacuation on children and their families.
- Evaluate intervention programs—at both a community and an individual level—using standard measures so that comparisons of efficacy can be made.

REFERENCES

Aldrich, G.H., & Van Baarda, Th.A. (1994). *Declaration of Amsterdam—The Declaration and Recommendations on the Rights of Children in Armed Conflict*. The Hague: International Dialogues Foundation.

American Psychiatric Association (1994). *Diagnostic and statistical manual of mental disorders* (4th ed.). Washington, DC: Author.

Ayalon, O. (1983). Coping with terrorism. In D. Meichenbaum & M. Jaremko (Eds.), *Stress reduction and prevention*. New York: Plenum.

Bracken, P.J., & Petty, C. (Eds.) (1998). *Rethinking the consequences of war*. London: Save the Children/Free Association Books.

Cairns, E. (1996). *Children and political violence*. Oxford: Blackwell.

Cairns, E., & Wilson, R. (1993). Stress, coping and political violence in Northern Ireland. In J.P. Wilson & B. Raphael (Eds.), *International handbook of traumatic stress syndromes*. New York: Plenum Press.

Dyregrov, A., Gjestad, R., & Raundalen, M. (2002). Children exposed to warfare: A longitudinal study. *Journal of Traumatic Stress, 15*, 59–68.

Dyregrov, A., & Raundalen, M. (1992, June). The impact of the Gulf War on the children of Iraq. Paper presented at the International Society for Traumatic Stress Studies World Conference, Amsterdam, The Netherlands.

Eth, S., & Pynoos, R. (1985). Psychiatric interventions with children traumatized by violence. In D.H. Schetky & E.P. Benedek (Eds.), *Emerging issues in child psychiatry and the law*. New York: Brunner/Mazel.

Fraser, M. (1974). *Children in conflict*. Harmondsworth: Penguin.

Freud, A., & Burlingham, D. (1943). *War and children*. New York: International University Press.

Goenjian, A.K., Karayan, I., Pynoos, R.S., Minassian, D., Nogarian, L.M., Steinberg, A.M., & Fairbanks, L.A. (1997). Outcome of psychotherapy among early adolescents after trauma. *American Journal of Psychiatry, 154*, 536–542.

Gupta, L., Dyregrov, A., Gjestad, R., & Mukanoheli, X. (1996, November). Trauma, exposure and psychological reactions to genocide among Rwandan refugees. Paper presented at the 12th Annual Conference of the International Society for Traumatic Stress Studies, San Francisco, CA.

Handford, H.A., Mayes, S.D., Mattison, R.E., Humphrey, II, F.J., Bagnato, S., Bixler, E.O., & Kales, J.D. (1986). Child and parent reaction to the Three Mile Island nuclear accident. *Journal of the American Academy of Child Psychiatry, 25*, 346–356.

Janoff-Bulman, R. (1985). The aftermath of victimization: Rebuilding shattered assumptions. In. C.R. Figley (Ed.), *Trauma and its wake*. New York: Brunner/Mazel.

Kalántari, M., Yule, W., & Gardner, F. (1990). Behavioural characteristics of Iranian Martyrs' pre-school children: Preliminary findings. *Bereavement Care, 9*, 5–7.

Kanagaratnam, P. (1996). *Child and soldier: Long-term effects of active participation in combat Tamils*. Unpublished Cand. Psychol. Thesis, University of Bergen.

Kinzie, J.D., Sack, W.H., Angell, R.H., Manson, S., & Rath, B. (1986). The psychiatric effects of massive trauma on Cambodian children: I. The children. *Journal of the American Academy of Child and Adolescent Psychiatry, 25*, 370–376.

Kinzie, J.D., Sack, W.H., Angell, R.H., & Clarke, G. (1989). A 3 year follow up of Cambodian young people traumatized as children. *Journal of the American Academy of Child and Adolescent Psychiatry, 28*, 501–504.

Korol, M., Green, B.L., & Gleser, G.C. (1999). Children's responses to a nuclear waste disaster: PTSD symptoms and outcome prediction. *Journal of the American Academy of Child and Adolescent Psychiatry, 38,* 368–375.

Liddell, C., Kemp, J., & Moema, M. (1993). The young lions—South African children and youth in political struggle. In L. Leavitt & N. Fox (Eds.), *The psychological effects of war and violence on children.* Hillsdale, NJ: Lawrence Erlbaum.

Mghir, R.W., Freed, W., Raskin, A., & Katon, W. (1995). Depression and post traumatic stress disorder among a community sample of adolescent and young adult Afghan refugees. *Journal of Nervous and Mental Disease, 183,* 24–30.

Milgram, R.M., & Milgram, N.A. (1976). The effect of the Yom Kippur war on anxiety level in Israeli children. *Journal of Psychology, 94,* 107–113.

Nader, K., Pynoos, R., Fairbanks, L., Al-Ajeel, M., & Al-Asfour, A. (1993). A preliminary study of PTSD and grief among the children of Kuwait following the Gulf crisis. *British Journal of Clinical Psychology, 32,* 407–416.

Pynoos, R. (1994). Traumatic stress and developmental psychopathology in children and adolescents. In R.S. Pynoos (Ed.), *Posttraumatic stress disorder: A clinical review.* Lutherville, MD: Sidran Press.

Richman, N. (1993). Annotation: Children in situations of political violence. *Journal of Child Psychology and Psychiatry, 34,* 1286–1302.

Rutter, J. (1994). *Refugee children in the classroom.* Stoke-on-Trent: Trentham Books.

Saigh, P.A. (1989). The validity of DSM-III posttraumatic stress disorder classification as applied to children. *Journal of Abnormal Psychology, 198,* 189–192.

Smith, P.A. (1998). *Psychological effects of war on children in Bosnia.* Unpublished doctoral thesis, University of London.

Smith, P., Perrin, S., Yule, W., Hacam, B., & Stuvland, R. (2002). War exposure and children from Bosnia-Hercegovina: Psychological adjustment in a community sample. *Journal of Traumatic Stress, 15,* 147–156.

UNICEF (1998). *Report of programme workshop in the area of psychosocial care and protection.* Nyeri, Kenya.

United Nations (1987). *Convention on the Rights of the Child (CRC).* New York: Author.

United Nations (1996). *Report of the UN Secretary-General on the impact of armed conflict on children (The Machel report).* New York: Author.

World Health Organization (1992). *The ICD-10 classification of mental and behavioral disorders: Clinical descriptions and guidelines.* Geneva: Author.

Yule, W. (Ed.) (1999). *Post traumatic stress disorder.* Chichester: Wiley.

Yule, W., Bolton, D., Udwin, O., Boyle, S., O'Ryan, D., & Nurrish, J. (2000). The long-term psychological effects of a disaster experienced in adolescence: I: The incidence and course of post traumatic stress disorder. *Journal of Child Psychology and Psychiatry, 41,* 503–512.

Yule, W., Smith, P.A., Perrin, S.G., Turner, S.W., Shapo, L., Bowie, C., & Dunn, G. (2001, December). The mental health of Kosovan Albanian child refugees in the UK. Paper presented at the 17th Annual Meeting of the International Society for Traumatic Stress Studies, New Orleans, Louisiana.

Chapter 11

Refugees and Internally Displaced People

Nancy Baron, Soeren Buus Jensen, and Joop T.V.M. de Jong

Millions of refugees and internally displaced people (IDP) reflect the human consequences of armed conflicts and disasters around the world. These individuals, families, communities, and societies suffer from conditions of war and violence, all of which can be considered human rights violations, including torture, rape, abductions, sexual violation, war wounds, deprivation of basic needs, ethnic cleansing, persecution and harassment, loss of home, loss of loved ones, premature death, and genocide.

> Soldiers came during the night and rounded up all the men in the village who were over 18 years old. They walked them into the darkness and repeated gunshots were heard. A truck drove away after the shooting and none of the men or their bodies were ever seen again. The families of these "missing" men and their communities were deeply affected.

When the *Universal Declaration of Human Rights (UDHR)* was adopted and proclaimed by the General Assembly of the United Nations on December 10, 1948, the concept of mental health was not mentioned. Yet the overall declaration of a human's rights could be interpreted as a set of preconditions for good mental health throughout the world. Refugees and IDP come from societal contexts where their human rights were not respected.

SCOPE OF THE PROBLEM

Demographics

The populations of refugees and IDP have grown enormously over the last decades. In 1960, there were an estimated 1.4 million refugees reported around the world. In May 2000, a United Nations General Assembly report stated that there were approximately 60 million displaced people worldwide. An estimated 11.5 million were refugees who had crossed international borders looking for safety. Between 17 and 25 million were internally displaced in their own countries due to armed conflict or generalized violence, and roughly 30 million were displaced by natural, environmental, or technological disasters.

Studies of the dynamic flow of uprooted populations confirm that groups may be refugees yesterday, repatriated today, and internally displaced tomorrow (Desjarlais, Eisenberg, Good, & Kleinman, 1995). For example, in 2001 statistics showed that 45% of the burden of refugees and IDP was in Asia. This included 3.5 million refugees and 1.2 million IDP from Afghanistan (UNHCR, 2002). Since the overthrow of the Taliban regime in Afghanistan, the number of displaced people in Asia greatly diminished. The burden within the African countries, however, remains more long-term and consistent, with statistics of 1996 and 2001 showing that at least 15 of the world's poorest countries each shared the responsibility for over 100,000 refugees (McFarlane & De Girolamo, 1996) (UNHCR, 2002).

Country of origin and country of exile are major factors in the life conditions and hopes for the future for refugees and IDP. The remainder of this chapter focuses primarily on adult refugees and IDP. (For a discussion focused on children, see Chapter 10.)

Variations in Conditions and Consequences for Refugees and IDP. Refugees and IDP have one major difference. **Refugees leave their native homeland** to go to another country due to war, violence, or disaster that either directly or indirectly threatens the safety of the individual, family, or community. **Internally displaced people (IDP)** may leave their *homes* for the same reasons, but **move to other locations within their own countries**.

> Susan is a southern Sudanese refugee. Ten years ago, a rebel group took control of her home area. After repeated aerial attacks on her village by the government, Susan's family fled to northern Uganda. They live in a rural settlement on land given to them by the Ugandan government and receive some support from the United Nations High Commission for Refugees [UNHCR]. Susan is now 12 years old and attends a school sponsored by a non-governmental organization. She has no memory of Sudan.

Her daily life as a refugee is similar to that of Kamal, a 12-year-old boy internally displaced 10 years ago. His family is part of a Muslim population who lived in the north of Sri Lanka for generations. Due to fighting between the government and rebels, the Muslim population was forced from their homes. The government gave them a safe piece of land on which to live. Kamal attends school sponsored by the government. His family receives food supplies from the Red Cross. He does not remember his village.

Other similarities and differences between refugees and IDP depend on the particular contexts. They are not a homogeneous group of people with a single set of social issues. People often become IDP due to violence and political unrest. They are often members of disenfranchised groups and, once displaced, are dependent on their existing governments to coordinate their security or support (e.g., Sri Lanka and Burundi). Yet, in many situations, their displacement stems from their relationship with their government. Within the United Nations, an Inter-Agency Standing Committee, in collaboration with the Secretary-General's office on IDP, established a series of *Guiding Principles on Internal Displacement* (United Nations Office for the Coordination of Humanitarian Affairs, 2000). The principles are based on international humanitarian law and human rights, and they aim to guide governments and humanitarian organizations toward the provision of adequate care and protection for the IDP. However, international law does not offer the same opportunities for protection and provision to IDP as it does to refugees. After leaving the borders of their countries, refugees have the advantage that UNHCR has a mandate to provide them with food, shelter, and health care, while IDP are dependent on their home government to support them directly or to request international assistance on their behalf. In recognition of the often desperate conditions of IDP, the UNHCR and other UN organizations have extended their assistance to IDP under certain conditions. In the year 2001, UNHCR took some responsibility for the care of 5.05 million internally displaced people (UNHCR, 2002). Despite guidelines and mandates, however, the adequate safety or sponsorship of refugees or IDP around the world is not ensured.

Losing one's home or living in an unfamiliar country without the support of family or community is difficult regardless of the circumstances, but the impact may differ depending on the context. For example, living in exile in the developing world may include the dire poverty and isolation of a camp, with full dependence on the United Nations for daily survival, while moving as a refugee to Europe or the United States of America will involve different hardships. The abundance or paucity of socioeconomic and employment opportunities in specific locations can influence psychosocial functioning and mental health, as can racial discrimination or other forms of social exclusion. However, relative poverty in Europe or

America, where there are social-welfare nets to assist people, is very different from the poverty of Africa, where starvation and disease pervade. For the refugee or IDP, regardless of location, "low socioeconomic status is a major risk factor for failure to adapt, cope, and achieve well-being in the new living environment" (Brody, 1994, p. 61).

In addition to the influence of economic status and living conditions, refugees and IDP share other psychological consequences. Both may be fearful and anxious in response to the loss of home, security, property, and loved ones. They are often distressed and angry about the circumstances or at the people who forced them from their homes. Both feel various degrees of helplessness and hopelessness. Responses may relate to feelings of permanence about their current situation. It is sometimes easier to have hope and imagine a return home when you remain in your own country than when you have moved to another country. Generally, it seems that IDP and refugees who go into exile as a community group more easily retain their cultural identity, traditions, and mores, as well as the natural support of family and community.

PSYCHOSOCIAL AND MENTAL HEALTH PROBLEMS OF REFUGEES AND IDP

Typical Problems in the Emergency Phase

The problems experienced by refugees and IDP change over time. In the emergency phase during and immediately following displacement, many people appear fearful, and psychosocial distress seems to be due to the experiences of the moment, worry about survival, and uncertainty of the immediate future. Though people have varying levels of symptoms of distress, most people concentrate their psychological energy on survival. For example, in Albania and Kosovo, during and immediately after the crisis of displacement, psychiatric emergencies due to trauma were few.

Levels of intensity or number of traumas experienced and extent of distress are related, but not in a one-to-one fashion. Some people are victims of extreme events without developing problems during the initial displacement, yet have symptoms of stress later, while others never have symptoms. Others may have symptoms at the beginning that later disappear. Some people experience what appear to be minor traumas, yet develop serious psychological reactions. Thus, simply experiencing an event does not necessarily trigger the symptoms of distress or more serious emotional reactions, like posttraumatic stress disorder (PTSD). Refugees and IDP who do become distressed often do not understand the relationship between their symptoms and the emotional trauma of their recent experiences.

Protective factors related to the individual, family, and community play a role in minimizing stress, aiding coping, and preventing PTSD and other disorders. For refugees, these protective factors include extended family involvement as a unit of mutual support, access to employment, human rights organizations' support and watchfulness, self-help groups for empowerment and sharing, small camps, freedom of cultural practice, and ability to frame problems in terms that transcend the immediate situation and give it meaning (Jablensky et al., 1994). The balance between number and severity of stressors and protective factors has an impact on possible traumatization, which might explain why some people develop reactions and others do not, even though they are exposed to the same events.

While the intensity, severity, and meaning of complaints immediately after a crisis may vary, the nature and types of symptoms seem quite consistent across cultures. Typical symptoms are similar to those reported by a focus group of southern Sudanese refugees soon after exile (Baron, 2002). They include feelings of fear and anxiety, physical pain (head, neck, back, chest, stomach, joints), shortness of breath and tightness in chest, loss of energy and motivation, change in temperament, estrangement from friends and family, disturbed sleep or nightmares, inability to make decisions, concentrate, or remember, lost faith and spirituality, inability to work, loss of interest in care of family and self, and change in interest in food or pleasure.

Help-seeking also varies. Often those who seek help do so from the natural systems that provided this help before the crisis. These natural helpers vary according to culture and can include extended family, religious or community leaders, traditional healers, physical or mental health facilities, or social service organizations.

Problems as the Years in Displacement Continue

As the years of displacement increase, there is a widening disparity in type of response. Most important to note is the resilience of refugees and IDP who experience traumatic events. Most cope adequately, creating a new life with varying levels of personal, social, and interpersonal change, even though they might experience periodic symptoms of distress. Some have alterations in personality, level of functioning, and quality of interpersonal relations. Others are unable to re-organize and re-stabilize their lives. Survivors seem to react to trauma, especially over time, in accordance with what it means to them. These meanings are socially, psychologically, culturally, and often politically framed (Summerfield, 1996).

Most often, after years in exile, the cumulative effects of the stress of their ongoing living situation seem to outweigh the memories of the initial traumatization. Van Der Veer (1995) writes that traumatization is usually not a specific traumatic event in the sense of an isolated incident or a set of events that have left painful scars for refugees. More often, it is an enduring, cumulative process that continues during exile because of distinct new events, in the native county and in the country of exile. It includes a chain of traumatic stressful experiences that confront the refugee with utter helplessness and interfere with personal development over an extended period of time.

A common pattern emerged in focus groups organized to discuss problems in refugee or displacement camps. Groups included refugees displaced for 1 to 18 years from Sierra Leone, Liberia, Southern Sudan, East Timor, and Eritrea, and with IDP in Burundi, Uganda, Cambodia, and Sri Lanka. The primary complaints always related to their present environment. The first problem to emerge was always inadequate food, and the next was either poor health care or the fear for their present security, followed by lack of quality education for the children (Baron, 2002). Repeatedly, refugees and IDP focused on survival fears rather than on past traumas experienced. The basis for these fears is not completely clear. Are they psychological reactions to the traumatic events experienced, exaggerations to elicit more assistance, or realistically-based fears about the reality of living in ongoing misery without security?

It has been suggested that refugee environments promote dependency or "learned helplessness" (Seligman, 1975), where people may give up the little control they do have. For example, Theodore and Elioto (1990) describe Afghan refugee men in long-term exile as experiencing

> the tragic psychopathological consequences of proud men becoming dependent on others for things they once handled well themselves. As a group, the men felt helpless, frustrated, angry and anxious. Their sense of helplessness in the face of brutality toward them and their families, coupled with the vulnerability they felt due to the destruction of their traditional self-reliance and pride, left many of them depressed, helpless, anergic, and demoralized (p. 57).

Harrell-Bond (1986), however, suggests that the "dependency syndrome" often observed among refugees is the result of the way in which aid is managed by humanitarian agencies. She believes that the method of giving makes a difficult life situation even worse.

The UNHCR, humanitarian organizations, and governments care for most displaced people. Each helping group has a limited budget, so the fears of refugees and IDP about survival are often real. For example, due to poor health care, sanitation, and nutrition during periods of displacement, child mortality can be as much as 60 times the expected rates (Toole & Waldman, 1993). Even with international laws mandating protection and provision, and with the best of moral intentions by all of the helpers, displaced people often live in inadequate life conditions, without comprehensive assistance. As an example, the UNHCR health budget in one refugee site, with almost a half a million refugees, had only $1.00 U.S. per person to spend per year. In this same site, refugees were provided with a diet of only 1700 calories per day. Diets are often unbalanced due to unavailability of stock, and refugees sell parts of their rations in order to survive. Most refugee health centers have limited medication supplies—often only aspirin and chloroquine. In some countries with large numbers of people who are HIV-positive, education programs effectively teach about the need to use condoms but are unable to provide adequate supplies. Refugees from Burma, Sierra Leone, and southern Sudan are terrorized by rebel groups while living in UNHCR-sponsored camps. Unfortunately, after surviving armed conflict, refugees or IDP may face new or similar life dangers in their new locations.

Cultural Presentation of Problems

Though refugees and IDP from around the world share similar problems, they experience and resolve them differently depending on cultural norms. In the developed world, autonomy and individualization are concepts for understanding and solving psychosocial problems. Individuals are expected to take responsibility for improving their own lives. Conversely, dependency and interdependency felt to be important in much of the developing world includes extended family or community as major sources of support and problem-solving. Yet, the responsibility for the care and maintenance of large extended families can also be a source of distress.

> *Steven is a 34-year-old Sudanese refugee. He has been living in a camp for five years. He has two wives and twelve children and is also responsible for his elderly mother and retarded sister. He is just able to feed his family from their food ration, a bit of farming, and the income made by one of his wives selling goods at the market. His youngest brother died of AIDS. Based on tradition, Steven must take full responsibility for the brother's two wives and eight children. He is encouraged by his senior wife to take the families into their home. She fears that the family will be punished by evil spirits if they do not provide full care for them.*

Variations in culture are also evident in the way people present their problems. For example, somatic complaints have different meanings depending on the culture. In the developed world, a headache might connote stress. In Asia, believing that the blood is hot or cold often refers to an emotional feeling. Within the developing world, stress and depression are often described as "thinking too much." In Africa, Asia, and Latin America, problems are often believed to be due to supernatural interference from a supreme being, evil eye, curses, ancestral or evil spirits, by a disturbed balance between heat and cold, or by trespassing on traditional taboos. Awareness of variations in meaning according to culture is critical to understanding problems and developing effective interventions for refugees and IDP.

Vulnerable Groups at Greatest Risk

In the context of substandard living conditions and the struggle with daily survival tasks, vulnerable individuals with special needs can become a burden to their families and communities (Desjarlais et al., 1995). Specific vulnerable groups include the disabled, mentally ill, mentally retarded, abandoned or orphaned children, unaccompanied minors, chronically ill, widows, and elderly without families. These populations often struggle the most to just survive.

> *Mary's last child, Rose, was born without problem in the refugee camp. At six months old, she developed a high fever. There was no available medication. Mary thought the child would die but she miraculously recovered. The child, however, was now different. Her development stopped, her head and body became rigid and she never walked or talked. She began to have seizures daily. When Rose was 6 years old, Mary's husband left the family, fearing that the child was possessed by evil spirits. Mary struggles for her family's survival. She finds it difficult to cultivate her fields since Rose needs constant care. The rest of her children must help and are unable to attend school. All are malnourished.*

Refugee and IDP women are at increased risk for gender-based violence. The aggressors can be soldiers, rebels, or the refugee and IDP men. For example, women in the former Yugoslavia were raped by government soldiers or rebels in an effort to terrorize the population. As they fled their homes and while living in the refugee camps, women from Sierra Leone were raped by rebels and soldiers. In the refugee camps in Kenya, large numbers of Somali refugee women were raped by local men or refugees while collecting firewood. Without question, gender-based violence provides added risk and stress for women.

Rates of Mental Health Disorders

Research efforts have tried to clarify the magnitude of mental health problems of refugees and IDP by studying the prevalence of functional distress, PTSD, and other mental disorders within populations in many different contexts. Most studies have been conducted with refugee rather than IDP populations.

Research is often initiated to look for the levels of PTSD within a trauma-exposed population. The resulting data are conflicting, with variations in frequencies of PTSD and other disorders reported. One reason for the variations may be real differences in the populations studied. For example, frequencies might be different in refugees in exile near their home country than in asylum-seekers in the Western world. Variations may also be due to selection factors., e.g., a clinical population of people seeking help in counseling centers, trauma clinics, or psychiatric institutions in the developed world, or countries in transition compared to community outreach clinics in the developing world.

In an effort to make a diagnosis, the DSM-IV or ICD-10 and various PTSD trauma scales are used. Studies often rely on the use of PTSD standardized scales, although they are often not culturally modified or tested, and cutoff scores vary. This problem was highlighted in an ongoing study in Burundi in a control survey (non-clinical population without services available). All participants had a history of at least one significant exposure to a traumatic event in 1993, with other exposures for some participants in subsequent years. When asked about the five most important complaints present on the day of the interview, about 30% reported a trauma-related complaint. Based on the 17-item PTSD scale, it could have been reported that about 15% had a PTSD cutoff score sufficient for PTSD. However, in further review of other mental health scales and a structured interview, the actual frequency of a PTSD-diagnosis was about 8%. This additional information showed that symptoms of depression and psychosis seemed to inflate the PTSD score (TPO-Burundi, 2002).

The variations in frequency of PTSD may also suggest that although we may see similar symptoms across the world that suggest PTSD, the meaning attributed to the symptoms may differ significantly. With these factors in mind, the following reviews some of the findings in the literature.

Rates of Mental Disorders in the General Population of Refugees and IDP. In a study of Cambodian refugees living in camps on the Thai-Cambodian border during the Khmer Rouge regime (1975–1979), 55% qualified for diagnoses of depression and 15% for PTSD (Mollica et al., 1993).

In a random sample of refugees, IDP, and post-conflict survivors, rates of PTSD were 37% in Algeria, 28% in Cambodia, 18% in Gaza, and 16% in Ethiopia (De Jong et al., 2001).

A study among Somali refugees in Europe reported that 38% suffered from PTSD, and an additional 60% from partial PTSD (Roodenrijs, Scherpenzeel, & De Jong, 1997).

In a study of refugees from Southeast Asia in the United States and Canada, Westermeyer (1989) found that 44% of Hmong adults in a 10-year follow-up in the United States suffered from chronic adjustment troubles (13%) and depressive symptoms (31%).

Rates of Mental Disorders in Refugees or IDP Seeking Mental Health Assistance. Among Cambodian, Hmong, Laotian, and Vietnamese psychiatric patients in the United States, Mollica, Wyshak, and Lavelle (1987) found that 50% of the patients suffered from PTSD. The diagnosis of PTSD was consistently associated with having another psychiatric diagnosis, primarily major affective disorder.

In a psychiatric inpatient unit in Denmark in 1987, about 95% of the refugee inpatients were asylum-seekers with PTSD reactions. At that time, there were relatively few and mainly political refugees in Denmark (Jensen, Schaumburg, Leroy, Boesen, & Larsen, 1989). Twelve years later, when the refugee population increased significantly and was no longer made up primarily of political refugees, an ongoing study showed that refugees in the psychiatric inpatient unit had a diagnostic profile similar to that of the native population. The frequency of PTSD among these refugee psychiatric patients was 8%.

A study examining diagnostic profiles of patients in psychiatric institutions in the former Yugoslavia found similar profiles of mental disorders before and during the war, with the exception of PTSD diagnoses. These appeared only during the latter period. The war-related PTSD diagnoses were reported for 15% of patients in Sarajevo (most active war zone), compared to 7% in Croatia and 0% in Macedonia (less active war zones) (Jensen, 1996).

A study of sexually violated men receiving counseling, all IDP and former prisoners from concentration camps in the former Yugoslavia, showed that 100% fulfilled the criteria for a PTSD diagnosis (Jensen & Loncar, 1996).

The diagnostic profile among southern Sudanese refugees (living in exile for more than 17 years) voluntarily attending community mental health clinics in northern Uganda showed the diagnoses to be about 70% psychosis, 20% depression, and 10% anxiety disorders including PTSD (TPO Uganda, 2001).

Rates of Mental Disorders among Vulnerable Subgroups within Refugee and IDP Populations. Prevalence rates for PTSD of 20% or more were found among torture survivors in the refugee camps in Gaza (El Sarraj, Punamäki, Salmi, & Summerfield, 1996).

A study of Bhutanese torture survivors living in refugee camps in Nepal and a matched control group of local Nepalese found that a diagnosis of PTSD was significantly more common in the tortured group (14%) than in the group not tortured (3%) (Shrestha et al., 1998).

Differences by Context.   Differences in findings between countries may be due to variations in culture, social factors, context, and time in history. For example, the level of PTSD is high in the Asian refugee population seeking psychiatric treatment in the United States (Mollica et al., 1987) and low in the African population seeking treatment in the refugee camps (TPO-Uganda, 2001).The rationale for the difference may be simple. Due to limited medication supplies, only refugees with psychotic disorders, major depression, and epilepsy are encouraged to seek medication treatment in the community-based mental health centers in Africa, while clinics in the United States may attract a different clientele.

Another complication in much of the research is that it takes an individual focus. In many developing countries, this is particularly problematic, since family and community are critical to understanding problems and designing interventions. "Traumatic experience needs to be conceptualized in terms of a dynamic, two-way interaction between the victimized individual and the surrounding society, evolving over time, and not only as a relatively static, circumscribable entity to be located and addressed within the individual psychology of those affected" (Summerfield, 1995, p. 19).

Most important to note is that the research shows that the majority of people do not develop PTSD or other major disorders even after traumatic exposure. They may experience various symptoms of distress, but most people are resilient and find ways to cope and avoid long-standing mental health consequences. This suggests the importance of studying resilience and coping to figure out what makes people *not* develop PTSD or other disorders.

EXISTING INTERVENTIONS FOR REFUGEES AND IDP

Natural Interventions

Similar to the research findings, experience shows that most refugees and IDP cope adequately with the distress caused by their displacement, traumatic experiences, and living conditions. Despite the distress, they are either able to activate an inherent ability to cope or they are able to utilize traditional methods of helping and support to establish a new life structure. De Jong (2000) states that coping with stress implies coming to terms with a new reality and trying to fit these new assumptions about the world with its harsh facts and with ourselves.

Normalizing the environment after a crisis appears to be important. In situations where traditional methods of coping, which include help from family and community, remain intact and retain their natural capacity to support their members and help them problem solve, people seem to adjust best (Baron, 2002). A range of protective factors helps minimize stress, improve coping, and prevent posttraumatic stress syndromes for refugees and IDP.

However, there is a percentage of the refugee and IDP populations that does suffer from symptoms of distress and might benefit from interventions. A few surveys have been completed that explain the problems reported by refugees and IDP seeking help. One was completed by staff working in programs for refugees and IDP from Sudan, Gaza, Tibet, Cambodia, Honduras, Algeria, Namibia, and Burundi. This survey found that the reasons people sought assistance, in order of importance, were health as most important and stress as the least:

- Health (sleep problems, headaches, body pain, epilepsy, neck pain, epigastric pain)
- Mood (sad, anxious, aggressive, nervous)
- Family (domestic violence, child problems, disharmony)
- Mental illness (psychosis)
- Substance abuse (alcohol and drugs)
- Social (lack of food, conflicts at work, poverty, unemployment)
- Cognitive (concentration, memory problems)
- Trauma
- Stress (stress, suicide, spirits) (De Jong, 2002)

With increasing frequency, psychosocial and mental health programs are established to assist refugees and IDP in situations where traditional methods are not available or may be ineffective due to the type and magnitude of the problems. The value of these interventions, as reported by the recipients, is often positive, but their effectiveness is not yet independently documented (Baron, 2002). Specific interventions designed for the specific problems of a particular population, using culturally appropriate methods that integrate natural healing styles and available resources, are expected to be the most useful.

Preplanning and Preparedness of Interventions

The main precondition for an appropriate intervention is the completion of a thorough assessment of needs and resources. A lesson learned from the large-scale psychosocial interventions in the last decade is that preplanning is necessary to be prepared for the inevitable crises. It is essential to have mental health and psychosocial disaster preparedness strategies in place in order to install a fast, qualified and comprehensive needs assessment.

Based on experiences in Bosnia-Herzegovina, Kosovo/Albania, and Rwanda, some common problems have been identified in the initial phase of interventions:

- Inadequate funds to quickly complete a systematic comprehensive emergency assessment.
- Lack of advance consensus within UN or UN-affiliated organizations about who was "in charge" and responsible for completing an assessment.
- A rush by multiple organizations with a variety of motives and qualifications into the crisis, collecting data from the same sources and often writing competing assessments for fund-raising purposes. These organizations often overburdened local professionals and international aid staff, who ended up spending a great deal of time giving information to the future "helping" organizations, which distracted them from more immediate work demands.
- Inexperienced professionals with little knowledge about the information that already existed in the field of psychosocial assistance to refugees and IDP. Some offered "help" based only on personal reasons or research opportunities.
- Lack of institutional memory in some international organizations. The documentation, staff, methods, and lessons learned from previous crises were not made available, so little was learned from previous crises.

Phases of Interventions

The design of intervention strategies is best when it comes from an assessment of the specific needs of the population of refugees and IDP. From crisis to crisis, there are similarities in the designs, but each still must take into account the specifics of culture and resources, as well as problems and needs as perceived and reported by the affected people. Each intervention has the best possible outcome if it begins with clear goals, aims, and purpose that connect to specific projected activities and a mechanism for monitoring and evaluating progress and outcome.

The immediate assessment of needs and resources often is carried out in the midst of the emergency phase. Although psychosocial and mental health issues are important, other emergency interventions, to help with such needs as adequate food and water, immediate medical care, and shelter/housing must be given priority in the acute phase. Even in this phase, however, it is possible to integrate a psychosocially sensitive approach in the way emergency aid is distributed. A United Nations report (2000) issued by the Secretary-General's office stated, "A major challenge for humanitarian agencies is to understand that the mental health consequences of emergencies can cause a level of distress that may hamper recovery as well as rehabilitation and to incorporate culturally appropriate psychosocial assistance programs in relief efforts, in cases of both war and natural disasters" (p. 4).

There are simple but important things to do even in the early phases of a crisis that can affect overall psychosocial well-being. Simple procedures for registration of people coming across the border, immediate systems for tracing and reconnecting people, use of respected community leaders to assist in assessment and in developing helping interventions, and provision of readily available and adequate food and health care, all promote feelings of mental well-being. Without them, the aid system may contribute to refugee and IDP stress. The majority of organizations implementing programs during the emergency phase are specialized in delivering concrete aid but not in mental health or psychosocial care. Many have recognized the importance of mental health, and have recently begun to add programs to their existing services in order to have a more holistic approach.

Mid- and long-term psychosocial and mental health interventions are only done by a small number of organizations that aim to create sustainable mental health structures in post-conflict countries. The international NGOs include the Association of Volunteers in International Service, German Development Organization, Handicap International, International Rescue Committee, Médecins Sans Frontières, Center for Victims of Torture, Save the Children Alliance, Transcultural Psychosocial Organisation, and World Vision, to name a few. Interventions may also be implemented by local NGOs. Financial and technical support can come from various donor countries and from UNICEF, UNHCR, and WHO.

Importantly, organizations need to coordinate with national mental health programming; however, these national services are rarely prepared to adequately handle the demands of conflict situations. National mental health assistance typically focuses on the management of institutions for the severely mentally ill living in urban areas, and there are usually few or no community mental health services. The more specialized international organizations, on the other hand, focus their interventions on assisting all areas of mental distress precipitated by war, as well as on traditional mental health areas. These interventions promote the use of local resources and follow a public mental health community-based approach. Though emergency response needs to be quick and efficient, sadly, history shows that most refugees and IDP do not return home quickly. As an example, the southern Sudanese have been refugees for more than 17 years, and the

Palestinians and Tibetans for more that 40 years. So emergency interventions must usually be seen as only a beginning and need to be integrated with mid- and long-term activities. Efforts in each phase of intervention must be coordinated to be effective for the beneficiaries and donors as well as to be cost-effective.

Systematic Organization of Interventions. Within each country, interventions need to be organized. A system of interventions can be developed according to the "6 Cs": Coordination, Collection of Systematic Data, Community Public Health Approach, Clinical Service Development, Capacity Building, and Supervision and Care for the Caretakers (Jensen, 2002).

Coordination. At the beginning of an emergency, it seems most effective when one UN organization or its delegate coordinates psychosocial and mental health providers. For example, this was done by the World Health Organization (WHO)/ Europe during the conflict in the former Yugoslavia, and it is also presently done by WHO in coordination with UNICEF in Kosovo. To be effective, this coordinating body must have full internal agreement and the power to require mandatory participation in regular meetings and sharing of information and coordinated field activities with NGOs and other UN organizations.

It is equally important to coordinate external efforts with local efforts, including those of the government ministries responsible for health, education, social welfare, and the like. In many of the developing countries, helping efforts must be coordinated with traditional healers and religious leaders, since they are responsible for mental health treatment.

In Guinea Conakry, once the home of half a million refugees, the government mandates that traditional healers are jointly responsible for mental health problems with the Ministry of Health. Healers exist throughout the country and in the camps, but formal mental health treatment is only available from three psychiatrists in one psychiatric hospital within the capital. Within the rural areas, the local healers, including those who specialize in mental health, are registered by the Ministry of Health and have a central office within the ministry.

Collection of Systematic Data. All helping groups, including the UN organizations, NGOs, and government, must work together to systematically collect initial data about refugee and/or IDP needs, and they must also continue mapping, monitoring, and documenting the mental health and psychosocial situation. Data can be gathered directly from the helping groups, community leaders, random samples of refugees and IDP, vulnerable groups, and those who have had specific traumatic experiences. All of the potential helping groups can use the same data to understand needs, coordinate existing resources, design projects, and write proposals. Since the population's needs change over time, data can also be used to update and upgrade projects to maintain effectiveness.

Community Public Health Approach. A community-oriented approach to mental health is believed to be the most cost-effective and potentially the most sustainable. Community leaders and local professionals are the best consultants to determine the most effective community approaches. The maximum number of people are helped and the service sustained when existing community structures are promoted and enhanced.

Clinical Service Development. The clinical services used within the community-oriented approach should be designed according to the needs, cultural orientation, and available resources of the population. Ideally, after assessment, a three-phase service delivery plan is designed that: 1) begins with a plan for meeting emergency needs, 2) continues with interventions to meet changing and ongoing needs, and 3) promotes the sustainability and maintenance of the services by the community for themselves.

As an example of matching services to needs, it was suspected that an increased risk of suicide might follow the apparent elevated rate of depression among refugees. Two studies with different long-term refugee populations had conflicting results. In the Thai-Cambodian border camps, which at that time had a population of 200,000, Mollica et al. (1994) found, in the space of a year, 35 suicide attempts per 100,000 and 2 deaths by suicide per 100,000. This rate of death by suicide is low compared to worldwide standards, so in this camp, specific suicide prevention interventions might not be necessary. In contrast, in 1999, a study examined the rates of death by suicide for Sudanese refugees living in camps in the north of Uganda. Suicide attempts were 46 per 100,000 per year. Suicide deaths were 11.5 per 100,000 for the total population and 25.2 per 100,000 for the adult population. Using World Health Organization data (Desjarlais et al., 1995) as a comparison, these Sudanese adults appeared to have one of the highest suicide rates in the world. Thus, a crisis intervention program that targeted at-risk adults was implemented. The suicide death rate dropped in the year 2000 by almost half, apparently due to the early interventions. The crisis teams were made up of specially trained community leaders, so the teams and the interventions were sustainable for as long as the problem persisted (Baron, 2002).

Capacity Building. Interventions require trained people for implementation. Most national health and social-welfare systems are not prepared for large-scale disasters, so there is usually need to train local people to effectively implement interventions. Often expatriate professionals are brought in as trainers, supervisors, and program developers. In the emergency phase, some expatriates provide the help themselves. To have sustainable care over the mid- and long-term, however, it is essential to provide training by local people who share the same culture, traditions, and language with the clients. It is important that training activities are adequate for the task, that they target immediate, mid-term, and long-term needs, and that they are grounded in existing local educational and training structures.

Training programs are most comprehensive when they cascade throughout the existing health, education, and government structures to communities, families, and individuals. However, mechanisms for doing this can differ depending on whether the situation pertains to refugees or to IDP. Local government structures are responsible for IDP in their own countries and so may be more motivated for training. Refugees, however, live in a foreign country. Though the central host government has theoretically accepted responsibility for their care, local governments in this situation often feel burdened by the refugees and may not be interested in building a capacity to care for them. Local government staff may be most motivated to attend when training also promotes the helping of the national population.

Training programs differ in developed countries compared to developing countries and countries in transition. In the developed countries, local professionals may have basic knowledge and skills for helping, but need training in transcultural issues so they can assist people from a wide variety of cultures. In most countries in transition, existing health professionals may benefit from training about modern reforms and the updating of their basic skills. In developing countries, there are usually few trained professionals. Training programs in these settings may need a two-phase process. In the immediate phase and in the mid-term, it is important to work with lay people and community leaders to build up a core group of resource people. In the longer term, the goal can shift to building more systematic training and educational institutions (Jensen & Baron, 2003).

Ongoing follow-up training and supervision is essential. Systematic supervision and training attached to existing institutions is more beneficial than "fly-in/fly-out" courses. Situations in which expatriate consultants are flown in for short-term training without follow-up and supervision often prove to have little long-term benefit. It is essential that all helpers, expatriate and local, are committed to assisting over the long term.

Care for the Caretakers.   Throughout this process, taking care of the caretakers is critical. Many local professionals and community helpers will have personally experienced traumatic events. Being exposed to additional traumatic experiences in their work puts some at risk of experiencing both direct and vicarious traumatization and thus becoming overwhelmed. Interestingly, however, in some situations, local workers report no additional stress. To the contrary, upon meeting their countrymen who have had worse experiences than they have, they report relief at their own situations (Prager, 2001). It remains important, however, that organizations offer support structures and training programs to promote awareness and self-care.

The risk of vicarious traumatization may be greatest for international aid workers. Many travel around the world from one conflict to another, often with a very limited network of support. In particular, UNHCR workers often live with much stress due to an overwhelming burden of responsibility for caring for refugees in exceedingly difficult circumstances with few resources. In UN posts throughout the world, workers from numerous countries are placed in isolated, often insecure locations. Many are without easy communication and are unable to visit their families frequently. Each posting may last as long as four years, and much longer for career workers. Many complain that their productivity is diminished by loneliness, isolation, fear for their own security, and more recently by financial cutbacks within the UN structure, which provokes job insecurity. All international organizations working in the field must be educated to the value of care for the caretakers and encouraged to provide their staff with emergency support, preventive measures, and follow-up (see also Chapter 14).

Levels and Content of Program Interventions.   The purpose of psychosocial projects can be described as promoting mental health and human rights through strategies that decrease the psychosocial *stressor* factors at different levels of intervention and enhance the existing psychosocial *protective* factors. The stressor factors in this context are the traumatic events and human rights violations experienced by the refugees and IDP. The protective factors relate to individual coping abilities, family strength and unity, social network, and ideological/political/religious consciousness.

The stratification of different levels of interventions allows us to create models that enable us to define the most appropriate intervention strategies for a target group, given available resources and presented needs (Agger, Jensen, & Jacobs, 1995). For the purpose of this chapter, different levels of program interventions are divided into nine categories (See Figure 11.1). The division is somewhat arbitrary and categories are interconnected. They

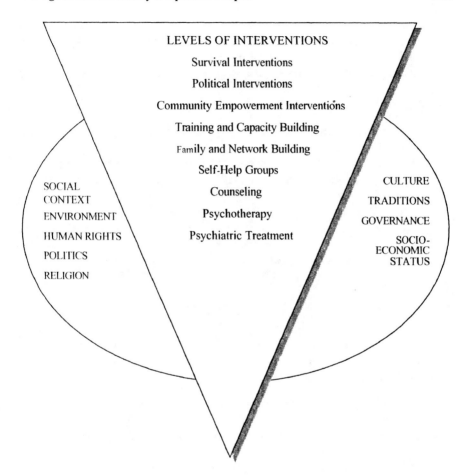

Figure 11.1. Psychosocial and Mental Health Intervention Levels.

are presented in descending order, with the interventions targeting the most people and requiring the least-trained staff presented first, and the interventions for the smallest number, but requiring the most-well-trained staff, presented last. Within each category, preventive versus curative interventions are specified. Lists of examples of some of the types of programs presently implemented in the field are outlined within each category. Each of these interventions is influenced by the context and by many existing community and societal factors, including those regarding human rights, governance, politics, environment, culture, traditions, socioeconomic status, and religion.

Survival Interventions (Preventive).   All helping efforts need first to ensure survival. The lack of adequate survival tools can cause extreme emotional distress. Types of survival interventions have an impact on emotional well-being. Methods used can either promote normalcy and empower people or promote helplessness and dependency. Examples of survival interventions:

- Helpers first request adequate food, shelter, security, and medical supplies from the responsible authorities.
- UN and NGO relief assistance staff is given psychosocial and mental health awareness training and taught methods they can use while distributing food and shelter to enhance the refugees' emotional well-being.
- The World Food Program utilizes food-for-work projects that promote self-reliance. Some programs also engage community leaders in assisting with food distribution to promote community empowerment. Other programs allow refugees to farm and independently feed their families to promote self-reliance and self-esteem.

Political/Policy Interventions (Preventive/Curative).   These interventions promote human rights, peace, democratization, conflict resolution, and reconciliation. They are critically important, since wars and violence are perpetuated by hatred and aggression within the same communities that hold the victims. Examples include:

- Advocacy for development and implementation of national mental health policies
- Education and training about human rights and children's rights
- Political advocacy to promote international tribunals for truth and justice
- Community dramas to relive previous atrocities and to discuss means of reconciliation
- Community sport and cultural activities to bring conflicting groups together
- Empowerment and reconciliation activities for widows of different ethnic groups

Community Empowerment Activities (Preventive/Curative).   These interventions promote community empowerment and self-help. Skills can be developed or taught that encourage communities to help themselves and to help their most vulnerable members, and to recreate normalcy within daily life. Examples of community empowerment interventions include:

- Psychosocial awareness education and development of helping skills for community leaders

- Psychoeducational workshops that teach communities about alcohol and drug abuse, childrearing, helping styles of communication, and other issues
- Promotion of collective traditional healing rituals and integration of psychosocial/mental health work with healers and healing churches
- Community education programs utilizing drama and storytelling that promote positive values, morals and self-help
- Community crisis intervention teams

Training and Capacity Building of Helpers (Preventive/Curative). Training is essential for all psychosocial and mental health helpers, including professionals, paraprofessionals, and government helpers. A cascade approach is often used for training to build knowledge and skills at all levels of helping. The training of local helpers builds the country's/community's capacity to care for itself. Examples of training and capacity-building interventions:

- Training a core group of helpers in psychosocial and mental health helping skills. The membership of this core group varies according to the country. In some developed countries and countries in transition, it contains professionally educated people. In developing countries, it also includes paraprofessionals.
- Awareness-raising and skills training of existing helpers like teachers, traditional healers, religious leaders, community leaders, and health workers
- Awareness training for communities
- Awareness training for UN, NGO, and government workers involved in development

Family and Network Building (Curative). These interventions promote the family and/or a network of supporters to help members who are vulnerable or have psychosocial and mental health problems. Examples of family-building and network-building interventions include:

- Engaging victimized families in the human rights movement
- Family counseling to assist a family member with a problem
- Traditional rituals that promote family cohesion

Self-Help Groups (Curative). Self-help groups are a sustainable method that encourages people with similar problems to help each other rather than depend on outside help. Participants share their feelings and experiences, and offer each other the wisdom that comes from being with others like themselves. For example, a common problem in camps is excessive alcohol abuse by the men. These men are idle, often feel miserable due to their lack of meaningful work, and develop feelings of impotence in regard to improving their lives or the lives of their loved ones. Self-help groups cannot change the reality of their situation; however, coming together to share feelings and examine the alcohol-related damage that is done to their lives and the lives of those they love is often the only way to provoke change. The influence of someone who truly understands the problem because they share the same misery is very powerful. Families who have had similar traumatic experiences, such as having a member abducted, murdered, or missing, can benefit through participation in groups with other families with similar problems. Self-help groups can be organized for ex-combatants, widows without extended family, survivors of gender-based violence, survivors of torture, families of the vulnerable, etc.

Counseling (Curative). The purpose of "counseling" is usually to assist an individual, family, or group to resolve emotional distress through talking in a supportive, confidential environment. The process of counseling differs according to context and culture. In some contexts, a counselor talks one-on-one with an individual and through support, encouragement, and insight empowers the person to find the means to help him or herself. In other contexts, the counselor empowers the family and community network to empower its distressed members.

The title of "counselor" is widespread and often controversial. People with wide variations in training and skill level all call themselves counselors. Goals may be the same, however, even if the level of training differs. Lack of trained professionals is a particular problem in the developing world, where there are few academic programs, professional organizations, or government guidelines for counseling. The title "social worker" is similarly confusing. In addition to providing counseling, social workers may also arrange material assistance and employment. Counseling interventions include:

- Paraprofessional counselors who provide crisis intervention, problem-solving, and supportive counseling for psychosocial and mental health problems to individuals, families, and groups
- Community-based counseling centers where services are provided by paraprofessional or professional counselors

Psychotherapy (Curative). The ability to provide psychotherapy requires extensive training and supervision. Within a post-conflict situation, people requiring this form of treatment are probably few. It may sometimes be necessary, however, when the person is unable to return to normal functioning after the experience of a traumatic event. In many developing countries, this level of treatment is not possible since the expertise is not available. Academic and training programs are growing in many world contexts. The therapist can target the individual, couple, family, or group.

> *At 16 years old, Abel was abducted and forced to join a group of rebels. He was tortured and forced to torture others. Finally, he was forced to kill one of his friends to prove his loyalty. After four years, he escaped and returned home. During his first year at home, he married and had his first child. However, he continually had nightmares. His fear of separation became so great that he refused to leave the house and would not allow his wife to leave the home for long periods of time. One night he beat his wife when she returned home after searching for firewood. Abel was referred to a community mental health clinic by his community leader. His therapist helped him to unravel the roots of his fear. He remembered the distress he felt when his mother and father died suddenly in his early childhood and left him in the care of a brutal uncle. Psychotherapy helped him to examine his history, understand and cope with his fears, and learn ways to improve his level of functioning and quality of life. His wife was also involved with him in couples therapy. She learned to understand his problems, and the couple worked cooperatively to help Abel change his behavior and improve their relationship.*

Some examples of psychotherapy interventions include testimony work, post-trauma therapy, therapy groups for children identified as traumatized, and therapy groups for survivors of violence.

Psychiatric Treatment (Curative).   Psychiatric medications are effectively used in developed countries and countries in transition with the small number of people suffering from a reactive psychosis, depression, or PTSD after a traumatic event, or for refugees or IDP who have other serious mental illnesses or epilepsy. In developing countries, the use of psychotropic medications by international groups working with refugees and IDP is sometimes controversial due to the question of future sustainability. The question is whether starting people on medications is ethical if upon their return home these medications may no longer be available. Many NGOs and UN groups believe, however, that the use of modern medications is a basic human right.

> *The first mental health clinic in the history of South Sudan was recently opened. One of the first patients was a 65-year-old man with a wild look in his eyes, who had not cut his hair or bathed in years. He lived by himself behind 15 years of high grass. His wife and daughter moved out years ago, and his son, who lived close by, tried to help him, but he refused all offers of food, fearing poison. His only contact with the world was to throw stones at people and count UN vehicles (though none existed in this area). A psychiatric nurse medicated him with a Haldol depot injection and chlorpromazine at night. Within 2 weeks of this treatment, he cut his hair, bathed, stopped throwing stones and cut a path to his house. Six weeks later his wife and daughter returned home and he had dinner at his son's home. He stopped counting UN vehicles, reporting that there were too few anyway.*

Psychiatric interventions include:

- Mobile mental health clinics within refugee and IDP camps
- Psychiatrists and psychiatric nurses trained in proper medication use for victims of war
- General practitioners and nurses trained to respond to psychiatric emergencies

NEED FOR RESEARCH AND COST-EFFECTIVENESS STUDIES

Greater understanding of hatred and aggression could prevent the cycles of violence that leave so many innocent people as victims, and provide peaceful means of mediation and reconciliation. Additionally, learning how some people who witness genocide and experience torture or other war crimes are able to "forgive" their perpetrators, or at least live "next door" to them without further conflict, is critical to designing long-lasting helping interventions. Without interventions that end hatred, violence erupts again and again.

Research has shown significant levels of PTSD and depression within refugee and IDP populations. However, most victims of war are resilient and cope with their traumatic experiences. Research to understand this natural resilience and effective coping is important. Once effective models are better understood, they can be integrated into programs designed for psychosocial helping and taught to those who are not coping.

There is little research that proves the effectiveness of organized psychosocial and mental health care for non-Western people. The accuracy of generalizing treatment outcome research findings from the West to populations outside the West is largely unknown (Sue, Zane, & Young, 1994). Even though an enormous literature has indicated that psychological treatment is generally effective in the West (Kopta, Lueger, Saunders, & Howard, 1999; Lambert & Bergin, 1994), the use of Western style psychotherapies outside the West is controversial. Research needs to determine empirically validated effective treatment techniques for non-Western people. Utilizing the results from this research, helping programs can be adapted to become even more effective.

Given the current trend among international aid donors to fund psychosocial and mental health care, it is essential to establish effectiveness information. It is theoretically possible that some of the current programs are even doing harm by focusing on vulnerable and traumatized individuals.

Additionally, it is important to compare the cost-effectiveness of helping refugees in the Western world to providing assistance to them within countries closer to their homes and cultures.

Though necessary, research is difficult to conduct within the context of conflict or war, or post-conflict. Violence can flare up at any moment, and follow-up measurements are hard to conduct since populations may be displaced again even after the end of an armed conflict. Preparing instruments for transcultural research is also a difficult task. Most accepted measurements must be translated and are not validated for refugee or IDP cultures. Comprehensive research results, however, will form a more informed basis from which effective interventions can be designed.

RECOMMENDATIONS

United Nations Guidelines

- Encourage equitable distribution of United Nations funds to all countries with refugees and IDP.
- Advocate for international guidelines and adequate levels of funds to fully provide for the protection of human rights and survival of refugees and IDP in all countries.
- Establish United Nations certification for NGO members who provide psychosocial and mental health assistance.
- Establish a United Nations-approved list of qualified mental health advisors/consultants.
- Establish institutional memory through a United Nations database, so that lessons learned in one crisis can be used in the next crisis.
- Establish formal United Nations guidelines for "best practices" for psychosocial and mental health work in emergency and long-term contexts.
- Promote quality assurance and effectiveness indicators as part of all United Nations-sponsored psychosocial and mental health programs.

Preplanning

- Include a mental health component in all emergency aid and ensure that prearranged funding is available for this component.
- Build sustainable community and government infrastructures for community mental health. Limit funds spent in emergencies to the management of crises, and retain most funds to be spent in mid- to long-term infrastructure and capacity building.

Coordination

- Coordinate mental health services and providers at all phases of planning and service delivery in order to provide continuity.

Capacity Building

- Encourage implementation of "Taking Care of the Caretakers" perspective and activities for all national and international aid workers.
- Establish systematic training programs nationally and internationally to promote psychosocial and mental health work with refugees and IDPs that includes training of UN staff, NGO workers, professionals, paraprofessionals, and those in related professions.
- Encourage relief and development organizations to integrate techniques that promote emotional well-being and empowerment into all aid work. Include assessment of these techniques in program evaluations.
- Promote interventions that utilize local human resources and culturally sensitive methods that empower individuals, families, and communities toward sustainable self-help.

REFERENCES

Agger, I., Jensen, S.B., & Jacobs, M. (1995). Under war conditions: What defines a psycho-social project? Emergency needs and interventions for victims of war. In I. Agger, S. Vuk, & J. Mimica, *Psycho-social projects under war conditions in Bosnia-Herzegovina and Croatia* (pp. 17–21). Brussels: ECHO.

Baron, N. (2002). Community based psychosocial and mental health services for southern Sudanese refugees in long-term exile in Africa. In J.T.V.M. de Jong (Ed.), *Trauma, war, and violence: Public mental health in a socio-cultural context.* New York: Kluwer.

Baron, N. (in press). Southern Sudanese refugees: In exile forever? In F. Bemak, R.C.-Y., Chung, & P. Petersen (Eds.), *Counseling refugees: A psychosocial approach to innovative multicultural interventions.* New York: Greenwood Press.

Brody, E. (1994). The mental health and well-being of refugees: Issues and directions. In A.J. Marsella, T. Borneman, S. Ekblad, & J. Orley (Eds.), *Amidst peril and pain: The mental health and well-being of the world's refugees* (pp. 57–69). Washington, DC: American Psychological Association.

De Jong, J.T.V.M. (2000). Psychiatric problems related to persecution and refugee status. In F. Henn, N. Sartorius, H. Helmchen, & H. Lauter (Eds.), *Contemporary Psychiatry: Vol. 2* (pp. 279–298). Berlin: Springer.

De Jong, J.T.V.M., Komproe, I.H., Van Ommeren, M., El Masri, M., Mesfin, A., Khaled, N., Van de Put, W.A.M., & Somasundaram, D. (2001). Lifetime events and posttraumatic stress disorder in 4 post-conflict settings. *Journal of the American Medical Association, 286*, 555–562.

De Jong, J.T.V.M. (2002). Public mental health and trauma in low-income countries: A model in times of conflict, disaster and peace. In J.T.V.M. De Jong (Ed.), *Trauma, war, and violence: Public mental health in a socio-cultural context*. New York: Kluwer.

Desjarlais, R., Eisenberg, L., Good, B., & Kleinman, A. (1995). *World mental health: Problems and priorities in low-income countries*. New York: Oxford University Press.

El Sarraj, E., Punamäki, R.L., Salmi, S., & Summerfield, D. (1996). Experiences of torture and ill-treatment and posttraumatic stress disorder symptoms among Palestinian political prisoners. *Journal of Traumatic Stress, 9*, 595–606.

Harrell-Bond, B. (1986). *Imposing aid*. London: Oxford University Press.

Jablensky, A., Marsella, A.J., Ekblad, S., Jansson, B., Levi, L., & Borneman, T. (1994). Refugee mental health and well-being: Conclusions and recommendations. In A.J. Marsella, T. Borneman, S. Ekblad, & J. Orley (Eds.), *Amidst peril and pain: The mental health and well-being of the world's refugees* (pp. 327–339). Washington, DC: American Psychological Association.

Jensen, S.B., Schaumburg, E., Leroy, B., Boesen, A.B., & Larsen, B.Ø. (1989). Refugees exposed to organized violence meet psychiatry: A comparative study of refugees and immigrants in a Danish county. *Acta Psychiatrica Scandinavica, 80*, 125–131.

Jensen, S.B. (1996). Mental health under war conditions during the 1991–1995 Yugoslavian war. *WHO Quarterly Statistics, 49*, 213–217.

Jensen, S.B., & Loncar, M. (1996). Sexually violated men. In S.B. Jensen (Ed.), *Mental health under war conditions in the countries of former Yugoslavia*. Copenhagen: WHO Report.

Jensen, S.B. (2001). Frontlines of mental health under war conditions. In I. Taipale (Ed.), *War and health*. London: Zed Books.

Jensen, S.B. (2002). In the aftermath of 11 September 2001: A European Perspective. *ESTSS Bulletin, 9*, 2–5.

Jensen, S.B., & Baron, N. (2003). Training programs for building competence in early intervention skills. In R. Ørner & U. Schnyder (Eds.), *Reconstructing early intervention after trauma*. London: Oxford University Press.

Kopta, S.M., Lueger, R.J., Saunders, S.M., & Howard, K.I. (1999). Individual psychotherapy outcome and process research: Challenges leading to greater turmoil or a positive transition? *Annual Review of Psychology, 50*, 441–469.

Lambert, M.J., & Bergin, A.E. (1994). The effectiveness of psychotherapy. In A.E. Bergin & S.L. Garfield (Eds.), *Handbook of psychotherapy and behavior change* (4th ed.) (pp. 143–189). New York: Wiley.

McFarlane, A.C., & De Girolamo, G. (1996). The nature of traumatic stressors and the epidemiology of posttraumatic reactions. In B. van der Kolk, A.C. McFarlane, & L. Weisaeth (Eds.), *Traumatic stress: The effects of overwhelming experience on mind, body and society* (pp. 129–155). New York: Guilford.

Mollica, R.F., Wyshak, G., & Lavelle, J. (1987). The psychosocial impact of war trauma and torture on South East Asian refugees. *American Journal of Psychiatry, 144*, 1567–72.

Mollica, R.F., Donelan, K., Tor, S., Lavelle, J., Elias, C., Frankel, M., & Blendon, R.J. (1993). The effect of trauma and confinement on functional health and mental health status of Cambodians living in Thai-Cambodian border camps. *Journal of the American Medical Association, 270*, 581–586.

Mollica, R.F. (1994). Southeast Asian refugees: Migration, history and mental health issues. In A.J. Marsella, T. Borneman, S. Ekblad, & J. Orley (Eds.), *Amidst peril and pain: The mental health and well-being of the world's refugees* (pp. 83–100). Washington, DC: American Psychological Association.

Prager, M. (2001). *TPO Kosova Annual Report*. Pristina: TPO.

Roodenrijs, T.C., Scherpenzeel, R.P., & De Jong, J.T.V.M. (1997). Traumatische ervaringen en psychopathologie onder Somalische vluchtelingen [Traumatic experiences and psychopathology among Somalian refugees in the Netherlands]. *Tijdschrift voor Psychiatrie, 98*, 3, 132–143.

Seligman, M. (1975). *Helplessness: On depression, development and death.* San Francisco: Freeman Press.

Shrestha, N.M., Sharma, B., Van Ommeren, M., Regmi, S., Makaju, R., Komproe, I., Shrestha, C., & De Jong, J.T.V.M. (1998). Impact of torture on refugees displaced within the developing world: Symptomatology among Bhutanese refugees in Nepal. *Journal of the American Medical Association, 280* (5), 1–6.

Sue, S., Zane, N., & Young, K. (1994). Research on psychotherapy with culturally diverse populations. In A.E. Bergin & S.L. Garfield (Eds.), *Handbook of psychotherapy and behavior change* (4th ed., pp. 783–820). New York: Wiley.

Summerfield, D. (1995). Addressing human response to war and atrocity. In R.J. Kleber, C.R. Figley, & B.P.R. Gersons (Eds.), *Beyond trauma: Cultural and societal dynamics* (pp. 17–30). New York: Plenum.

Summerfield, D. (1996). The impact of war and atrocity on civilian populations: Basic principles for NGO interventions and a critique of psycho-social trauma projects, relief and rehabilitation network. *Network Paper 14.*

Theodore, L.O., & Elioto, J. (1990). Afghanistan in 1988: Stalemate. *Asian survey and monthly review of contemporary Asian affairs.* Los Angeles: University of California Press.

Toole, M.J., & Waldman, R.J. (1993). Refugees and displaced persons: War, hunger and public health. *Journal of the American Medical Association, 270,* 600–605.

Transcultural Psychosocial Organisation (TPO)—Uganda (2001). *Annual review of client statistics.*

Transcultural Psychosocial Organisation (TPO)—Burundi (2002). *Report on preliminary analysis of research.*

United Nations General Assembly Economic and Social Council (2000). *Report of the Secretary-General on strengthening of the coordination of emergency humanitarian assistance of the United Nations.*

United Nations High Commissioner of Refugees (2002). Statistics for 2001. Web site www.unhcr.ch/statistics.

United Nations Office for the Coordination of Humanitarian Affairs (2000). *Guiding principles on internal displacement.*

Van der Veer, G. (1995). Psychotherapeutic work with refugees. In R.J. Kleber, C.R. Figley, & B.P.R. Gersons (Eds.), *Beyond trauma: Cultural and societal dynamics* (pp. 151–168). New York: Plenum.

Westermeyer, J. (1989). *Psychiatric care of migrants: A clinical guide.* Washington, D.C: American Psychiatric Press.

Chapter 12

Former Combatants

Brian Engdahl, Purnaka de Silva, Zahava Solomon and Daya Somasundaram

Our focus is on psychosocial and health problems experienced by former combatants. **We include all who have actively participated in war, including former members of regular military units, militants, rebels, resistance fighters andguerrillas, and former prisoners of war (POWs).** We summarize what is known about their psychosocial problems and describe potential interventions at multiple levels. Recognition of war-related psychosocial problems waxes and wanes after wars, and so does attention paid to combatants' psychosocial needs (Solomon, 1995). Combatants may experience immediate psychosocial problems, long-term psychosocial problems, or both, as consequences of their involvement in armed conflict. Interventions may occur immediately after, or long after, their traumatic experiences.

NATURE AND SCOPE OF THE PROBLEM

There have been, and continue to be, so many wars and war-like events that the number of people having participated in armed conflicts is vast. For example, Zwi (1991) counted 127 wars and more than 20 million war-related deaths in the world since World War II. The number of surviving ex-combatants is many times greater. Millions have been captured during conflicts in this century. Stenger (2002) reported that there are 42,800 living American POWs. In the brief Indo-Pakistani War of 1971, more than 76,000

Pakistanis were captured. Worldwide, the number of former POWs is many times these figures.

Combatants are exposed to many stressors during wartime; chief among them are physical hardships and threats to life itself. POWs experience additional stressors, including isolation and loss of freedom, malnourishment and disease, and even torture. Civilian resistance against foreign occupation and opposition against suppressive regimes can be particularly traumatic. Unlike military veterans, who act on behalf of the government, civilian resistance fighters and so-called "dissidents" primarily act on their own initiative. They often lack protection under international conventions or democratic legal systems. They not only have to face danger from those they oppose, but often also disapproval and even rejection by family members, and from other civilians who fear retaliation. One former rebel noted that he would love to go back to his village, but that he could never live there, as he knew the "look in the people's eye" when they saw him (De Silva, 2000).

Stressful Aspects of Recruitment and Training

Apart from exposure to specific life-threatening events and the resultant spectrum of problems noted later in this chapter, sociocultural aspects of warfare also have an impact on combatants. Political violence that attacks societal structures (e.g., "roundups" or "stop-and-search" of civilians) can serve to draw civilians into guerrilla warfare. Witnessing or hearing about atrocities can brutalize people even before they experience combat. Against this backdrop, in most societies recruits undergo further physical and psychological brutalization through combat training. Physically arduous training is used to develop combat skills. At the psychological level, morality and conscience are attacked through dehumanizing and demonizing "the enemy," by which means killing is not only sanctioned, but justified. War-related narratives are constructed to support this process. Distinctions between right and wrong are blurred, and peacetime morality is set aside. Behavior comes under the control of the commanding officers. Individual identities are submerged, isolated from social influences, yielding cohesive units that support the organization's objectives.

To illustrate how socialization in a combat environment is an important aspect of the stressors of war, we present the following story of the recruitment of a teenage girl in a civil war (University Teachers for Human Rights, 2000). For a discussion of psychosocial concerns specific to child soldiers, please see Chapter 10.

Kala was forcibly recruited by the Liberation Tigers of Tamil Eelam (LTTE) in Northern Sri Lanka. She and her classmates had been frequently accosted by LTTE recruiters, who also pressured teachers and families to persuade all students to join the LTTE. Kala and her friends were walking home when LTTE members in a vehicle stopped them. They were told, "We lost 400 comrades in the Kilinochchi battle and we are going to replace them, or else the Sri Lankan Army will retake it and their sacrifice will be wasted." They were forced into the vehicle and driven to a base filled with about 1000 other females. Kala was made the deputy leader of a group of eight. Kala approached girls on sentry duty who were from her school and told them of her group's wish to go home. The sentries allowed the eight to escape through the jungle. At one house a family gave them tea and directions. They eventually returned home.

An LTTE agent in Kala's area threatened to re-abduct her, so she fled to a neighboring village, returning after he was transferred out. The LTTE surrounded her school, pressuring the students to join. Kala was given mixed messages. She was told she need not have escaped, because the LTTE leader had withheld approval for her to undergo training. Supposedly, only those above 18 were to be trained, and others sent home. Another rumor suggested that all escapees would be captured and sent back, when in fact the LTTE did not pursue escapees; the LTTE maintained that the leader had rejected them.

Kala returned to the camp. She and many others felt homesick, but tried to forget about it and be militants. Others cried inconsolably and so were separated from the group. Kala was soon pressed into combat duty by the LTTE. Many months later she returned to her home village, but experienced adjustment problems. There was no knowledgeable professional help available. Support from family, friends, and the community was key to her re-entry to civilian life. However, the ongoing conflict in her country poses a threat to her ability to function optimally.

Powerful propaganda often captures plausible realities; people may be told that the enemy is determined to wipe them out, making no distinction between civilians and militants. Themes of sacrifice, courage, and martyrdom may be introduced. Elements of pseudo-legality are often used by resistance movements; their conscription methods are not purely physical. People conscripted in this manner may develop guilt, rage, and profound mistrust and fear of authority and society.

Gender Factors

Although military service may help liberate some women from sexist societies, women in the military more often experience denial of status and promotion, as well as disproportionate harassment and sexual abuse within their own armed forces, and when captured. Research on emotional vulnerability to military-related traumatic stressors among female military personnel reveals great variability. American female peacekeepers deployed to Somalia exhibited posttraumatic stress disorder [PTSD] rates that were no higher than those observed in male counterparts (Litz, Orsillo, Friedman, Ehlich, & Batres, 1997). On the other hand, American female personnel deployed to the Persian Gulf were three times as symptomatic as men with respect to PTSD (Wolfe, Sharansky, & Reed, 1998). Much of this difference can be explained by the fact that female troops had to cope with sexual harassment and assault in addition to the other war-related stressors of the Persian Gulf War. It appears that the risk of psychological distress among female military personnel may have less to do with gender per se and more to do with the severity, duration, and unique aspects of each distinct deployment. Therefore, it is currently an open question whether women in the military are at greater risk than men to experience deployment-related short- or long-term psychological distress.

Women may be kidnapped (or offered "protection") and forced to serve as combatants, servants, "wives," or members of so-called "suicide squads" (United Nations Division for the Advancement of Women, 1997). In Sri Lanka, at least a third of the press-ganged recruits were females from the Tamil community (Somasundaram, 1998). Raised in a patriarchal society, they had no experience of physical contact sports or the rough-and-tumble of fistfights. Therefore, their combat training heavily emphasized physical training and psychological conditioning to promote aggression against the enemy (de Silva, 2000). Many of these female fighters were viewed as more frightening than men, appearing to lack a threshold for cessation of aggression, particularly when conducting interrogations.

Vulnerable Populations

Even if people want to flee, there is often nowhere to go. Recruitment may be targeted toward vulnerable population segments, such as school children. The UN is presently devoting attention to the widespread problem of child soldiers (United Nations, 2000a). It provides recommendations for their demobilization and rehabilitation. Everyone involved—both the recruiters and the recruited—may become trapped in different ways in a "war machine" that becomes a systematized part of life. Many join because family members have fought and died. Those who are socioeconomically disadvantaged are very vulnerable, perceiving military service as a way out of unemployment and poverty.

Brutalization Through Killing

The psychosocial impact of training such as that described above is magnified through actual combat, as well as acts of cruelty, torture, and killing through massacres and other abusive acts that are not part of "traditional" warfare. Willfully taking another human life is always a special event; its intensity varies across perpetrators. The first killing may be seen as "breaking in" the combatant; often a senior has to initiate the new recruit into the act. One rebel fighter likened killing to driving a car, where at first one is unsure and rather shaky, but after a period of practice, it is as easy and unthinking an action as pressing the clutch, engaging the gear, and pressing the accelerator. Certain groups (i.e., terrorists) may have been conditioned to extremes of action, and may therefore be particularly affected by their experiences. Such sophisticated conditioning programs often make psychosocial interventions more difficult and time consuming.

IMPACT/EFFECTS OF COMBATANT EXPERIENCE

Most combatants and POWs experience short-term stress reactions; many of them recover. Others have longer-lasting problems. The effects of war trauma differ because each combatant's experience of war is different, and wars themselves differ in how many people are exposed to which kinds of events. Therefore, war-related psychosocial problems differ by conflict, and by combatants' characteristics and their roles within a given conflict. Who was the enemy? How far from home did the fighting occur? What were the physical hardships endured in combat? The meaning or context of the conflict is important as well. Was the war won or lost? Or neither? To what extent were combatants' ideals realized or disappointed? When morale among combatants is high, stress reactions tend to be fewer, and vice versa. How was the war appraised by the population and the combatants in the aftermath? When social support for ex-combatants is high, there are fewer chronic stress reactions.

War-related stress disorders not only compromise mental health, but also negatively affect quality of life and economic functioning (Fairbank, Ebert, & Zarkin, 1999). Ex-combatants may cause secondary traumatization to others by bringing violence into their own families and communities after the war. Participation in armed conflict is associated with postwar family violence and involvement in the criminal justice system, including arrests for violent crimes (Kulka et al., 1990). Interpersonal attachments, dependency, and spiritual beliefs may also be affected by war. War-related trauma can even be "transported" across generations (Danieli, 1998). For example, many of the leaders accused of war crimes in the former Yugoslavia experienced traumatization as children during WWII. Among American Vietnam veterans with PTSD, those whose fathers had served in combat in previous wars had more severe PTSD symptoms, more survivor guilt, less current social support, and were more likely to experience panic disorder and drug abuse (Rosenheck & Fontana, 1998). And the persistent resurgence of ethnic conflicts such as those in Nigeria can in part be attributed to cycles of violence that cut across generations (Odejide,

Sanda, & Odejide, 1998). Living and fighting in war zones may force rebels and their adversaries to become trapped in the "combat mode" (De Silva, 1995), which can become an impediment to peacemaking, perpetuated by mistrust in the good faith of enemies and/or the political process. A focus on "war trauma" is understandable in relatively brief conflicts, but what happens when wars go on for years, even decades? In such cases, social-developmental aspects may assume greater explanatory and rehabilitation importance. The breakdown of normal social and economic structures may affect more people and may have greater impact than experiencing specific traumatic events (Bendana, 2000). Even in successful peace processes like that in Northern Ireland, paramilitaries may cling to their "combat mode," reluctant to part with their weapons—to the detriment of formal peace agreements (such as the 1998 Good Friday Peace Agreement). This reluctance to give up weapons may stem in part from socialization in the culture of armed struggle, central to the combat training process.

Regarding specific psychological/psychiatric effects narrowly defined by ICD-10 (WHO, 1992) and the DSM-IV (American Psychiatric Association, 1994), the most frequent effects include acute stress disorder (ASD) in the short run, and PTSD in the long run. Both disorders are discussed in detail elsewhere in this volume. Additional disorders include depression, anxiety disorders, and substance abuse. Conversion and somatization disorders may also occur, and may be more likely to be observed in non-Western cultures (Engdahl, Jaranson, Kastrup, & Danieli, 1999). The prevalence of some of these effects is described below.

Military Veterans

Among Israeli veterans of the Lebanon war, 16% of those who did not experience an acute combat stress reaction had PTSD one year after the war. Those who did experience acute combat stress reactions had a PTSD prevalence of 59% one year after the war (Solomon, Weisenberg, Schwarzwald, & Mikulincer, 1987). In a large epidemiologic study in the US Kulka and colleagues (1990) found that two-thirds of the men and women who served in Vietnam reported serious readjustment problems. Among those with high combat exposure, alcohol abuse, depression, and antisocial behaviors were frequent. Thirty-one percent of the men and 27 percent of the women developed PTSD. They reported high levels of occupational instability, divorce, homelessness, and distress in family members. A direct link between combat exposure and a wide spectrum of physical diseases was also demonstrated in this group (Boscarino, 1997). Further insights into the psychosocial effects of military trauma are highlighted elsewhere in this volume by Friedman and colleagues. In an Australian study of Vietnam veterans, O' Toole and colleagues (1996) found that 12 to 21 percent developed PTSD. They also reported greater health service usage and more health problems. Ayalew and Dercon (2000) studied Ethiopian ex-combatants with disabilities. The most frequently reported primary disability was "mental illness."

Prisoners of War

Psychiatric disorders among this population are high and represent the most enduring and debilitating effects of POWs' war experiences. Kozaric-Kovacic, Folnegovic-Smalc, and Marusic (1993) diagnosed PTSD in 34% of a group of Croatian POWs. Jukic, Dodig, Kenfelj, and De Zan (1997) examined over one thousand Croatian soldiers and civilians held in Serbian detention camps. PTSD rates as high as 86% were observed in certain POW groups. In a sample of American POWs of World War II and the Korean War, Engdahl, Dikel, Eberly, and Blank (1997) reported that over half met lifetime criteria for PTSD, and 30% met current PTSD criteria, even 40 to 50 years after the traumatic events. Solomon, Neria, Ohry, Waysman, and Ginzburg (1994) reported a 20-year follow-up of Israeli combat veterans and POWs. Anxiety symptoms were especially frequent and persistent among POWs; fewer than half of those with lifetime PTSD had recovered some 20 years after the POW experience. POWs had more severe problems in functioning at home, at work, and in the military than did other Israeli veterans.

Rebels and Resistance Fighters

There are few studies of these groups. More than 50 years after WWII, Hovens and colleagues (1998) found that Dutch resistance veterans had high rates of health and mental health problems. Those with anxiety symptoms had more medical problems than those who had none. Problem onset was often preceded by an apparently symptom-free interval, often of many decades. Many of them had been able to function socially and professionally for a considerable time, but had to retire early because of mental and physical health problems. Norwegian resistance fighters arrested and held in German concentration camps had significantly poorer physical and mental health than the general population (Strom, 1968). In Nicaragua, 82 wounded ex-combatants, representing both sides of the conflict, were assessed nearly five years after their injuries (Hume & Summerfield, 1994). Although many had PTSD, social dysfunction better predicted the need for psychological help than did a PTSD diagnosis. Identification with the social ideals being defended by the war effort was psychologically bolstering.

Availability of appropriate training and work was a major determinant of long-term psychosocial outcomes.

INTERVENTIONS

National and International Level of Intervention

At the national and international level of intervention, psychosocial problems among ex-combatants may be reduced through *adherence to relevant international agreements.* Observance of the *Geneva Convention Relative to the Treatment of Prisoners of War* (United Nations, 1949), and its Protocols of 1977, has reduced short- and long-term suffering among combatants who fall into enemy hands; in terms of loss of POW lives, there have been no disasters comparable to that of WWII. When allowed to play its role, the International Committee of the Red Cross (ICRC) has helped immeasurably in guaranteeing POWs' rights: to be treated in a humane manner, to send and receive mail, to receive relief parcels, to speak to an objective party about grievances, and to be repatriated in a humane way (Beaumont, 1996). In cases where nations block ICRC involvement, other human rights monitoring organizations, the media, and international public opinion may play important roles. The establishment of international war crimes tribunals offers additional hope of curbing maltreatment of future POWs.

Governmental Policy

Governmental policy can help overcome stigmatization and aid in the healing process. The problem of reluctance to seek proper treatment because of resignation, avoidance behavior, survivor guilt, and societal indifference is characteristic of many survivor groups, including ex-combatants. Many governments and militant/rebel groups are reluctant to acknowledge that their veterans may have mental health problems. To admit this might require payment of compensation and provision of treatment, or lead to questioning of the war effort, negatively affecting troop or social morale.

The Dutch, and more recently the Americans, have passed laws establishing benefits including medical and mental health care for ex-resistance fighters and POWs, respectively. In the United States, the major boost for POW services began with a 1981 *Former POW Act* (Public Law 97-37), offering health exams and certain benefits to all POWs. Using repatriation records and the help of veterans' service organizations, POWs were contacted and offered exams, medical care, and mental health care. Research was authorized that helped establish links between maltreatment in captivity and later medical and psychiatric disorders; accordingly, compensation and treatment have been granted for these conditions.

Even though many POWs experienced significant health problems following repatriation, most had not sought help until the exams were offered. As Elias (1986) put it, survivors must often be "beckoned to help themselves." This reluctance may be, in part, a direct effect of captivity experiences, creating a mindset of passivity, resignation, or survivor guilt, leading some to question whether they deserve benefits of any kind. Further, many POWs felt abandoned by their government when they were taken captive ("we were expendable") and reject governmental aid efforts. Some report that health care providers attended to combat injuries but ignored psychiatric problems. Still others perceive that they were treated with indifference and rejection by society due to their status as "soldiers who surrendered to the enemy" when, in fact, nearly all were ordered to surrender by their commanding officers. For many, the authorization and award of a "POW Medal" that honors them has played a significant part in their healing.

Societal Level of Intervention

At the societal level of intervention, attitudes toward the war and toward combatants can influence psychosocial health and recovery. Despite war's many negative effects on a society, qualities of human decency remain, including the desire for peace and reconciliation. Mental health providers must accordingly widen their focus of attention. Simply treating individuals or groups is insufficient. Cycles of violence at a group or societal level can be broken by giving these qualities of human decency fuller rein (Agerbak, 1996). Mental health providers, along with peace groups, can work to open democratic space conducive to further intervention. During war (especially civil conflicts), societies often become deeply divided. The middle ground can evaporate due to such polarization, and its reestablishment must be actively promoted. A key element in the early phase is the initiation of internal debate, where the claims of the warring parties are subjected to peer review, using the simple device of critical evaluation and accountability. It is inaccurate (and could hinder recovery efforts) to assume that "the people" totally support one side or another. Ambiguous stances may be more common (and realistic) than polarized positions. Reconciliation should be vigorously pursued through intensive information drives and sound public relations campaigns among the population.

International organizations may be centrally involved in programs of awareness and action targeting ex-combatants when appropriate, as in Mozambique. There, a Commission for Reintegration coordinated support from organizations such as the European Union, the United Nations Developmental Program, and the World Bank. However, it is preferable for these intervention programs to be developed locally, using NGO input and support where appropriate (Summerfield, 1996). Indigenous practitioners can be trained in psychosocial interventions targeted at groups and individuals (Shackman & Reynolds, 1996), and many psychosocial problems can be addressed by trained non-professional volunteers. For example, with help from European NGOs, 70 Nicaraguan psychologists and social workers have trained 1,100 such volunteers (Metraux & Aviles, 1991).

An example of a reasonably successful approach to reintegration and rehabilitation of ex-combatants is provided by Eritrea:

> With only modest outside assistance, Eritrea demobilized and re-integrated 54,000 soldiers through a process labeled Mitias, a name referring to a traditional mutual-help system in which the community gives a helping hand to someone starting a new life. Mitias was staffed by veteran fighters who handed out the demobilization money and assisted ex-combatants with job placement, training, securing farmland and loans, and psychosocial counseling. Particular difficulty was noted in assisting those requiring psychosocial help. The 20 trained staff members could not serve all those in need. More than half who came were women with pronounced symptoms of stress and depression (Bruchaus & Mehreteab, 2000). Gender-specific factors operating after the trauma were noted. Economic problems were faced by most ex-combatants. Yet, specific problems also arose—particularly family and mental health problems—because female ex-fighters often resisted pressure to return to submissive behavior and traditional roles (Bruchhaus & Mehreteab, 2000). Nonetheless, surveys showed that a firm basis for security, economic growth, and human development was laid through a combination of human resources, material resources, and self-reliance (Bruchhaus & Mehreteab, 2000).

Service Coordination and Capacity Building

Societies face many concerns in postwar recovery, among them the rehabilitation of ex-combatants. The interventions described in this chapter may be collectively referred to as "rehabilitation" (United Nations, 2000b). Public safety is often a first priority, followed by relief services (food, water, health, shelter, etc.). Safety is a complex problem (United Nations, 2000b). It must be viewed from the community-at-large perspective. On the one hand, ex-combatants must lay down their arms to end the cycle of violence so that rebuilding a peacetime society can begin in earnest. On the other hand, the sense of danger and mistrust that fueled the war in the first place makes it very difficult for ex-combatants to relinquish their weapons unless they have confidence that it is really safe to do so.

The rebuilding of the physical and social infrastructure is an obvious need. Soldiers need to be demobilized and reintegrated into civilian society along with other war-affected groups (e.g., returning refugees and internally displaced people), who usually outnumber the ex-combatants. Given scarce resources, policy-makers face a dilemma: how to balance targeted support to ex-combatants and support for other war-affected or generally disadvantaged groups. In countries such as Mozambique, it has even been argued that certain groups of ex-combatants should receive no special support, as they were the ones who "created all the havoc." On the other hand, history demonstrates that society benefits when it provides ex-combatants the means to reintegrate themselves (United Nations Department of Peacekeeping Operations, 1999). However, as a rule they should not be regarded as a social group of their own for too long; the sooner they are seen to be members of the general community, the better for themselves and for society. Ongoing programs that last too long may actually raise tension instead of reducing it (Lundin, Chachuia, Gaspar, Guebuza, & Mbilana, 2000). To make reintegration programs more appealing to civil society, they could ultimately be opened to all members of the community.

Social Organizations, Education, and Family
Self-Help Networks

Many ex-combatants feel estranged and alienated from their environment. In post-conflict environments, ex-combatants are often overwhelmed, confused, and in need of support. They may be extremely sensitive to how others describe, define, or make attributions about the event, and the role the combatant played. Ex-combatants' experiences are consensually validated or invalidated by their families and society. They often return home after the most powerful emotional experiences of their lives to find little acknowledgement and much misunderstanding by their families and society at large (Johnson et al., 1997). The degree to which a social community holds a shared view of a conflict and its participants predicts the well-being of its members. Reconciliation between ex-combatants and their society should be vigorously pursued (United Nations, 2000b). Existing positive publicity about the peace process and reintegration should be reinforced, especially in situations where the public is not sympathetic towards the ex-combatants. Community elders, tribal chiefs, and various organizations, such as the media, churches, and community groups, should be encouraged to participate in these efforts.

In many countries, ex-combatants participate in service organizations. Their conventions provide opportunities for them to gather, along with their families, military groups, community leaders, and the media to recognize, honor, and support the veteran and the veteran's family. During these occasions, family members have made ceremonial presentations of poems, essays, or other gifts related to the veterans' war experiences and the impact they have had upon them. Family members share experiences and feelings with others, many for the first time. Such ceremonies compartmentalize the review of the trauma and allow previously shattered relationships to be symbolically transformed, reestablishing connections with family and society (Johnson, Feldman, Lubin, & Southwick, 1995). Ceremonies also have value for ex-combatants who settle in communities new to them. These veteran service organizations also participate in public education efforts, providing education to local schools about combatants' experiences, and actively promote the general welfare of their communities.

Community and Family Level Interventions

In the immediate aftermath of war, many effective activities are action-oriented and short-term. Helping ex-combatants cope with war-related psychological distress requires attention to their material existence and social well-being, as these aspects are intertwined. An environment conducive to the re-establishment of trusting relationships is highly desirable. Materials for training providers and for public education in such situations have been developed (Lundin, 1998; Parong, 1998) and can be adapted for use in new situations. Treatment strategies typically are most effective when they use local sources of social, cultural, and organizational support. Demonstrable cultural sensitivity during contact and a willingness to listen, along with a knowledge of the operational context, are other invaluable elements for successful intervention programs. For further recommendations, see the *Draft Guidelines for International Trauma Training* (ISTSS, 2002). Educational efforts throughout school systems aimed at reducing aggression and increasing tolerance can be vital and are underway in such places as the Bosnian Federation (Pupavac, 2000), where entire schools are providing rehabilitation programs as a matter of course. These programs emphasize the promotion of good relations among the peoples of Yugoslavia, although their effectiveness remains to be demonstrated. Psychoeducation (Allen, Kelly, & Glodich, 1997), directed at the entire community and covering the effects of trauma and methods of coping, can be a cost-effective approach to assist ex-combatants, families, and communities adjust in the aftermath of war. Spouse and family involvement is strongly encouraged. As demonstrated by studies of secondary traumatization, spouses and other family members of traumatized veterans are often indirect casualties who can benefit from such intervention.

The following vignette illustrates eight important aspects of meaningful and cost-effective psychosocial interventions for ex-combatants. *Local treatment providers were used.* They were initially *trained by consulting experts.* They in turn *trained other providers,* extending their impact in a cost-effective manner. They used *culturally-tailored intervention approaches* (healing rituals) with which they were familiar and which the combatants found acceptable and meaningful. These approaches incorporated selected *cost-effective Western interventions* (therapy offered at the group level), as well as *social and community re-integration* (an emphasis on return to productive employment). Finally, *basic indicators of effectiveness* (decreases in alcohol use and nightmares, increases in employment) were recorded. This vignette is provided by a local female lay counselor working in northern Africa in the Transcultural Psychosocial Organization (TPO) project among 170,000 Sudanese refugees:

> *In 1998, one of the ex-rebel groups who had abducted, killed, or raped our refugees gave up fighting. Their commander came to me and asked for help. He told me he was crazy, but that the other ex-rebels were even crazier. They were drunk most of the time, beat their wives, and three of them had set their own hut on fire when they got frustrated. After a few sessions with me, the commander felt much better, and he asked me to visit his former colleagues. He said that they were scared to meet people, and that they did not want to talk to anybody. So he sat on the back of my moped and we drove to their huts. But whenever they heard the sound of the motorbike, they ran into the jungle. Since he knew them and knew how to find them, after a few weeks we had the group of 12 men together. They all had similar problems. They feared the soldiers and the hatred of the community, used alcohol and drugs, suffered from nightmares and flashbacks, had broken families, and felt that they had no future.*
>
> *So we first had some group sessions in which we discussed the past and their atrocities. We also did relaxation exercises. We discussed the dangers of alcohol and drugs in the same way as we do in the Alcohol Anonymous groups in the camps. After 2 or 3 months, all except two stopped drinking and felt much better. But some were still suffering from nightmares and flashbacks. Our TPO trainer instructed us in a specific relaxation-based psychotherapy that we in turn used with these ex-combatants. The group members felt much better, and the total number of nightmares they reported per week dropped from nine to five, and later to two. After another month we decided that we did not need to talk further, and we started to discuss how they could build up their lives. Some got tools and seeds to start a vegetable garden, one took up fishing, and one learned how to make baskets.*
>
> *Some sent a letter to TPO requesting training to help other ex-rebels. Eight completed a five day training workshop: five were ex-rebels, two were women who had been raped by rebels, and one was a community leader. During the first day of the training, the two women sat on one edge of a bench trying not to touch any of the rebels. By the third day, after sessions on community participation in psychosocial helping, stress and its management, mental health, coping skills, and personal growth,*

they looked like one family. Later on, one of the women did a cleansing ritual with a rebel who raped her. It is a ritual we use when the victim and the perpetrator are both known. The man and the woman stand apart and eat at both ends of the intestine of a goat, gradually approaching each other. When they get closer to each other, the intestine is cut, signifying reconciliation.

A second vignette is drawn from Mozambique, where a 25-year-old ex-soldier was quoted:

"When I came home after the war, my father took me to the house of a traditional doctor. That was done because in my area there is a tradition saying that 'When someone leaves the military life, coming home, in the first place, before eating anything, your father has to take you to the house of a traditional doctor to treat your head, so it may stop going round as it used to do, in the army'. That means a ceremony has to be performed, to slow down the rhythm [of] the heart as it used to beat when in the bush, in order to become normal again" (as cited in Lundin et al., 2000).

Ritualized processes of reintegration into community life usually include three specific aspects. First is the treatment of the ex-combatant: a symbolic act that may be broadly categorized as a cleansing ritual is often helpful. Such rituals may include actual cleaning (e.g., a ritual bath, a sweat-lodge ceremony). He or she reacquires a civilian identity and puts aside the military identity of "a killing machine." This promotes the reconciliation of the ex-combatant with the self. Second, a collective social perception that now he or she "is a person again" is developed. The community, family, and even ancestors are given the message that a "lost child" is back home. Third, forgiveness is asked for the wrongdoing committed during the conflict. To clean and to be cleaned after an armed conflict is vital in restoring the social order in communities in which individuals live close together and must depend on each other for survival. The psychological character of these rituals often helps alleviate hard feelings in the community and also benefits the individual.

Clinical Treatment

Recently, more efforts have been made to reduce the risk of long-term stress disorders by intervening before or soon after war trauma exposure. Such efforts include stress management programs, debriefing, and frontline treatment. The literature based on American veterans treated via psychotherapy and pharmacotherapy 10–30 years after the Vietnam War is voluminous. The interventions noted above are reviewed by Fairbank and colleagues (see Chapter 4) and Friedman and colleagues (see Chapter 14).

Comprehensive treatment programs for ex-combatants exist in many nations (Engdahl & Fairbank, 2001), but most have not been systematically studied. In one of the few treatment-outcome studies among prisoners taken during wartime, Drozdek (1997) assigned 120 refugees from the former Yugoslavia now living in the Netherlands to either six months of group psychotherapy, nonsystematic pharmacotherapy, or a combination of the two. Mental health treatment was initiated within three months of release from the prison camps. Psychotherapy incorporated psychodynamic and abreactive (trauma discussion) components. All treatments (i.e., group therapy and drugs, group therapy alone, or drugs alone) yielded positive short-term effects, with continued positive effects observable three years later.

Providers dealing with the psychosocial needs of ex-combatants the world over have developed approaches based on their experience and training. Their task is especially difficult because the psychosocial needs of ex-combatants are often denied, as well as under-recognized, under-served, or both. Even in state military forces there is a lack of services and trained personnel geared to the care of ex-combatants. For example, the British armed forces possess only one small specialized unit, belonging to the Royal Navy, for the treatment of combat-related mental health problems. In developing countries, military health leaders may officially state that combatants only suffer physical injuries. Off the record, they may acknowledge a lack of capabilities to deal with the psychological effects of armed combat. A further hindrance to recognition and intervention is the pervasive stigma directed toward people who develop combat-related mental health problems. They are often viewed as cowards, as weak, or—in many countries, worse still—as mentally ill. Unfortunately, stigmatization of affected combatants only keeps their problems underground; they suffer in silence and often experience severe impairments in social and economic functioning.

War-Related Medical Conditions

Both medical and psychosocial problems deserve attention in those so affected, as each problem area can worsen the other. Combatants wounded in war may be twice as likely to experience psychosocial problems as non-wounded former combatants (Kulka et al., 1990). It is crucial to address war injuries that may lead to psychosocial problems in their own right, particularly head injuries and chronic physical handicaps, such as the loss of a leg with no hope of an adequate prosthesis. Untreated diseases and the effects of malnutrition experienced during war also need to be recognized. Sutker, Winstead, Galina, and Allain (1991) contrasted POWs and combat veterans; the POWs had not only more mental health problems, but also increased cognitive deficits that the authors attributed to captivity weight loss. Successful recovery and societal reintegration is less likely in those with untreated war-related medical conditions.

RECOMMENDATIONS

- Restore the social fabric by promoting group and individual healing in war-torn societies through appropriate programs in the areas of disarmament, demobilization, and reintegration.
- Adhere to relevant international agreements, including the *Geneva Convention Relative to the Treatment of POWs* (GPW) and its 1977 Protocols, to reduce suffering among combatants and POWs. Extend the GPW to prohibit repatriation of POWs against their will.
- Inform legislators in affected countries and representatives of donor nations about psychosocial problems faced by ex-combatants, and encourage funding of services that include outreach and research.
- Pursue vigorous reconciliation between ex-combatants and their society/community through intensive information drives and sound public relations campaigns. Develop public information and civic education materials, and use the most effective channels for their timely dissemination (UN, 2000b).
- Develop special programs for ex-combatants during resettlement and rehabilitation that are community-based and part of general postwar rehabilitation efforts.
- Provide special care, socioeconomic assistance, and pensions, plus access to any general reintegration support programs for disabled ex-combatants. Care for them as disabled citizens, not disabled ex-combatants.
- Take into account the special needs of female ex-combatants in rehabilitation efforts such as child care, employment and economic development, and mental health.
- Aim interventions at rebel/paramilitary/militant fighters *and* members of state security forces, in cases of internal conflict/civil war (e.g., Mozambique).
- Train and use indigenous practitioners in psychosocial interventions whenever possible. Involve, as appropriate, community elders, tribal chiefs, and organizations such as the media, churches, and community groups in rehabilitation efforts.

Recommendations for Future Research

- Study problems associated with reintegrating ex-combatants into a society, particularly those from formerly opposing parties. Evaluate the effectiveness of various approaches to reintegrating ex-combatants into societies that have limited resources. Develop situation-specific intervention programs that include integral research components.

- Study war-related health and psychosocial problems among ex-combatants, including ill-defined and poorly understood symptom complexes observed in many ex-combatants (i.e., joint pain, fatigue, headaches, memory loss, skin problems, etc.). ~

REFERENCES

Agerbak, L. (1996). Breaking the cycle of violence: Doing development in situations of conflict. In D. Eade (Ed.), *Development in states of war* (pp. 26–32). London: Oxford.

Allen, J.G., Kelly, K.A., & Glodich, A. (1997). A psychoeducational program for patients with trauma-related disorders. *Bulletin of the Menninger Clinic, 61*, 222–239.

American Psychiatric Association (1994). *Diagnostic and statistical manual of mental disorders* (4th ed.). Washington, D.C.: Author.

Ayalew, D., & Dercon, S. (2000). "From the gun to the plow": The macro- and micro-level impact of demobilization in Ethiopia. In K. Kingma (Ed.), *Demobilization in sub-Saharan Africa* (pp. 132–172). London: MacMillan.

Beaumont, J. (1996). Protecting prisoners of war, 1939–1995. In B. Moore & K. Fedorowich (Eds.), *Prisoners of war and their captors in World War II* (pp. 277–298). Oxford: Berg.

Bendana, A. (2000). *Demobilization and reintegration in Central America: A peacebuilding perspective*. Managua: Centro de Estudies Internacionales.

Boscarino, J.A. (1997). Diseases among men 20 years after exposure to severe stress: Implications for clinical research and medical care. *Psychosomatic Medicine, 59*, 605–615.

Bruchhaus, E.M., & Mehreteab, A. (2000). "Leaving the warm house": The impact of demobilization in Eritrea. In K. Kingma (Ed.), *Demobilization in sub-Saharan Africa* (pp. 95–131). London: MacMillan.

Danieli, Y. (Ed.) (1998). *International handbook of multigenerational legacies of trauma*. New York: Plenum Press.

De Silva, P.L. (1995). The efficacy of "combat mode": Organisation, political violence, affect and cognition in the case of the Liberation Tigers of Tamil Eelam. In P. Jeganathan & Q. Ismail (Eds.), *Unmaking the nation: The politics of identity and history in modern Sri Lanka* (pp. 176–190). Colombo: Social Scientists Association.

De Silva, P.L. (2000). Sri Lankan futures: Conflicts, alternatives and twenty-first century possibilities. In R. Munck & P.L.D Silva, (Eds.), *Postmodern insurgencies: Political violence, identity formation and peacemaking in comparative perspective* (pp. 167–200). London: Macmillan.

Drozdek, B. (1997). Follow-up study of concentration camp survivors from Bosnia-Herzegovina: Three years later. *Journal of Nervous and Mental Disease, 185*, 690–694.

Elias, R. (1986). *The politics of victimization: Victims, victimology, and human rights*. New York: Oxford.

Engdahl, B.E., Dikel, T., Eberly, R.E., & Blank, A. (1997). Posttraumatic stress disorder in a community sample of former prisoners of war: A normative response to severe trauma. *American Journal of Psychiatry, 154*, 1576–1581.

Engdahl, B., & Fairbank, J. (2001). Former prisoners of war: Highlights of empirical research. In E. Gerrity, T. Keane, & F. Tuma (Eds.), *The mental health consequences of torture and related violence and trauma* (pp. 133–142). New York: Kluwer Academic/Plenum Publishers.

Engdahl, B., Jaranson, J., Kastrup, M., & Danieli, Y. (1999). Traumatic human rights violations: Their psychological impact and treatment. In Y. Danieli, E.C. Stamatapoulou, & J. Dias (Eds.), *The Universal Declaration of Human Rights: Fifty years and beyond* (pp. 337–356). Amityville, New York: Baywood.

Fairbank, J.A., Ebert, L., & Zarkin, G.A. (1999). Socioeconomic consequences of traumatic stress. In P.A. Saigh & J.D. Bremner (Eds.), *Posttraumatic stress disorder: A comprehensive text* (pp. 180–198). Boston: Allyn and Bacon.

Hovens, J.E., Op Den Velde, W., Falger, P.R., De Groen, J.H., Van Duijn, H., & Aarts, P.G. (1998). Reported physical health in resistance veterans from World War II. *Psychological Reports, 82,* 987–996.

Hume, F., & Summerfield, D. (1994). After the war in Nicaragua: A psychosocial study of war-wounded ex-combatants. *Medicine and War, 10,* 4–25.

International Society for Traumatic Stress Studies (ISTSS) (2002). *Draft guidelines for international trauma training.* www.istss.org/Guidelines.html.

Johnson, D.R., Feldman, S.C., Lubin, H., & Southwick, S. (1995). The therapeutic use of ritual and ceremony in the treatment of PTSD. *Journal of Traumatic Stress, 8,* 283–296.

Johnson, D.R., Lubin, H., Rosenheck, R., Fontana, A., Southwick, S., & Charney, D. (1997). The impact of the homecoming reception on the development of PTSD. *Journal of Traumatic Stress, 10,* 259–277.

Jukic, V., Dodig, G., Kenfelj, H., & De Zan, D. (1997). Psychical difficulties in former prisoners of detention camps. *Collegium Antroplogicum, 21,* 235–242.

Kozaric-Kovacic, D., Folnegovic-Smalc, V., & Marusic, A. (1993). Psychological disturbances among 47 Croatian prisoners of war tortured in detention camps. *Journal of the American Medical Association, 270,* 575.

Kulka, R.A., Fairbank, W.E., Hough, R.I., Jordan, B.K., Marmar, C.R., & Weiss, D.S. (1990). *Trauma and the Vietnam War generation: Report of findings from the National Vietnam Veterans Readjustment Study.* New York: Brunner/Mazel.

Litz, B., Orsillo, S., Friedman, M., Ehlich, P., & Batres, A. (1997). Posttraumatic stress disorder associated with peacekeeping duty in Somalia for US military personnel. *American Journal of Psychiatry, 154,* 178–184.

Lundin, I.B. (1998). Mechanisms of community reception of demobilized soldiers. *African Journal of Political Science, 3,* 104–118.

Lundin, I.B., Chachuia, M., Gaspar, A., Guebuza, H., & Mbilana, G. (2000). "Reducing costs through an expensive exercise": The impact of demobilization in Mozambique. In K. Kingma (Ed.), *Demobilization in sub- Saharan Africa* (pp. 173–212). London: MacMillan Press.

Metraux, J.-C., & Aviles, A. (1991). Training techniques of non-professionals: A Nicaraguan preventive and primary care programme in mental health. In M. McCallin (Ed.), *The psychological well-being of refugee children: Research, practice and policy issues* (pp. 226–243). Geneva: International Child Catholic Bureau.

Odejide, A.O., Sanda, A.O., & Odejide, A.I. (1998). Intergenerational aspects of ethnic conflict in Africa: The Nigerian experience. In Y. Danieli (Ed.), *International handbook of multigenerational legacies of trauma* (pp. 373–386). New York: Plenum.

O'Toole, B.I., Marshall, R.P., Grayson, D.A., Schureck, R.I., Dobson, M., French, M., Pulvertaft, B., Meldrum, L., Bolton, J., & Vennard, J. (1996). The Australian Vietnam Veterans health study: II, Self-reported health of veterans compared with the Australian population. *International Journal of Epidemiology, 25,* 319–330.

Parong, A.A. (1998). Caring for survivors of torture: Beyond the clinic. In J.M. Jaranson & M.K. Popkin (Eds.), *Caring for victims of torture: An international perspective* (pp. 229–242). Washington, D.C.: American Psychiatric Press.

Pupavac, V. (2000). From statehood to childhood: Regeneration and changing approaches to international order. In M. Pugh (Ed.), *Regeneration of war-torn societies* (pp. 134–156). London: MacMillan.

Rosenheck, R., & Fontana, A. (1998). Warrior fathers and warrior sons: Intergenerational aspects of trauma. In Y. Danieli (Ed.), *International handbook of multigenerational legacies of trauma* (pp. 225–242). New York: Plenum.

Shackman, J., & Reynolds, J. (1996). Training indigenous workers in mental-health care. In D. Eade (Ed.), Development in states of war (pp. 69–77). Oxford: Oxfam.

Solomon, Z. (1995). Oscillating between denial and recognition of PTSD: Why are lessons learned and forgotten? *Journal of Traumatic Stress, 8*, 271–282.

Solomon, Z., Neria, Y., Ohry, A., Waysman, M., & Ginzburg, K. (1994). PTSD among Israeli former prisoners of war and soldiers with combat stress reaction: A longitudinal study. *American Journal of Psychiatry, 151*, 554–559.

Solomon, Z., Weisenberg, M., Schwarzwald, J., & Mikulincer, M. (1987). Posttraumatic stress disorder in frontline soldiers with combat stress reaction: 1982 Israeli experience. *American Journal of Psychiatry, 144*, 448–454.

Somasundaram, D. (1998). *Scarred minds: The psychological impact of war on Sri Lankan Tamils.* Colombo: Vijitha Yapa Bookshop.

Stenger, C.A. (2002). *American Prisoners of War in WWI, WWII, Korea, Vietnam, Persian Gulf, Somalia, Bosnia, Kosovo, and Afghanistan.* Washington, DC: Dept. of Veterans Affairs Advisory Committee on Former Prisoners of War.

Strom, A. (Ed.) (1968). *Norwegian concentration camp survivors.* New York: Humanities Press.

Summerfield, D. (1996). Assisting survivors of war and atrocity: Notes on "psycho-social" issues for NGO workers. In D. Eade (Ed.), *Development in states of war.* (pp. 85–89). London: Oxford.

Sutker, P.B., Winstead, M.D., Galina, Z.H., & Allain, A.N. (1991). Cognitive deficits and psychopathology among former prisoners of war. *American Journal of Psychiatry, 148*, 67–72.

United Nations. (1949). *The Geneva Convention Relative to the Treatment of Prisoners of War.* New York: Author.

United Nations Department of Peacekeeping Operations (1999). *Disarmament, demobilization and reintegration of ex-combatants in a peacekeeping environment: Principles and guidelines.* New York: Author.

United Nations Division for the Advancement of Women (1997). *Gender-based persecution.* New York: Author.

United Nations (2000a). *Report of the Secretary-General to the Security Council on children and armed conflict.* New York: Author.

United Nations (2000b). *The role of United Nations peacekeeping in disarmament, demobilization and reintegration: Report of the Secretary General.* New York: UN Security Council.

University Teachers for Human Rights–Jaffna (UTHR–Jaffna) (January, 2000). *The scent of danger* (Information Bulletin No.23), pp. 9–12.

Wolfe, J., Sharkansky, E., & Reed, J. (1998). Predictors of PTSD symptomatology among US female Persian Gulf War personnel. *Journal of Interpersonal Violence, 13*, 40–57.

World Health Organization (WHO) (1992). *International classification of diseases* (10th revision). Geneva: Author.

Zwi, A.B. (1991). Militarism, militarization, health and the third world. *Medicine and War, 7*, 262–268.

Chapter 13

Natural and Technological Disasters

Daya Somasundaram, Fran H. Norris, Nozomu Asukai, and R. Srinivasa Murthy

Disasters are very common. Worldwide, earthquakes, floods, cyclones, landslides, technological accidents, and urban fires occur daily. They tend to occur suddenly, without much warning, and cause massive destruction, sometimes killing or injuring large numbers of people within a short time. In 1999 alone, natural disasters killed over 60,000 people in Turkey, 10,000 people in India, and 25,000 people in Venezuela (United Nations General Assembly Economic and Social Council [UNGAESC], 2000). Disasters disproportionately strike the poor, socially deprived, and marginalized, and their consequences may be more serious and long-lasting in these groups. Similarly, disasters affect developing nations more adversely than developed nations. However, these groups and nations may have the fewest resources or facilities to cope with the aftermath of disasters.

It is now recognized that disaster survivors will need food, shelter, and other relief measures, as well as long-term rehabilitation facilities. It is also generally acknowledged that financial aid is needed for the survivors to recover. Year after year, international relief agencies and nongovernmental organizations (NGOs) find themselves stretched to the limit to meet these basic needs of disaster-stricken populations (UNGAESC, 2000). Yet food, shelter, and material goods constitute only the "tip of the iceberg" with regard to disaster victims' needs. Disaster-stricken communities often experience disruption of family and community life, work, normal networks, institutions, and structures. Loss of motivation, dependence on relief, hostility, and despair can sometimes develop in members of the community exposed to disasters. As much as we work to provide emergency relief and look after survivors' basic needs, their right of access to health care has to be recognized, including care for mental health as well as physical health. Mental health problems will cause difficulties in normal functioning, working capacity, relationships, and family life. As the report from UNGAESC (2000, p. 14–15) points out, "A major challenge for humanitarian agencies is to understand that the mental health consequences of emergencies can cause a level of distress that may hamper recovery as well as rehabilitation and to incorporate culturally appropriate psychosocial assistance programmes in relief efforts, in cases of both war and natural disasters. Member States may wish to encourage increased international attention to this issue." This is precisely the purpose of this chapter, as well as this volume as a whole.

Broadly, this chapter is divided into four parts. We begin with a general discussion of the epidemiology, definitions, and characteristics of disasters (Nature and Scope). Then we describe how disasters unfold in time and highlight the personal characteristics and social dynamics that appear to be most important in understanding the recovery process (Effects). In the third section, we review methods of providing assistance to disaster victims (Interventions), and then we conclude by describing actions that policymakers, communities, families, and individuals can take to foster post-disaster mental health (Recommendations).

NATURE AND SCOPE OF DISASTERS

Epidemiology

On average, natural and technological disasters kill 50,000 people each year. An additional 74,000 are seriously injured, 5 million are displaced from their homes, and over 80 million are affected in some way. We have adjusted the statistics presented in the *World Disaster Report* (International Federation of Red Cross and Red Crescent Societies, 1999) to include only the effects of earthquakes, floods, high winds, landslides, technological accidents, and urban fires. Thus these statistics do *not* include the effects of drought or famine or war. No area of the world is immune from these events. Averaging 197 disasters per year, Asia leads the rest of the world, followed by the Americas at 111 disasters, Europe at 77, Africa at 61, and Oceania at 18. Although some developed countries, such as the United States, are quite vulnerable to disasters, developing countries are disproportionately exposed. De Girolamo and McFarlane (1996) estimated that the ratio of disaster victims in developing countries to disaster victims in developed countries is 166:1. Fatalities average 13:1 (International Federation of Red Cross and Red Crescent Societies, 2002). There is every reason to believe that this imbalance will only get worse in the foreseeable future. Increasing industrialization, urbanization, decaying infrastructures, and deforestation are among the factors that place many of the world's countries at increased or increasing risk (Quarantelli, 1994).

The involvement of an individual and community in a given disaster will depend on where they are in reference to the site of maximum impact. At the epicenter, where the disaster strikes, many may die or be severely injured or maimed. A little farther out, survivors may have felt the full impact and experienced the terror but not suffered major injury. More peripherally, witnesses may have seen the disaster, experienced fear, and taken shelter, while most will have heard of the event only second-hand or through the media. Nonetheless, some in the community may have relatives or friends who are dead or injured, or they may take part in rescue and relief efforts. All these grades of exposure or involvement may give rise to a variety of psychological responses. Although people who have directly experienced losses, threat to life, and injury will be most strongly affected psychologically, lesser effects may extend to the community at large.

Definitions

Almost all definitions of disasters emphasize their collective nature. In contrast to many other potentially traumatic events, such as criminal victimization or life-threatening accidents, disasters create stress for many people simultaneously. Noting that previous definitions variously emphasized the agents themselves (e.g., hurricane, earthquake), the physical impact of such agents (e.g., quantified damages), the social impact (e.g., losses and social disruption), socially constructed perceptions of crisis, and political phenomena (e.g., declarations), Quarantelli (1985) defined disaster as a **"consensus-type crisis occasion where demands exceed capabilities." This definition of disaster as "an imbalance in the demand-capability ratio"** is particularly useful because it reminds us that the consequences of disasters follow not only from the needs of disaster-stricken populations but also from the ability of communities to meet those needs. Thus, to understand disasters, we must evaluate the capabilities and resources of stricken individuals and communities, just as we evaluate the objective characteristics and impact of physical agents. And, to lessen the severity of disasters, we must bolster resources, just as we attempt to prevent or mitigate the actual physical impact of agents such as floods, high winds, and earthquakes. Moreover, if we understand that the "capabilities" side of the disaster equation includes psychological and social resources as well as material resources, we also understand that intervention efforts directed solely at replacing the latter will undoubtedly fail.

Characteristics

Current schemes (e.g., Bolin, 1985; Green, 1982; Quarantelli, 1985) for classifying and describing disasters de-emphasize specific agents and emphasize characteristics of the experience and/or crisis occasion that have more adverse consequences for resources and mental health. From a psychological perspective, the *extent of terror and horror* associated with the event is critical. Following events as varied as the Mt. St. Helens eruption (Murphy, 1985), the Buffalo Creek dam collapse (Gleser, Green, & Winget, 1981), Hurricane Paulina in Mexico (Norris, Perilla, Ibañez, & Murphy, 2001), and the 1997 Polish flood (Norris, Kaniasty, Inman, Conrad, & Murphy, 2002), disaster victims who experienced injuries, bereavement, or threat to life were shown to be at higher risk for poor psychological outcomes. Rescue and recovery workers may be severely exposed to horrific sights even if they escape the terror and threat to life associated with the disaster itself. Transportation accidents, for example, often require prolonged contact with mass death because of the need to recover, identify, transport, and bury human remains (Ursano & McCarroll, 1994).

A very important dimension along which disasters vary is the *impact ratio*, which refers to the proportion of the population that is affected rather than to the absolute number of victims (Green, 1982). This is important because it determines the ability of the community to respond and the extent to which it will need outside help. In a study of 10 counties in eastern Kentucky (Appalachia), USA, affected by the same flood (e.g., Phifer & Norris, 1989), community destruction, defined as the number of victims to non-victims in the respondent's county of residence, predicted increases in depression, anxiety, and somatic symptoms even when the effects of personal loss were controlled. The victims who fared most poorly were those who experienced high levels of personal loss in combination with high levels of community destruction.

Disasters vary in their *rapidity of onset* and *predictability*, attributes that affect how long people have to act or prepare for the ensuing event. For example, flash floods and earthquakes often occur with very little warning, whereas there is often a substantial warning period before riverine floods and hurricanes. Warning systems and the mass evacuations they allow have saved countless lives and, undoubtedly, have prevented an even greater number of physical injuries. Given that personal injury, threat to life, and bereavement are among the strongest predictors of post-disaster psychological distress, we may also infer that warning, preparedness, and evacuation greatly reduce the trauma potential of disaster agents.

Unfamiliarity also appears to heighten the impact of disasters. Prior experience or training appears to lessen the stressfulness of recovery efforts for disaster workers (e.g., Ersland, Weisath, & Sund, 1989; Ursano & McCarroll, 1994). The same advantage sometimes appears to hold for primary disaster victims (Norris & Murrell, 1988). Possibly, experienced victims are simply more prepared for the event and better equipped to reduce their risk of being exposed to the more traumatic elements of disaster (terror and horror). People who have experienced disasters in their communities often show higher levels of hazard preparedness in ways such as having a plan for their household and keeping basic supplies on hand (Norris, Smith, & Kaniasty, 1999).

Another important attribute is the *duration of the crisis*. Sometimes, disasters happen and pass, but at other times, the threat persists. After the nuclear accidents at Three Mile Island and Chernobyl, residents remained fearful about the long-term effects of exposure to radiation and the possibility of future accidents (Baum, Fleming, & Davidson, 1983; Bromet, 1995; Weisaeth, 1994). Similarly, prolonged chronic stresses caused by displacement and conflict can produce, in time, psychological effects. Prominent are development of feelings of hopelessness, despair, or depression.

Finally, classification schemes have almost always distinguished between disasters of *natural versus technological origin*. Human-caused events such as dam collapses and industrial accidents "represent in the eyes of victims a callousness, carelessness, intentionality, or insensitivity on the part of others" (Bolin, 1985). In developed countries, technological disasters are frequently followed by lasting disputes and litigation concerning the allocation of blame. Such antagonisms further separate, fragment, and politicize the community (Edelstein, 1988; Kroll-Smith & Couch, 1993). Probably due to these factors, technological disasters appear to have more adverse consequences for mental health (Baum, 1987; Green & Solomon, 1995; Weisaeth, 1994). However, the distinction between natural and technological disasters may be fading because victims of the former often attribute their suffering, at least in part, to decisions made by humans. When beliefs about causal factors move away from nature toward human agents, community divisions become more likely to surface (Kaniasty & Norris, 1999; Rochford & Blocker, 1991).

EFFECTS OF DISASTERS

Temporal Dimensions of Disaster Impact

Because disasters are events that unfold over time, it is often useful to differentiate the temporal dimensions of (1) pre-impact, (2) impact, and (3) post-impact phases (e.g., Freedy, Resnick, & Kilpatrick, 1992) in considering the effects of these events. Each phase will have its own stresses, which are manifest in the individual as well as in the social realm.

The *pre-impact period* will consist of a threat and warning phase. Ideally, before a disaster strikes, there should be adequate warning through the mass media and locally through mechanisms such as loudspeakers. Some disasters, like earthquakes, may not allow time for warnings. Authorities, helping agencies, and community organizations can theoretically help to prepare for the disaster by taking protective actions and, if necessary, evacuating the population to safer areas. The form of preparation will depend on the type of disaster, its expected severity, and the resources of the community. Training of community level workers also can be done in advance. When a disaster is probable or imminent, residents may experience generalized fear and worry, anxiety, disturbed sleep, and agitation. Families and friends should try to support and help one another to prepare for the disaster by storing food and other supplies, building protective shelters, or leaving in an organized way, if possible. Right before the disaster is a period of high arousal, apprehension, and fear. Panic can occur but is not common. Whereas some people will take urgent action to protect themselves and others, some individuals may deny or ignore the imminent danger, thus exposing themselves to risk.

At present, the superiority of their warning systems and preparedness may be among the strongest advantages that more developed countries have over less developed countries (UNGAESC, 2000). However, slow onset and predictability do not necessarily translate to greater preparedness or trauma reduction, because potential victims do not always believe or heed such warnings even if they receive them or have real options for avoiding the events. In a study of 777 adults for whom evacuation was at least suggested by authorities prior to hurricanes Hugo (South Carolina, USA, 1989) or Andrew (Florida, USA, 1992), 58% did not evacuate (Riad, Norris, & Ruback, 1999). Among those who did not evacuate, the most common reason was that they had believed that the hurricane was not a serious threat. A smaller but notable percentage indicated that they lacked the resources that would have allowed them to evacuate (e.g., money, transportation, someplace to go).

The *impact stage* is when the disaster strikes. There may be deaths, injuries, and destruction. The duration will vary with the type of disaster, from seconds in the case of earthquakes to minutes or hours for a cyclone or industrial accident, to days and weeks for floods. There is heightened arousal and attention with scanning of the environment for cues for safety or escape. Survival or self-preservation is the chief goal. Most people will behave appropriately to protect themselves and significant others. Family-oriented behavior, intense concern and frantic searching for those not accounted for, and hierarchical roles of caring, with men protecting the women and the women caring for the children, is often seen. There may be clinging onto others seeking the reassurance experienced in sharing the terror. When there has been little or no warning, traumatic shock will be a prominent effect of the impact. Rarely there may be intense panic or paralysis of action that inhibits and delays the person's response.

A sense of helplessness against powerful forces, including feelings of ineffectiveness and inadequacy, may cause the traumatic imprinting of the impact in vivid detail. Later, during recovery, the traumatic event may be repeatedly re-experienced as recurrent, intrusive recollections, images, or dreams to be given meaning and assimilated by the individual. A sense of abandonment may be a powerful and frightening component of the feeling of helplessness. The person or group may feel forsaken by God and humanity. Children who are separated from their parents may especially feel that trusted, good, and protective people have deserted them. Even adults can lose their sense of being safe and invulnerable or of having others who care for them. The yearning for relief and rescue is intense. Prayers, rosaries, or mantras may be repeated incessantly. The victims are sometimes dazed, numbed, and passive; they may show acute stress reactions or inappropriate apathetic and automatic behavior. Usually this *disaster syndrome* is transient, giving way to hyperactivity or to appropriate activity. But in a few cases, it may persist as a numbing of general responsiveness and avoidance behavior. Other people, however, may exhibit great heroism by rescuing those whose lives are in danger, helping and assisting those who are injured, and initiating relief operations.

The *post-impact phase* can be divided (a) into the immediate recoil, relief, or emergency phase and (b) the longer rehabilitation and reconstruction phase. During the recoil period, survivors sometimes initially experience euphoria at having survived in the face of death and destruction. Often such feelings are accompanied by a temporary breakdown of social barriers of class or caste, the forgetting of old quarrels, the sharing of experiences, and elation regarding the altruistic responses of those helping and caring. In contrast, there can be disruption of services, breakdown in community functioning, and complete chaos. This is the period when emergency operations have to be launched for rescue, first aid, and provision of basic needs like water, food, shelter, clothing, health care, and communication. Sometimes, indigenous leaders arise who serve to organize their community's recovery.

Mrs. K. couldn't sleep the night of July 9th, 1997. Although local officials reported that the rising river would not threaten her community in southeastern Poland for at least another 48 hours, she was too anxious to sleep. She and her husband, both in their late sixties, lived on the top floor of a concrete and boxy apartment building. It was easy to see from the tenth floor the cresting waters of the Odra River. The day before she had insisted that her husband haul all the way to their apartment all items of any value from their basement storage carrel. Neighbors who saw it made fun of her and called her panicky. Early that morning, she began to hear a noise, like a "whisper of an incoming sea wave." She peeked through the window and saw a shiny narrow tongue of water coming straight into her building followed by a rushing wave. She and her husband rushed to wake residents on the lower floors and to help them move their belongings to higher floors. About that time, the water hit the building with a terrifying sound and she felt the entire structure shaking. She has never forgotten that sensation, and that rumbling sound and the shaking still wake her up almost every night. A few people managed to run out of the building, but the water entered the stairwell very quickly and soon all the ground-floor apartments were submerged in the dirty water up to their ceilings.

Electric power was down, the phones were down; soon they would obviously shut down water and the natural gas that most people used for cooking. Mrs. K. felt that the residents had to get organized. She went out onto her balcony, leaned over the railing, and summoned her husband to relay her directives: Everybody should go back to their apartments, the rescue efforts would come much later; they should do something useful in the meantime! Men—start catching water in the bathtubs and other containers, women—take out all the fresh and frozen meat and other perishables and start cooking. Cook everything; just boil it. They should not waste any time. Some people at first were amused and thought that "grandma" must be crazy, but they followed her directions anyway. About five hours later, the gas was shut off.

It took two days to evacuate the building. Helicopters lifted some people up, and boats took the others. During all that time Mrs. K. and her husband coordinated the efforts of their "stairwell community." She devised the plan of who should be evacuated when. She asked all the pet owners to have their pets use a designated and clearly marked space on the roof for their sanitary needs. She had parents of school-age children search their apartments for blackboard chalk to write messages on the roof for the pilots. Whenever there was a drop of goods (e.g., food, water, medicine) from the helicopters, the person intercepting the bag would first take it to Mrs. K., who supervised the distribution. She was one of the last people to leave the building; strapped in a floating device, Mrs. K. was evaluated by boat. She still has "shivers" when talking about it. Six months later, when a researcher arrived in the neighborhood to study the flood, most people immediately directed him to "the stairwell of that older lady who made everybody cook."

In the longer period that follows, the reality of loss, death, and destruction, the unalterable facts of changes in community and personal life, and the prolonged issues of restitution and recovery must be faced. With the passage of time, decline in attention and breakdown of informal support networks, as well as withdrawal of relief and professional assistance, all contribute to grief, anger, and a sense of disillusionment in those affected. Particularly potent in this context is the attitude of others who may now be likely to make the victims feel that they should have recovered and no longer be in need of special interest or support. In some people, psychological distress may be delayed. The explanation is that during acute emergencies, physical safety, treatment of injuries, food, and shelter take priority while emotional problems are suppressed or ignored. Once there is some reduction in the acute stress, the psychological problems may come to the forefront. Psychological reactions for some survivors include symptoms of posttraumatic stress disorder (PTSD), anxiety, or depression, family and marital discord, relationship problems, alcohol and drug abuse, and psychosomatic complaints (for a review of the psychological consequences of disasters, see Green & Solomon, 1995).

Reconstruction involves taking inventory of the destruction and loss, re-establishing a sense of reality, working through the traumatic experience, and adaptation at the individual and community level. Although most communities recover in a reasonable amount of time, this process may be prolonged in some communities, sometimes taking years, sometimes never resolving, and sometimes leaving some individuals within those communities mentally scarred and disabled. If the devastation and damage overwhelm recovery efforts and reconstruction cannot be completed, reminders, inconveniences, and hardships remain, making psychological recovery more difficult. Rehabilitation and resettlement may bring about permanent changes in cultural values, economic structures, and religious and political beliefs. A new chapter in the life of the community may begin with the end of the disaster.

Factors That Influence Disaster Recovery

Disaster recovery is complex because it depends upon severity of exposure, availability of aid, individual vulnerability, and community level dynamics. First and foremost among predictors of recovery is the severity of the person's exposure and losses (Freedy, Resnick, & Kilpatrick, 1992; Freedy, Shaw, Jarrell, & Masters, 1992). Such losses may include not only the obvious losses of objects (housing, personal belongings) but also of personal characteristics (self-esteem, trust, perceived safety), energies (time, money), and conditions (employment). Economic resources in the form of employment, loans for rehabilitation, resettlement, and rebuilding, or funds for mere existence are of crucial importance in determining posttraumatic adaptation. Attitudes and responses toward victimized individuals can further influence adaptation. When there is adequate social support, and where opportunity structures are in place or created for the affected population to participate in their own rehabilitation and reconstruction, the recovery is usually good for that community as a whole, although some individuals may develop lasting problems. Below we will highlight a few of these factors and dynamics.

Personal Characteristics: At-Risk Groups. Although some distress is quite normal immediately after disasters, most people do not develop more serious, lasting disturbances. Some groups have been found to be more vulnerable to experiencing more lasting effects of disasters than others. Whereas men may be more exposed to trauma related to rescue and recovery, women may be disproportionately exposed to other disaster-related stressors, particularly those that are secondary or vicarious, because of the centrality of home and family in their lives (Gleser, Green, & Winget, 1981; Solomon, Bravo, Rubio-Stipec, & Canino, 1993). After disasters, women generally show higher rates of PTSD, anxiety, and depression than do men (De La Fuente, 1990; North et al., 1999; Shore, Tatum & Vollmer, 1986; Steinglass & Gerrity, 1990). Some recent evidence suggests that the difference between men's and women's outcomes after disasters is greater in societies or groups that foster traditional views of masculinity and femininity, such as Mexico, than in societies that adhere to these traditions less rigidly, such as in African-American culture (Norris et al., 2001). The report from UNGAESC (2000) stressed the need to integrate a gender perspective in humanitarian assistance activities.

Age has attracted a considerable amount of research attention. Studies in the U.S. that have included the full range of adult ages have generally found middle-aged persons at greater risk than either older adults or younger adults for disaster-specific symptoms (e.g., Gleser, Green, & Winget, 1981), in part because they are most likely to experience chronic stressors, such as parenting, financial, or occupational stress (Thompson, Norris, & Hanacek, 1993). However, the strength and even the direction of age effects may vary depending upon the social, cultural, economic, and historical context of the exposed setting (Norris et al., 2002). In children, as in adults, there is a variable rate of traumatic stress following degrees of exposure to danger (Green et al., 1991; LaGreca, Silverman, Vernberg, & Prinstein, 1996; Shannon, Lonigan, Finch, & Taylor, 1994). Witnessing extreme violence, particularly to their parents, is likely to cause serious traumatic stress among children. The report from UNGAESC (2000) stressed the importance of providing assistance to children and older adults during all phases of emergencies.

Ethnicity has received less attention than have gender and age, but a few studies have found that persons who are ethnic minorities fare more poorly after disasters than their counterparts, presumably because of their lower resources (Palinkas, Russell, Downs, & Peterson, 1992; Perilla, Norris, & Lavizzo, 2002).

Persons with prior psychiatric histories are likely to show post-disaster psychiatric conditions as well. Although there are few data that address whether psychiatric cases are differentially vulnerable to the *effects* of disasters, prospective studies clearly show that pre-disaster symptoms are the best predictors of post-disaster symptoms (e.g., Phifer & Norris, 1989; Smith, Robins, Przybeck, Goldring, & Solomon, 1986). For more information on risk factors for PTSD, see Chapter 2.

Community Dynamics: The Mobilization and Deterioration of Social Support.   The ability of social support to protect mental health has been demonstrated repeatedly. The fact that so many people are in need simultaneously complicates the role of social support in disaster-stricken communities (see Kaniasty & Norris, 1997; 1999). Disaster victims often find it difficult to maintain supportive relationships just when they need them the most. The initially heightened level of helping and concern seldom lasts for the full length of the recovery process. Because disasters affect entire networks, the need for support may simply exceed its availability, causing expectations of support to be violated. Relocation, and even death in the most severe cases, removes important others from victims' supportive environments. Physical fatigue, emotional irritability, and scarcity of resources increase the potential for interpersonal conflicts and social withdrawal. Moreover, as time passes, supportive networks may become saturated with stories of and feelings about the event. Consequently, victims and their supporters begin to minimize or downplay the importance of sharing their emotions or may even escape interacting. Thus, over time, social relationships are strained, and this causes psychological distress for many survivors.

In addition, it is common for conflicts to arise after disasters because of actual or perceived inequities in the distribution of aid. When communities function well, the most support will go to those who need it the most. Typically, however, need is not the only determinant of received support. In some cultures and settings, patronage systems still predominate, and consequently the amount of help received may be determined more by whom one knows than by what one needs. Often, racial and ethnic minorities and persons of lower socioeconomic status receive less help than other victims who have comparable levels of need, placing them at greater risk for continuing losses and psychological distress (Kaniasty & Norris, 1995).

Cultural Variations in Effects

Health professionals must be sensitive to the varying ways in which distress may be expressed or displayed cross-culturally. Although many human emotions are experienced universally, they may take different forms. A finding commonly noted in the cross-cultural psychiatry literature (e.g., Kirmayer, 1996) is the predominance of somatic symptoms in non-Western societies. Too much reliance on "Western" definitions of post-traumatic stress may cause important expressions or idioms of distress to be missed. Idioms of distress are folk categories that are used by people in many different ways to explain a wide range of problems. For example, in studies of disasters and trauma in Latin America, several culturally-specific idioms of distress have been identified. In Jenkins' (1996) work with Salvadoran refugees, *el calor* (the heat) stood out as a particularly salient form of bodily experience. Likewise, studies of Puerto Rican trauma victims have shown that *ataques de nervios* (acute episodes of emotional upset and loss of control) are very important to consider (Guarnaccia, Canino, Rubio-Stipic, & Bravo, 1993). Yet another example from Latin America is *susto*, which literally means "the fright" (e.g., Hough, Canino, Abueg, & Gusman, 1996; Kirmayer, 1996). Spanish-speaking persons often attribute a wide range of symptoms to a frightening experience and thus name their resulting discomforts after the *susto* they believe is the cause. *El susto* tends to be recognized in retrospect, after symptoms bring about the recollection of a traumatic experience. *Susto* is more the explanation than the illness itself, since the latter is manifested in different ways, including weakness, sadness, fatigue, and fearfulness.

> *In 1992, Carmen Sanchez's family was among several Mexican families living in Homestead, Florida that were unable to evacuate the area even though they knew Hurricane Andrew was approaching. Carmen's family and four other families took shelter in one small trailer. In order to hold the trailer safely in place under the force of massive wind gusts, the men found a truck door and tied it to the trailer's roof. Although weighted down by the heavy truck door, the trailer was rocked by wind. At one point, the air conditioning unit became dislodged from the window. Santiago, Carmen's 45-year-old uncle, grabbed the air conditioner but then found himself being sucked out of the window as well. The men in the trailer quickly grabbed Santiago and pulled him back inside. Once safely inside the trailer, Santiago was quiet and his face was discolored.*
>
> *In the weeks following the hurricane, Santiago refused to eat and became very skinny. He became confused, disoriented, and was unable to sleep. He became*

apathetic and depressed. He also suffered from diarrhea and other stomach ailments. When it would start to rain, he would lock himself indoors and refuse to leave his home. Carmen and her family recognized this as susto or fright sickness. Literally, susto refers to the loss of one's soul from one's body due to fright. In order to help her uncle, Carmen sought the aid of a folk healer, who performed a ceremony known as the barrida or sweeping. The folk healer brushed Santiago with herbs and recited ritual prayers. In addition, the folk healer and other people from the community talked to Santiago in order to pull his frightened soul back into his body. Following several repetitions of this ceremony, Santiago was healed from susto.

INTERVENTIONS

· Perhaps the most important lesson to be learned from the research summarized in the previous section is that the stress precipitated by catastrophic disasters is often long-lasting. Thus the response to a disaster must include ongoing attention to the psychosocial aspects of the event as part of the overall emergency response—for without mental health being established first or concurrently, reconstruction efforts may not be of much benefit. In developing an overall integrated scheme for rehabilitation, it is essential to take a systems approach, acknowledging that individuals, families, communities, and political forces each influence the others. Moreover, different types of interventions are called for during different phases of the event.

It is traditional to talk about three types of prevention (Caplan, 1964). *Primary prevention* aims to lower the rate of *new* cases of mental disorder by counteracting harmful situational circumstances before they have had a chance to produce illness, or by strengthening individual-based resources. With regard to the aims of this chapter, we can think of primary prevention interventions as those that attempt to reduce the prevalence or trauma potential of disasters in the future (and thus correspond to the pre-impact phase).

Secondary prevention is initiated at the early stages of crisis and targets those most at-risk. The assumption of secondary prevention is that by identifying problems early, more serious psychosocial problems can be avoided. Secondary prevention programs generally attempt to expand the reach of the mental health system by using both individual-based and system-based resources effectively. Interventions that take place in the aftermath of disasters (impact and post-impact phases) often have such secondary prevention goals.

Tertiary prevention resembles individual rehabilitation in that it is initiated after damage has occurred, but it differs from individual rehabilitation in being large enough in scale to reduce the prevalence of disorder in the population. Most disaster survivors will recover successfully, but a minority of persons may require more formal or professional level mental health care. Specialized psychotherapeutic interventions will not be discussed in this chapter; information on them is provided in Chapter 4. In this section, we will focus on primary and secondary prevention strategies that apply to disaster mitigation and recovery.

Pre-Impact Interventions: Trauma Prevention and Hazard Preparedness

Although floods, earthquakes, and hurricanes may not be preventable, much of the destruction they cause can be avoided by appropriate policies and plans at the societal level. This is even more true for human-caused (or technological) disasters. In many cases, it is discovered after the fact that building codes had been ignored, communities had been located in dangerous areas, warnings had not been issued or followed, or plans had been forgotten. Serious attention should be paid to prevention in the future as we develop a better understanding of disasters: how and why they occur, their effects, and how best to manage their short- and long-term mental health consequences. The report from UNGAESC (2000) emphasized the need to strengthen disaster preparedness and early warning systems at the country and regional level and cited collaborative efforts in Ethiopia and Vietnam as examples.

At the community level, interventions that provide adequate warning and information about evacuation procedures are particularly important. As noted previously in this chapter, such actions not only save lives but also protect mental health by reducing exposure of the public to the most traumatic elements of disasters (injury, threat to life, and bereavement). Almost any community can benefit from developing strategies and procedures for warning and evacuating people when it is appropriate. There is no one simple formula for how to do this, because any plan must take into account the probable threats (e.g., volcano, hurricane, chemical plant), resources (e.g., transportation, shelter), attitudes (e.g., understanding of risk, fear of looting, trust in authorities), social networks (e.g., informal communication channels), economic realities (e.g., willingness to leave land to which there is no title), and communication infrastructures (e.g., ability to reach people by television or radio) of the area involved. There are even creative examples available of plans and exit routes developed using narratives of indigenous communities: for instance, the *Just in Case* program developed by researchers in Puebla and Mexico City, Mexico for a community that has lived at the base of the volcano *Popocatepetl* (*Popo*) for centuries. It is believed in this community that *Don Gregorio*, the local name for the volcano, will warn the local villagers if he is about to erupt. But *just in case* Don Gregorio doesn't oblige, the community now also has a civil defense plan. For example, each family has been given a clear, sealable bag to protect their valuable papers—and on it is imprinted the evacuation route and procedures.

Previous research suggests that intervention efforts can also be effective in enhancing family and individual disaster preparedness. Hazard-preparedness is a multi-dimensional behavior (Faupel, Kelley, & Petee; 1992; Mulilis & Lippa, 1990; Norris et al., 1999) involving *proactive strategies* (e.g., having escape plans, keeping supplies on hand), *vigilance* (e.g., remaining alert to potential hazards), and *reactive strategies* (e.g., boarding windows, evacuating). Though disaster preparedness is difficult to promote, beliefs that people can influence their own chances of surviving can lead to precautionary acts (Mulilis & Duval, 1995). Consequently, at least in developed countries, programs that attempt to educate citizens to change those behaviors that place them at risk undoubtedly constitute the most widely used prevention approach.

Impact and Post-Impact Interventions: Community Development, Crisis Counseling, and Psychoeducation

In the immediate aftermath of disasters, interventions focus on the management of the crisis. Although such interventions take place within a specific community context, the planning for them is often initiated at societal and policy levels. In the United States, for example, the federal government provides funding and technical support for post-disaster mental health interventions and has often taken the lead in promoting local planning efforts. As an example of this, we reproduce the "salient points for disaster management" published by the Emergency Services Branch of the U.S. Substance Abuse and Mental Health Administration in 1994.

- No one who experiences the event or sees the event is untouched by it. Individuals find comfort and reassurance when told that their reactions are normal and understandable. Therefore, mental health workers have to educate people about common disaster stress reactions, ways to cope with stressors, and available resources to respond to their needs. Relief from stress, ability to talk about the experience, and passage of time usually lead to the reestablishment of equilibrium. Most people pull together and function during and after a disaster, but their effectiveness is diminished.
- Loss of natural buffers in the community is less visible. Mental health interventions should seek to reestablish linkages between individuals and groups through outreach, support groups, and community organizations.

- Disaster mental health services must be uniquely tailored to the communities they serve. Such programs are most effective if workers indigenous to the community and to its various ethnic and cultural groups are integrally involved in service delivery.
- Survivors respond to active interest and concern.
- Interventions must be appropriate to the phase of disaster.

Community level interventions aim to foster community competence and ownership of problems and solutions. Mary Harvey (1990) may be among the most vocal advocates for the use of a system level perspective in the aftermath of disaster. In her view, trauma emanates from profound powerlessness. The emphasis for intervention, then, should be on empowerment, meaning such interventions need to emphasize strengths, mobilize the community's capabilities, and help the community to become self-sufficient. Too much reliance on outside professionals can amplify a community's trauma. According to Harvey, one of the major tasks of a community crisis response is to identify existing resources and resource gaps: "What's there? What isn't? Can we fill the gap?" It is critical to make use of existing resources, i.e., to include any individual, setting, and hidden resource that can be affirmed and integrated into the response plan. Likewise, Van Den Eynde and Veno (1999) argue that caregivers' roles in the aftermath of disasters must be to facilitate rather than to direct, to encourage the development of new organizational skills, to support community action, and explicitly to resist a "victim community" approach in favor of a "competent community" approach. In a community-centered intervention, the community itself plays an active role in shaping the intervention. The most appropriate post-disaster intervention may be one that aims to build the community's capacity to make informed choices, while recognizing that those choices and responsibility for recovery remain the community's own. No one post-disaster intervention strategy can fit all communities, cultures, or contexts. However, there are methods, tools, and materials that communities can use to characterize and assess their own psychosocial needs.

In the aftermath of disasters, crisis counseling is probably the most common intervention. This strategy often blurs boundaries between community and individual level interventions because crisis programs tend to be enacted at the community level but are targeted at individual level change. Although crisis intervention encompasses a wide range of activities directed toward persons experiencing acute distress, it most often takes the form of making individual or group counseling quickly and easily available to victims. As a strategy for prevention, crisis intervention is particularly appropriate when (a) the event cannot be prevented and

(b) the at-risk population is readily identified and available for interventions. Disasters, by their collective and uncontrollable nature, provide an ideal setting for crisis intervention. Numerous authors (e.g., Cohen, 1985; Myers, 1989; Seroka, Knapp, Knight, & Starbuck, 1986) have advocated the use of crisis intervention following disasters to prevent the development of psychopathology and have offered useful guidelines for such services.

One such guideline is that crisis counseling programs should assume a proactive posture rather than a reactive one in identifying persons in need of services. This posture involves active case-finding and outreach services in the community. Outreach is needed because many people who need help may not seek it. A reluctance to use formal assistance may reflect an emphasis on independence and "carrying one's own weight" or a belief that one should rely on one's family for care and support. In most communities and locales, a traditional "office" approach in which the clients are self-referred will not be effective after disasters.

Likewise, crisis intervention programs must be tailored to the cultural and community context (for in-depth discussion of these intervention issues, see Danieli, Rodley, & Weisaeth, 1996; de Jong, 1995; Gist & Lubin, 1999). Many cultures attach stigma to receiving psychological help. Whereas some cultures encourage the expression and sharing of feelings (Wierzbicka, 1994), others discourage public expression of emotion and the seeking of emotional support (Ellsworth, 1994).

> In September 1999, an accident at the Tokai-Mura Nuclear Fuel Processing Facility exposed 69 workers directly to radiation and forced persons living near the facility to evacuate from their homes. Psychologists at Sophia University were asked to provide psychological assistance to the community. They provided consultation services and seminars for local helping professions, such as public health nurses, school teachers, and counselors, some of whom were victims themselves. The services they provided were designed to fit Japanese culture in several ways. First, the seminars were titled "Helping Children," because the consultants reasoned that people would be less resistant to this topic than one described as dealing with their own mental health issues. Also, the purpose of the seminar was described as "information provision," rather than "emotional support" or "debriefing," because seeking information is considered more culturally appropriate than sharing feelings or seeking emotional support. Yet the seminar was actually designed to provide an environment where such support would be received along with the information provided. By eliminating the threat of stigma, the consultants provided an effective means to provide crisis intervention in Japan (Inamoto & Konishi, 2000).

Sometimes, crisis counseling differs from corrective therapy more in timing and scope than in orientation. One lesson that appears to be very difficult to learn is the irrelevance of mental health programs to persons who have more immediate and basic needs. Lois Gibbs' (1982) story is illustrative: Following the first crisis at Love Canal, New York (an infamous case of residential toxin exposure; see Gibbs, 1982), the local mental health clinic arrived on site and set up a display to offer services. According to Gibbs, a resident and grass-roots organizer, the "beaming" Mental Health Center sign alienated most of the residents. People avoided these professionals to protect their images and reputations. Gibbs believed those professionals were desperately needed, but that they should have been more sensitive to community attitudes and needs. As others (e.g., Faberow, 1978) have also noted, outreach efforts to victims are most effective when they take the form of assisting them with the variety of practical problems that arise during the impact period, such as needs for housing, insurance settlements, medical care, material aid, and social services. Some people are more likely to accept help for such "problems in living" than to accept help for "mental health problems." Practical, resource-oriented help may be every bit as important for the preservation or restoration of mental health.

Though retaining a focus on mental health, Gist and Stolz's (1982) intervention following the Hyatt disaster differed greatly from the provision of on-the-spot, brief psychotherapy that has characterized many crisis counseling programs. Following the dramatic "skywalk" disaster at the Hyatt Regency Hotel in Kansas City, Missouri, where an internal "bridge" collapsed, killing more than one hundred people and injuring many more, these authors, along with others in their community, enacted a "three-fold community-wide response" (p. 1137). First, support groups were initiated by community mental health centers in every part of the metropolitan area. Second, trauma-related training was provided to both psychologists and natural caregivers (e.g., ministers) in the area. Third, the media were engaged to publicize the availability of services, to describe typical psychological reactions to disaster, and to communicate that these reactions were normal reactions to abnormal situations that should be accepted and discussed with friends and colleagues. In the month following the skywalk's collapse, 500 persons participated in support groups, and 200 professionals attended training programs. Gist and Stolz believed that the aggressive media campaign freed those at risk from the stigma of seeking psychological help. Empirical data are lacking, but the authors built a good case for the success of the intervention.

In many ways, the Kansas City program could stand as a model for crisis counseling initiatives. Particularly appealing was the effort to normalize rather than to pathologize distress. The fit between the goals of the program and the community's needs and resources was excellent. As for the generalizability of the model, it is important to recognize that Kansas City's communication and general infrastructure of goods and services were left intact. The media would be more difficult to exploit in settings where electricity is lacking and communication systems are impaired. However, as the following case study illustrates, similar psychoeducational approaches can be used even after larger-scale disasters. As this example shows, primary care physicians often serve as the first point of referral for the care of mental health needs of adults and very young children, while teachers are key in identifying the mental health needs of school-age children. Many communities will need to designate some individuals to be community health workers. Such persons will disseminate information and stimulate and support community efforts.

> A supercyclone hit the Orissa coast of India on October 29, 1999. The wind force was more than 250 kms per hour, creating sea waves 20 to 30 feet high. This disaster affected over 15 million people living in 12 districts, killing 10,000 and leaving millions homeless. The most striking aspect of this disaster was the extensive damage to the trees, animals, and houses. A series of studies of individuals in the disaster zone showed that 65% had mental health problems, of which 25% were severe. Visits by specialists confirmed the high level of psychosocial problems and psychiatric symptoms in the population. Against this background, the number of mental health resources available in the whole state was extremely small. There were only 31 psychiatrists and even fewer clinical psychologists and psychiatric social workers.
>
> This disaster was important for causing the psychosocial problems of the affected population to be recognized. A specific program to meet the needs of the population was initiated that had the following components:
>
> 1. A simple information booklet, written at an accessible level for all the affected population, which described how people could take care of their own health by measures that are within their reach.
> 2. A more detailed booklet, prepared for all categories of community level workers to provide support and information on first-aid and referral procedures and to stimulate community support systems.
> 3. A program of training in mental health care developed for primary care physicians.
> 4. A manual developed for teachers to help them provide mental health care to affected children.

This discussion has focused on the provision of services to survivors, but it should be noted that disaster workers themselves experience considerable trauma. This observation has led some practitioners to develop intervention strategies especially tailored for emergency-service personnel. The best-known of these may be Critical Incident Stress Debriefing (CISD; Mitchell, 1983). A critical incident is defined as "any situation faced by emergency service personnel that causes them to experience unusually strong emotional reactions which have the potential to interfere with their ability to function either at the scene or later" (Mitchell, 1983, p. 36). To defuse the stress, group meetings and structured discussions are held that emphasize normal responses to abnormal events. Typically, these meetings take place within one to three days after an incident. Following the 1989 San Francisco earthquake, for example, Armstrong, O'Callahan, and Marmar (1991) modified and expanded CISD into a Multiple Stressor Debriefing Model for use with Red Cross volunteers and personnel. CISD has found wide acceptance by the professional mental health community, but well-controlled studies documenting its effectiveness are generally lacking. See Chapter 14 for a more detailed discussion of interventions for civilian and field personnel.

RECOMMENDATIONS

In accord with the previous discussion we make the following recommendations for disaster management:

Recommendations for Policy-Makers

- Increase global access to technologies that provide advance warning of many disaster agents, e.g., floods, hurricanes, volcanic eruptions.
- Develop international/national/provincial plans for a mental health-oriented response to disasters that establish collaborative relationships among formal emergency management agencies, public health agencies, and citizen's groups.
- Develop culturally appropriate interventions that educate the public about disaster preparedness. Like other behavioral interventions, campaigns to educate the public about disaster preparedness must focus on specific suggestions and will be most effective if they successfully communicate that the behavior is necessary (vulnerability), that the behavior is effective (controllability), that the recipient of the message has the skills needed to perform the behavior (self-efficacy), that others expect the recipient to act (norms), and that the behavior will show a concern for the welfare of others (moral obligation). Different aspects of the message might be emphasized (e.g., norms, moral obligation) or de-emphasized (controllability) as culturally appropriate for the community involved.
- Support research on the effects of disasters. Following most disasters, research gets a very low priority. To date, few disaster-focused interventions have been evaluated empirically and fewer still have met standards of rigorous research (Burkle, Bolton, & Watson, 2001).

Recommendations for Disaster Managers

- *Provide accurate and consistent information.* The importance of accurate, trustworthy, easily understood, and consistent information about the disaster and its consequences, especially if there are continuing threats, cannot be overemphasized.
- *Train rescue and relief workers to provide psychological first aid.* Regardless of their specific duties, rescue and relief workers should be sensitive to survivors' psychosocial needs. Workers must interact with survivors in a caring and supportive way and attempt to provide reassurance, basic information, and referrals to helping agencies.
- *Educate health care providers, teachers, and community workers about mental health.* Basic knowledge about mental health, simple interventions, and ways to identify and refer problematic cases is helpful to both the workers and the community as a whole. A manual such as the WHO/UNHCR *Mental Health of Refugees* (De Jong & Clark, 1992) that has been adapted to the local cultural context can be used.
- *Educate the public.* The affected population will need clear information about normal reactions to stress, what to do and not to do, and when and where to seek help. Pamphlets, such as *Coping with Stress*, produced by the Royal Children's Hospital and Prince Henry Hospital following the Ash Wednesday fires in Australia, can be used for this purpose. Where feasible, various media can also be engaged to help with this task.
- *Initiate crisis intervention services.* Various professionals and paraprofessionals from inside or outside the community can be called upon to provide services and support to survivors as well as first-line rescue and relief workers. Although needs vary depending upon the nature of the disaster, such services might include (a) crisis counseling, (b) debriefing of workers, (c) assistance in notifying families regarding death of kin and helping them with identification of bodies, (d) establishing links between disaster services and pre-existing helping structures, and (e) organizing self-help, support, or community action groups.
- *Establish integrated, ongoing services.* In situations where ongoing, specialized mental health care is needed and available, it may be useful to establish a center where multidisciplinary teams can work together to intervene on behalf of individuals, families, or the community as a whole. The team might include psychiatrists, psychologists, counselors, social workers, nurses, creative therapists, relaxation therapists, alcohol and drug therapists, or occupational therapists.
- *Involve the community and identify their strengths.* To be effective, any such program must involve the participation of the local population in an

active and decision-making role rather than in a dependent, "victim" role. Local skills and resources have to be tapped and utilized if the community is to gain a sense of accomplishment and fulfillment in the reconstruction process.

- *Provide meaning.* Provision for the cultural working-through of the shared traumatic experience, in the form of periodic reminders of the loss and reiteration of its meaning, will be helpful. Community gatherings, meetings, and religious ceremonies will allow for communal release of feelings and coming to terms with the collective trauma. Such gatherings help people to define and interpret their experiences, to establish social links, and to plan for the future.

Recommendations for the Community

No one set of recommendations will apply to all communities cross-culturally. It is important that the activities match the cultural context and needs of the group (De Jong, 1995; De Vries, 1995). The best way to assure this is to involve the community in evaluating its own needs and typical ways of behaving and determining which actions are most suitable (Figley, Giel, Borgo, Briggs, & Haritos-Fatouros, 1995). We offer these suggestions as starting points for discussion but emphasize that community groups will need to tailor them to their own particular contexts.

- *Grieve and sing together.* Grief resolution should occur at the personal, family, and community levels. Collective grieving expresses solidarity and facilitates unity and collective action. Such activities should be organized initially on a weekly basis, then a monthly basis, and later annually. Folk songs and devotionals that describe the tragedy and its impact provide another way for communities to share their grief. Such actions may increase the cohesiveness of the community and motivate participants to initiate collective action.
- *Meet.* Group meetings are important activities in which the community as a whole participates. Participants think and brainstorm about various themes for rebuilding the community. This not only helps them to come to terms with the reality of loss but also helps them to identify and discuss local problems and initiate collective action toward such goals as rebuilding school or roads, restoring power or water, or providing access to medical care. Encourage survivors to share their success stories (coping with loss) with others in group meetings. This will make them feel good and may benefit others. Such forums may also provide a way to stay informed about the relative needs of network members.

- *Hold rallies.* This conveys solidarity and strength and sensitizes administrative bodies that can address delays in restoration, rebuilding, relocation, or compensation.
- *Work together toward achievable, specific goals.* Clearing the bushes to create a playground for children, putting up a hut for a school, or devising a plan for providing food for survivors who are disabled or dependent brings communities closer together.
- *Be inclusive.* Involve religious leaders, opinion leaders, and village members in all these activities. Reach out to people who might feel isolated or marginalized. Consider ways of canvassing the community to learn of the needs of others.
- *Seek and provide accurate information.* Uncertainty can create much stress. Create mechanisms for keeping the community informed about problems and progress. Sensitize the group about rumors and discuss ways to handle them as a group.

Recommendations for Families

- *Keep the family together.* Sending women, children, and the aged to far-off places for the sake of safety can be anxiety-producing for them and other family members. If a family member must be separated or hospitalized, keep him/her informed about the safety of the others. Get information about his/her condition as often as possible.
- *Have family members talk* about their experiences, losses, and feelings with one another.
- *Contact relatives* outside the disaster zone to ease their fears and mobilize support.
- *Enact rituals and other meaningful activities* such as prayers or preserving the belongings of a lost family member.
- *Resume normal activities* to provide a sense of stability and provide important ways for network members to stay informed about the needs of other members.
- *Handle conflict appropriately* to minimize increases in negative encounters due to the strain, fatigue, and irritability that may follow trauma. Be tolerant, but help family members direct their anger into appropriate channels.

Recommendations for Individuals

- *Seek accurate information* and do not believe in rumors that go around during such times.
- *Establish daily routines* as early as possible to help you feel in control of the situation.

- *Talk and listen.* Though all of you have had the same experience, it will do you good to talk about the disaster, your experiences, and your feelings with family members and friends. Tell others you understand how they feel.
- *Seek and give comfort.* Touching and comforting your family members, especially children and old people, is beneficial to you and others.
- *Get to know others.* Even in temporary dwellings it is good to be with known community people, i.e., people from your own village. Consider organizing the new community, if someone else has not done so.
- *Join or initiate rituals.* Rituals, like prayers or mourning, are very helpful; so join or initiate such rituals. If you have lost family members, perform the last rites, and bid them farewell.
- *Work.* If you are unhurt, take part in the rescue, relief, and rehabilitation operations. Work is a good tonic for healing.
- *Relax and recreate.* Take time every day to relax. Go for a walk, exercise, listen to music, visit the temple, sing or pray, and invite others to join you.
- *Accept your limitations.* Make time for yourself and recognize that it may be weeks or months before you are able to function at your usual level of efficiency.

ACKNOWLEDGEMENT: The authors wish to thank Krzysztof Kaniasty, Professor of Psychology at Indiana University of Pennsylvania, for the story about the Polish lady who made everyone cook.

REFERENCES

Armstrong, K., O'Callahan, W., & Marmar, C. (1991). Debriefing Red Cross disaster personnel: The Multiple Stressor Debriefing Model. *Journal of Traumatic Stress, 4*, 581–594.

Baum, A. (1987). Toxins, technology, and natural disasters. In G. VandenBos & B. Bryant (Eds.), *Cataclysms, crises, and catastrophes: Psychology in action* (pp. 9–51). Washington, DC: APA.

Baum, A., Fleming, R., & Davidson, L. (1983). Natural disasters and technological catastrophe. *Environment and Behavior, 15*, 333–354.

Bolin, R. (1985). Disaster characteristics and psychosocial impacts. In B. Sowder (Ed.), *Disasters and Mental Health: Selected Contemporary Perspectives* (pp. 3–28). Rockville, MD: National Institute of Mental Health.

Bromet, E. (1995). Methodological issues in designing research on community-wide disasters with special reference to Chernobyl. In S. Hobfoll & M. De Vries (Eds.), *Extreme stress and communities: Impact and intervention* (pp. 307–324). Dordrecht, The Netherlands: Kluwer.

Burkle, F., Bolton, P., & Watson, P. (2001). *Disaster-related mental health interventions: Review of the published literature.* White River Junction, VT: National Center for Posttraumatic Stress Disorder.

Caplan, G. (1964). *Principles of preventive psychiatry.* New York: Basic Books.

Cohen, R. (1985). Crisis counseling principles and services. In M. Lystad (Ed.), *Innovations in mental health services to disaster victims* (pp. 151–160). Rockville, MD: National Institute of Mental Health.

Danieli, Y., Rodley, N., & Weisaeth, L. (Eds.) (1996). *International responses to traumatic stress: Humanitarian, human rights, justice, peace and development contributions, collaborative actions, and future initiatives.* Amityville, New York: Baywood Publishing.

De Girolamo, G., & McFarlane, A. (1996). The epidemiology of PTSD: A comprehensive review of the international literature. In A. Marsella, M. Friedman, E. Gerrity, & R. Scurfield (Eds.), *Ethnocultural aspects of posttraumatic stress disorder: Issues, research, and clinical applications* (pp. 33–86). Washington, D.C.: APA.

De Jong, J. (1995). Prevention of the consequences of man-made or natural disaster at the international, the community, the family, and the individual level. In S. Hobfoll & M. De Vries (Eds.), *Extreme stress and communities: Impact and intervention* (pp. 207–227). Dordrecht, The Netherlands: Kluwer.

De Jong, J., & Clark, L. (1992). *WHO/UNHCR Mental health training manual.* WHO: Geneva.

De La Fuente, R. (1990). The mental health consequences of the 1985 earthquakes in Mexico. *International Journal of Mental Health, 19,* 21–29.

De Vries, M. (1995). Culture, community and catastrophe: Issues in understanding communities under difficult conditions. In S. Hobfoll & M. De Vries (Eds.), *Extreme stress and communities: Impact and intervention* (pp. 375–393). Dordrecht, The Netherlands: Kluwer.

Edelstein, M.R. (1988). *Contaminated communities: The social and psychological impacts of residential toxic exposure.* Boulder, CO: Westview.

Ellsworth, P. (1994). Sense, culture, and sensibility. In S. Kitayama & H. Markus (Eds.), *Emotion and culture: Empirical studies of mutual influence* (pp. 23–50). Washington, D.C.: American Psychologcial Association.

Ersland, S., Weisaeth, L., & Sund, A. (1989). The stress upon rescuers involved in an oil rig disaster. "Alexander L. Kielland" 1980. *Acta Psychiatrica Scandinavica Supplementum, 80,* 38–49.

Faberow, N. (1978). *Training manual for human service workers in major disasters.* Washington, DC: U.S. Government Printing Office (DHEW Publication No. ADM 77–538).

Faupel, C., Kelley, S., & Petee, T. (1992). The impact of disaster education on household preparedness for Hurricane Hugo. *International Journal of Mass Emergencies and Disasters, 10,* 5–24.

Figley, C., Giel, R., Borgo, S., Briggs, S., & Haritos-Faturos, M. (1995). Prevention and treatment of community stress. In S. Hobfoll & M. De Vries (Eds.), *Extreme stress and communities: Impact and intervention* (pp. 489–497). Dordrecht, The Netherlands: Kluwer.

Freedy, J., Resnick, H., & Kilpatrick, D. (1992). Conceptual framework for evaluating disaster impact: Implications for clinical intervention. In L. Austin (Ed.), *Responding to disaster: A guide for mental health professionals* (pp. 3–23). Washington, DC: American Psychiatric Press, Inc.

Freedy, J., Shaw, D., Jarrell, M., & Masters, C. (1992). Towards an understanding of the psychological impact of natural disasters: An application of the Conservation Resources stress model. *Journal of Traumatic Stress, 5,* 441–454.

Gibbs, L. (1982). Community response to an emergency situation: Psychological destruction and the Love Canal. *American Journal of Community Psychology, 11,* 116–125.

Gist, R., & Lubin, B. (1999). *Response to disaster: Psychosocial, community and ecological approaches.* New York: Brunner/Mazel.

Gist, R., & Stolz, S.B. (1982). Mental health promotion and the media: Community response to the Kansas City hotel disaster. *American Psychologist, 37,* 1136–1139.

Gleser, G., Green, B., & Winget, C. (1981). *Prolonged psychosocial effects of disaster: A study of Buffalo Creek.* New York: Academic Press.

Green, B. (1982). Assessing levels of psychological impairment following disaster: Consideration of actual and methodological dimensions. *Journal of Nervous and Mental Disease*, *170*, 544–552.

Green, B., Korol, M., Grace, M., Vary, M., Leonard, A., Gleser, G., & Smitson-Cohen, S. (1991). Children and disaster: Age, gender, and parental effects on PTSD symptoms. *Journal of the American Academy of Child and Adolescent Psychiatry, 30*, 945–951.

Green, B., & Solomon, S.D. (1995). The mental health impact of natural and technological disasters. In J. Freedy & S. Hobfoll (Eds), *Traumatic stress: From theory to practice* (pp. 163–180). NY: Plenum Press.

Guarnaccia, P., Canino, G., Rubio-Stipec, M., & Bravo, M. (1993). The prevalence of ataques de nervios in the Puerto Rico disaster study. *The Journal of Nervous and Mental Disease, 181*, 157–165.

Harvey, M. (1996). An ecological view of psychological trauma and trauma recovery. *Journal of Traumatic Stress, 9*, 3–23.

Hough, R., Canino, G., Abueg, F., & Gusman, F. (1996). PTSD and related stress disorders among Hispanics. In A. Marsella, M. Friedman, E. Gerrity, & R. Scurfield (Eds.), *Ethnocultural aspects of posttraumatic stress disorder: Issues, research, and clinical applications* (pp. 301–340). Washington, D.C.: APA.

Inamoto, E., & Konishi, T. (2000, November). The psychological response of residents in the aftermath of the radiation accident at Tokai-Mura, Ibaraki Prefecture, Japan. Paper presented at the annual meeting of the International Society for Traumatic Stress Studies, San Antonio, Texas.

International Federation of Red Cross and Red Crescent Societies (1999). *World disaster report.* Dordrecht, The Netherlands: Martinus Nijhoff.

International Federation of Red Cross and Red Crescent Societies (2002). *World disasters report 2002.* Bloomfield, CT: Kumarian Press, Inc.

Jenkins, J. (1996). Culture, emotion, and PTSD. In A. Marsella, M. Friedman, E. Gerrity, & R. Scurfield (Eds.), *Ethnocultural aspects of posttraumatic stress disorder: Issues, research, and clinical applications* (pp. 165–182). Washington, D.C.: APA.

Kaniasty, K., & Norris, F. (1995). In search of altruistic community: Patterns of social support mobilization following Hurricane Hugo. *American Journal of Community Psychology, 23*, 447–477.

Kaniasty, K., & Norris, F. (1997). Social support dynamics in adjustment to disasters. In S. Duck (Ed.), *Handbook of personal relationships* (2nd edition) (pp. 595–619). London, UK: Wiley.

Kaniasty, K., & Norris, F. (1999). Individuals and communities sharing trauma: Unpacking the experience of disaster. in R. Gist & B. Lubin (Eds.), *Psychosocial, ecological, and community approaches to understanding disaster* (pp. 25–62). London: Brunner/Mazel.

Kirmayer, L. (1996). Confusion of the senses: Implications of ethnocultural variations in somatoform and dissociative disorders for PTSD. In A. Marsella, M. Friedman, E. Gerrity, & R. Scurfield (Eds.), *Ethnocultural aspects of posttraumatic stress disorder: Issues, research, and clinical applications* (pp. 165–182). Washington, D.C.: APA.

Kroll-Smith, J.S., & Couch, S. (1993). Technological hazards: Social responses as traumatic stressors. In J.P. Wilson & B. Raphael (Eds.), *International handbook of traumatic stress syndromes* (pp. 79–91). New York: Plenum Press.

La Greca, A., Silverman, W., Vernberg, E., & Prinstein, M. (1996). Symptoms of posttraumatic stress in children after Hurricane Andrew: A prospective study. *Journal of Consulting and Clinical Psychology, 64*, 712–723.

Mitchell, J. (1983). When disaster strikes...The critical incident stress debriefing process. *Journal of Emergency Medical Services, 8*, 36–39.

Mulilis, J., & Duval, S. (1995). Negative threat appeals and earthquake preparedness: A person-relative-to-event (PrE) model of coping with threat. *Journal of Applied Social Psychology, 25*, 1319–1339.

Mulilis, J., & Lippa, R. (1990). Behavioral change in earthquake preparedness due to negative threat appeals: A test of protection motivation theory. *Journal of Applied Social Psychology, 20*, 619–638.

Murphy, S. (1985). Health and recovery status of victims one and three years following a natural disaster. In C. Figley (Ed.), *Trauma and its wake, Vol II.* (pp. 155). New York: Brunner/Mazel.

Myers, D. (1989). Mental health and disasters: Preventive approaches to intervention. In R. Gist & B. Lubin (Eds.), *Psychosocial aspects of disaster* (pp. 190–228). New York: John Wiley & Sons.

Norris, F., Kaniasty, K., Inman, G., Conrad, L., & Murphy, A. (2002). Placing age differences in cultural context: A comparison of the effects of age on PTSD after disasters in the U.S., Mexico, and Poland. *Journal of Clinical Geropsychology, 8*, 153–173.

Norris, F. & Murrell, S. (1988). Prior experience as a moderator of disaster impact on anxiety symptoms in older adults. *American Journal of Community Psychology, 16*, 665–683.

Norris, F., Perilla, J., Ibanez, G., & Murphy, A. (2001). Sex differences in symptoms of PTSD: Does culture play a role? *Journal of Traumatic Stress, 14*, 2001.

Norris, F., Smith, T., & Kaniasty, K. (1999). Revisiting the experience-behavior hypothesis: The effects of Hurricane Hugo on hazard preparedness and other self-protective acts. *Basic and Applied Social Psychology, 21*, 37–47.

North, C., Nixon, S., Shariat, S., Mallonee, S., McMillan, J., Spitznagel, E., & Smith, E. (1999). Psychiatric disorders among survivors of the Oklahoma City bombing. *Journal of the American Medical Association, 282*, 755–762.

Palinkas, L., Russell, J., Downs, M., & Peterson, J. (1992). Ethnic differences in stress, coping, and depressive symptoms after the Exxon Valdez Oil Spill. *The Journal of Nervous and Mental Disease, 180*, 287–295.

Perilla, J., Norris, F., & Lavizzo, E. (2002). Identifying and explaining ethnic differences in PTSD six months after Hurricane Andrew. *Journal of Social and Clinical Psychology, 21*, 28–45.

Phifer, J., & Norris, F. (1989). Psychological symptoms in older adults following natural disaster: Nature, timing, duration, and course. *Journal of Gerontology, 44*, 207–217.

Quarantelli, E. (1985). Social support systems: Some behavioral patterns in the context of mass evacuation activities. In B. Sowder (Ed.), *Disasters and mental health: Selected contemporary perspectives* (pp. 122–136). Rockville, MD: National Institute of Mental Health.

Quarantelli, E. (1994). *Future disaster trends and policy implications for developing countries.* Newark, DE: Disaster Research Center.

Riad, J., Norris, F., & Ruback, B. (1999). Predicting evacuation following two major disasters: The roles of risk perceptions, social influence, and resources. *Journal of Applied Social Psychology, 29*, 918–934.

Rochford, B. & Blocker, T. (1991). Coping with "natural" hazards as stressors. *Environment and Behavior, 23*, 171–194.

Seroka, C.M., Knapp, C., Knight, S., Siemon, C.R., & Starbuck, S. (1986). A comprehensive program for postdisaster counseling. *Social Casework: The Journal of Contemporary Social Work, 67*, 37–45.

Shannon, M., Lonigan, C., Finch, A., & Taylor, C. (1994). Children exposed to disaster: I. Epidemiology of post-traumatic symptoms and symptom profiles. *Journal of American Academy of Child and Adolescent Psychiatry, 33*, 80–93.

Shore, J., Tatum, E., & Vollmer, W. (1986). Evaluation of mental effects of disaster, Mount St. Helens Eruption. *American Journal of Public Health, 76*, 76–83.

Smith, E., Robins, L., Przybeck, T., Goldring, E., & Solomon, S. (1986). Psychosocial consequences of a disaster. In J. Shore (Ed.), *Disaster stress studies: New methods and findings* (pp. 49–76). Washington, DC: American Psychiatric Press.

Solomon, S.D., Bravo, M., Rubio-Stipec, M., & Canino, G. (1993). Effect of family role on response to disaster. *Journal of Traumatic Stress, 6*, 255–269.

Steinglass, P., & Gerrity, E. (1990). Natural disasters and post-traumatic stress disorder: Short-term versus long-term recovery in two disaster affected communities. *Journal of Applied Social Psychology, 20*, 1746–1765.

Substance Abuse and Mental Health Services Administration (1994). *Disaster response and recovery: A handbook for mental health professionals.* Washington, D.C.: U.S. Department of Health and Human Services.

Thompson, M., Norris, F., & Hanacek, B. (1993). Age differences in the psychological consequences of Hurricane Hugo. *Psychology and Aging, 8*, 606–616.

United Nations General Assembly Economic and Social Council (2000). *Strengthening of the coordination of emergency humanitarian assistance of the United Nations.* New York: Authors.

Ursano, R., & McCarroll, J. (1994). Exposure to traumatic death: The nature of the stressor. In R. Ursano, B. McCaughey, & C. Fullerton (Eds.), *Individual and community responses to trauma and disaster: The structure of human chaos* (pp. 46–71). Cambridge: Cambridge University Press.

Van Den Eynde, J., & Veno, A. (1999). Coping with disastrous events: An empowerment model of community healing. In R. Gist & B. Lubin (Eds.), *Response to disaster: Psychological, community, and ecological approaches* (pp. 167–192). Philadelphia, PA: Taylor & Francis.

Weisaeth, L. (1994). Psychological and psychiatric aspects of technological disasters. In R. Ursano, B. McCaughey, & C. Fullerton (Eds.), *Individual and community responses to trauma and disaster: The structure of human chaos* (pp. 72–102). Cambridge: Cambridge University Press.

Wierzbicka, A. (1994). Emotion, language, and cultural scripts. In S. Kitayama & H. Markus (Eds.), *Emotion and culture: Empirical studies of mutual influence* (pp. 133–196). Washington, D.C.: American Psychological Association.

Part IV

United National Personnel

UNSECOORD: PROCTECTING THE PROTECTORS

The conditions under which staff members of the United Nations system have carried out their duties have changed drastically over the past few years. Consequently, the General Assembly[1] has asked the office of the United Nations Security Coordinator (UNSECOORD) to take on the responsibility for coordinating the daily security of field operations for the organizations of the United Nations system as well as designated officials, including officials working in the areas of stress counseling and security training.

More specifically, UNSECOORD has been given the mandate to develop a comprehensive United Nations policy pertaining to: management of critical incident stress, taking into account gender-related issues; a rapid response to traumatic events and critical incidents (e.g. hostage-taking, evacuation, death of a staff member under malicious circumstances); and providing appropriate stress defusing/debriefing and counseling to all affected staff. At the same time, UNSECOORD was also assigned the task of establishing and providing stress management training to all staff worldwide, preparing relevant stress management training materials for use by staff in the field, and chairing an inter-agency working group on stress management.

To this day, and given its very limited resources, UNSECOORD has done its very best to meet the needs of staff in the field. Stress counseling and stress management training have been integrated into the security management training program designed by UNSECOORD and offered to all staff working within the UN system. More specifically, the stress-awareness training component included in the security management

---

[1] Resolutions of the United Nations General Assembly *A/55/494, A/56/469.*

training program aims at enabling UN personnel to recognize and deal with stress and its symptoms. Traditionally, a qualified mental health professional (e.g. a psychologist or a counselor) has been in charge of stress awareness and stress management training.

Rapid response to traumatic events and critical incidents has thus far been provided and supervised by the UNSECOORD team, in coordination with field personnel (e.g. designated official, field security officer, staff counselor,[2] or locally/regionally recruited mental health professionals). With its two stress counselors,[3] UNSECOORD continues to develop training materials and to design an intervention model that can be implemented in the field, one with flexibility for cultural or other specificities.

By way of illustration, from September 1998 up to January 2002, UNSECOORD has sent its staff on 17 missions to 28 different countries. Eight additional missions to 16 countries were planned as well for 2002. Eighteen missions to 39 countries are anticipated in 2003. Each mission team consists of three people (two security coordination officers and one stress counselor) who do stress awareness training and security management training, and are available for individual or group consultations as well.

UN staff service to humanity exacts a high price on the welfare of these individuals. It is now time to protect the protectors. Organizations have a duty of care towards their staff. The commitment of the General Assembly to provide stress management assistance worldwide is an important step forward.

UNSECOORD welcomes all efforts to promote knowledge about stress. In *Trauma Interventions in War and Peace*, the ISTSS has called upon a host of scholars, researchers, and practitioners and has come up with an authoritative overview of traumatic stress, its determining factors, and its consequences. The book provides the reader with all the key elements needed to comprehend the multifaceted aspects of traumatic stress.

Researchers, clinicians, and policy-makers will find an up-to-date account of what has been done and published in the area of posttraumatic stress. Numerous suggestions pertaining to new research areas are here to be explored, and recommendations are included as well. Of particular importance to UNSECOORD is the chapter dealing with UN peacekeepers and civilian field personnel. The authors have presented a

---

[2] As of 2 February 2000, qualified staff counselors have been posted to East Timor (UNTAET), Lebanon (UNIFIL), and Kosovo (UNMIK). In addition, another staff counselor is being appointed to Sierra Leone (UNAMSIL). These staff counselors work in coordination with the UNSECOORD stress counseling focal point.

[3] It is worth mentioning that the UNSECOORD Stress Counseling Unit will eventually comprise five stress counselors on a full-time basis.

conceptually-driven discussion regarding the distinctiveness of the stressful experiences of UN professionals, the traumatizing events they are likely to face, and the *slowness* that has characterized civilian institutions and agencies in acknowledging and addressing theses issues. The suggestions concerning future areas of research and the recommendations that are made here are, to say the least, in touch with reality.

DIANA RUSSLER
Deputy United Nations Security Coordinator
Office of the United Nations Security Coordinator

Chapter 14

UN Peacekeepers and Civilian Field Personnel

Matthew J. Friedman, Peter G. Warfe, and
Gladys K. Mwiti

This chapter is unlike any other in this volume. Instead of addressing traumatic stress among people who require UN assistance because of social circumstances or humanitarian emergencies, we focus on the needs of UN personnel charged with providing such assistance. Although this is a massive topic, we attempt to succinctly review the nature of the stressors experienced by these individuals, their potential psychological impact, the consequences of institutional failure to address such adverse exposure and responses, what can be learned from the relevant literature, and what intervention models to consider. We provide illustrative case examples, identify important gaps in our current knowledge, and generate a series of recommendations.

Due to space constraints, we discuss UN peacekeepers and civilian field personnel in the same chapter. By civilian field personnel, **we refer to staff both of parent UN organizations (e.g., UNHCR, WHO, UNICEF, etc.) as well as to staff of non-governmental organizations (NGOs)**. This category includes humanitarian personnel responding to acute refugee or disaster emergencies, human rights officials gathering evidence on crimes against humanity, or social service providers dealing with human misery (e.g., social deprivation; social injustice; aggression and injustice against women; child abuse; religious or ethnic repression; or discrimination against disabled individuals or the elderly). Despite some overlap, there are important distinctions to be drawn between these two large heterogeneous sets of UN operatives. There have been approximately 35 deployments of peacekeeping forces since 1948. There is an emerging scientific literature on the psychological impact of such assignments. Military officials from many nations have made these concerns a high priority, and there are a number of interventions that have begun to be tested.

The picture is quite different for civilian field staff. Indeed, recognition has been slow that UN responsibilities may have adverse psychological consequences which may deleteriously affect both functional performance and long-term adjustment. There is a sparse scientific literature, little official national or international attention to this problem, and virtually no institutional resolve to address these consequences systematically. With the exception of one recent report concerning NGO humanitarian personnel (Eriksson, Van De Kemp, Gorsuch, Hoke & Foy, 2001), the literature cited here is extrapolated from pertinent research with professionals who work with other trauma survivors such as emergency medical personnel, disaster responders, police, firefighters, or mental health professionals.

NATURE AND SCOPE OF THE PROBLEM

Stressors and Potentially Traumatizing Events

Table 14.1 lists the kinds of stressors that may be encountered by UN personnel in the course of their duties. The nature of the assignment will obviously affect the risk of exposure to certain stressors. For example, UN peacekeepers are more likely to struggle with ambiguous rules of engagement, frustration from the need to maintain neutrality (especially in the face of threats, harassment, and taunting), and hostility of the host country. Civilian field personnel may be more likely to experience hopelessness and guilt due to their inability to change the external situation (e.g., starvation), inability to meet personal expectations for success, or a sense of powerlessness vs. denial in the face of unremitting demands by the massive number of people requesting assistance. Both groups may experience personal vulnerability (e.g., attacks, kidnappings, or hostage situations) as well as exposure to the acute consequences of war, disasters, human carnage, or deprivation; they are likely to witness the ongoing suffering of the populations they have been tasked to assist or protect, the ongoing violence or abuse, and boredom, inactivity, and uncertainty in the midst of danger. A final set of stressors, the most preventable, includes shock from the lack of pre-deployment preparation, and distress due to sudden separation from the safety and familiarity of the home environment. Let us provide a few illustrative examples of these stressors.

Table 14.1. Stressors and Potentially Traumatizing Events Experienced by UN Personnel

Personal Vulnerability, Attacks, Kidnapping, Kept as Hostage, Sexual Assault

Encountering the Acute Consequences of War, Disasters, Human Carnage, Starvation, Deprivation

Exposure to Emotional Suffering of Populations Assisting

Witnessing Ongoing Trauma, Violence, or Abuse

Ambiguous Rules of Engagement for Peacekeepers

Frustration from the Need to Maintain Neutrality in the Face of Threats, Harassment & Taunting (Peacekeepers)

Hopelessness/Guilt Due to Inability to Change External Situation (Civilian Field Personnel)

Inability to Meet Personal Expectations for Success (Civilian Field Personnel)

Hostility of Host Country/Environment

Sudden Detachment/Separation from Familiar/Safe Environment

Shock due to Lack of Pre-deployment Preparation

Powerlessness vs. Denial in the Face of Unremitting Demands

Boredom/Inactivity/Uncertainty in the Midst of Danger

Swedish soldiers deployed to peacekeeping operations in Congo, Lebanon, Cyprus, and Bosnia reported cognitive and emotional stressors. *Cognitive stressors* included: overstimulation alternating with periods of deprivation; too much information at certain times in contrast to too little information at other times; uncertainty; unpredictability; hard choices vs. no choices; and ambiguous rules of engagement. *Emotional stressors* included: threats of death or injury; loss of close colleagues; resentment, anger, and rage; boredom; and moral conflicts (Lundin & Otto, 1992).

Individual American peacekeepers deployed to Somalia reported the following specific stressful incidents: being shot at, driving a truck in a convoy behind a vehicle blown up by a land mine, experiencing intense fear while riding in a convoy under attack, and witnessing severe starvation, dying children and the bloody aftermath of an attack in which he or she could have been killed (Litz, 1996).

NGO humanitarian personnel reported a number of stressors in which they were personally exposed to life threatening situations that were experienced as very distressing. The most frequent events of this sort included: being threatened with serious physical harm; being shot at; being chased by a group or individual; sustaining damage to home or office by bombing or shelling; and witnessing death, injury, or destruction of property (Eriksson et al., 2001).

Humanitarian aid workers in Goma, Zaire in 1994 had to function in a situation in which they were exposed to people dying by the thousands due to dehydration, children sitting for hours uncomprehendingly beside their mothers who had just died, and the daily visual, olfactory, and emotional reminders of such enormous suffering because disposal of dead bodies was such a massive logistical challenge that the same dead bodies often remained in the same location for days or weeks (Smith, Agger, Danieli, & Weisæth., 1996). "The conditions in the camps were unnerving to relief workers not only because of the crowding, the smells, the filth and the bodies, but because no one was able to fill a small percentage of the need" (Smith et al., 1996, p. 401).

During the siege of Sarajevo in 1992, humanitarian workers were exposed to threats to their own lives or well-being, such as random violence from sniper fire, food shortages, uncertainty whether the city would or would not be occupied, and total disruption of civil life. Paradoxically, these incessant dangers promoted a sense of intense bonding, compassion, and warmth among humanitarian workers who shared the same risks as the people they had come to help (Smith et al., 1996).

Distinctiveness of Stressful Experiences of UN Professionals

The stress and trauma literature has focused, for the most part, on the emotional impact of overwhelming stressors on exposed individuals. The intensity, persistence, uncontrollability, and unpredictability of the events described above may sometimes have profound emotional consequences. UN personnel deployed to a war zone, disaster site, refugee camp, scene of crimes against humanity, or region marked by injustice or deprivation are exposed to severe and overwhelming stressors even though they may not have suffered the personal loss of loved ones, home, community, or way of life experienced by the people they have come to assist.

In addition, the responsibilities of civilian field workers and peace-keepers, by their very nature, make this work extremely difficult. Listening to people talk about suffering, child abuse, or lack of basic needs, or witnessing continued violence, injustice, or state terrorism may also be very stressful for field personnel because they cannot intervene to improve the situation (Litz, Orsillo, Friedman, Ehlich, & Batres, 1997). In short, UN and NGO personnel face a unique set of potential psychological problems in addition to those shared with the people they are assisting.

It is important to emphasize that since this book is about the impact of traumatic stressors that is our major focus. To put this chapter into its proper context, however, it should be understood that in practice, there are other common but significant stressors with which peacekeepers must contend. Indeed, according to Dr. Christen Halle, Chief of the UN Department of Peacekeeping Operations (DPKO) Medical Support Services, these non-traumatic stressors may constitute the greatest concern for the majority of peacekeepers. They include understimulation, boredom, separation from loved ones (already mentioned) as well as the guilt and frustration of being unable to support the partner at home when s/he must contend with

Table 14.2. Potential Consequences of Institutional Failure to Address Stressful Aspects of UN Peacekeeping/Civilian Field Assignments

To UN/NGO Personnel
  Emotional Distress During Deployment
  Alcoholism and Drug Abuse/Dependence
  Insensitivity to the Needs of Others: Numbing, Dissociation, Hostility, Cynicism
  Burnout
  Persistent Psychological Distress
  Posttraumatic Stress Disorder
  Persistent Functional Impairment
To UN and NGO Missions
  Performance Deficits and Inefficiencies
  Attrition of Trained Personnel
  Increased Costs
  Success of the Mission in Jeopardy

difficult problems, and the limited chance to achieve what could have been achieved during the deployment because there was little or no opportunity to do so (C. Halle, personal communication, 2001).

Consequences of Institutional Failure to Address this Problem

As noted earlier, while the military establishments of many UN member nations have recognized the deleterious impact of extreme stressors experienced during peacekeeping, civilian institutions and agencies have been much slower to acknowledge and address these problems. Thus, some UN or NGO personnel may become so emotionally distressed that they develop acute and/or chronic psychological symptoms that may impair their functional capacity in the field or at home. The institutional costs of this problem include decreased productivity, low morale, attrition of trained personnel, and higher monetary expenses, all of which jeopardize the successful completion of the mission as well as the reputation of the UN or NGO as an effective organization that can achieve its stated aims.

Table 14.2 lists adverse consequences to the individual and to UN and NGO missions when the emotional impact of mission-related stressors is not addressed. Although there is clearly a relationship between individual and institutional problems, we believe it useful to address them separately, because separate preventive strategies must be considered at both the individual and institutional level.

Consequences to the Individual

The assignments of peacekeepers and civilian field personnel are challenging and difficult. Bearing witness to the suffering of fellow human beings is a part of the job. Responding emotionally to such sights, sounds, and smells is a normal human reaction. Indeed the sensitivity and compassion generated by such feelings can sometimes promote a sense of purpose and dedication that not only enhances the determination of UN or NGO personnel to carry out their assigned duties, but may also elevate the quality of their performance in the field.

On the other hand, strong emotional reactions to mission-related stressors can also have adverse psychological consequences. Such reactions may be acute emotional responses that occur only in the field of operations. Other responses may persist long after repatriation and, in some cases, may result in persistent psychological or functional problems.

Peacekeepers and civilian field workers experience a variety of acute reactions that may be divided roughly into *intrusive* and *avoidance* reactions (Smith et al., 1996). These reactions develop from the enormity of mission-related demands to ameliorate the suffering of war-zone survivors, refugees, disaster victims, and others who require assistance. Multiplying the suffering of one severely traumatized person by the comparable distress of hundreds or thousands of similarly affected individuals may produce a spectrum of intrusive reactions including feelings of helplessness, horror, frustration, anger, guilt, and enmeshment.

Intrusive Reactions.   Peacekeepers have reported fear, helplessness, horror, a sense of vulnerability, frustration, anger, guilt, conflict over the demand to maintain neutrality, fear of losing control over their aggressive impulses, and moral/spiritual confusion (Egge, Mortensen, & Weisæth, 1996; Litz, 1996; Lundin & Otto, 1992; Orsillo, Roemer, Litz, Ehlich, & Friedman, 1998; Weisæth, Mehlum, & Mortensen, 1996).

Another set of intrusive reactions is related to a loss of personal boundaries (enmeshment) between UN or NGO personnel and the local population. Enmeshment is an insidious process in which relief workers over-identify with the victims of humanitarian crises, social deprivation, injustice, or interpersonal abuse, and lose both their objectivity and their capacity to intervene effectively (Smith et al., 1996).

In the most extreme manifestation of intrusive reactions, UN or NGO personnel will themselves begin to have mental images, nightmares, or other mental representations of traumatic events experienced—not by themselves, but by the people whom they have been sent to assist. This phenomenon has been called *vicarious traumatization, secondary traumatization,* or *compassion fatigue* (Figley, 1995; McCann & Pearlman, 1990). A comprehensive guide to the growing number of publications on this psychological process among helping professionals can be found elsewhere (Stamm, 1997). It should also be noted that very little of this literature has focused on the unique problems of peacekeepers or civilian field personnel. Rather it is based on observations of police, firefighters, emergency medical personnel, disaster workers, or mental health practitioners who have worked in the security of a stable or peacetime environment. Yet, UN and NGO personnel must cope not only with the suffering of others, but also in some cases carrying out their responsibilities in an environment where their own personal safety is at risk.

Avoidance Reactions. It can be very difficult to maintain one's psychological equilibrium when faced with the intense personal and vicarious responses mentioned earlier. One way to minimize their impact is through a variety of behavioral or psychological strategies. At a conscious or behavioral level, personnel may avoid thoughts, feelings, people, or places that will evoke such feelings. In practice, such a strategy in its extreme results in the avoidance of the very people and situations they have been sent to assist (Danieli, 1984). The less conscious psychological strategy for minimizing intrusive emotions is called *psychic numbing*. This mechanism automatically suppresses intense emotional feelings. While this provides some degree of relief, a high price must be paid for numbing. Numbed personnel are incapable of empathy and other emotional acknowledgments of the suffering of others. In short, the personal protective strategies of behavioral avoidance or psychic numbing may seriously impair humanitarian workers from performing as they can and must. It makes them insensitive to others and affects their judgment, since they are liable to misjudge situations by minimizing their danger, urgency, or severity.

A related avoidant strategy is *dissociation* (Smith et al., 1996), which involves an altered perception of one's environment or oneself. During dissociation people feel detached from the world and themselves. Such a mechanism can markedly impair one's ability to recognize dangerous situations or to elicit normal emotional responses. Dissociation impairs both judgment and performance.

Fear, helplessness, and horror may also be transformed into hostility and cynicism (Smith et al., 1996). Such emotional redirection can be protective, can permit personnel to carry out their assignments, and can evolve into a lifelong reaction pattern that will prove extremely maladaptive after completion of the assignment, repatriation, and return to family.

Finally, another common avoidant strategy is misuse of alcohol or other drugs that will blunt the impact of intolerable mission-related intrusive emotional reactions.

Burnout is a problem that may afflict previously competent individuals who have lost either their motivation or capacity to perform as before. We distinguish it from the performance deficits discussed previously that are due to mission-related traumatic stressors, because burnout is well-recognized as a problem that may occur in the safest work setting. It is related to generic work-related problems such as poor management, excessive demands, and/or inadequate rewards. Burnout affects individual performance and morale as well as the collective productivity and efficiency of the mission in general.

> *After recruitment and a brief orientation, Dr. Waters (a fictitious composite) had been sent to head a medical support unit in a refugee-camp situation. In the midst of insecurity, refugee need, and much suffering, the few humanitarian workers lived in a secured compound, a small haven that provided much-needed peace. However, away from friends, family and familiar social life, there was much boredom and many attempts to alleviate it. Besides the boredom, the suffering of so many in the refugee camp, the regular outbreaks of cholera, fighting, and killings that went on among the refugee factions, and limited communication with the outer world soon began to affect the workers.*
>
> *At first, Dr. Waters was very optimistic, and he immersed himself in his work as supervisor of both expatriate and local medical staff. Although difficult, the work was an invigorating challenge. However, soon he started facing the realities around him. He was bone-tired many days, disturbed by the massive suffering all around him, and feeling increasingly helpless because his contribution did not seem to make much difference, since people continued to die from cholera faster than they could be buried. Several of his staff also contracted the illness. There was no hope of obtaining more fresh water for the camps. Refugees were arriving in such numbers as to overrun litter disposal, garbage collection, and construction of latrines. Then the rains came, and the children and the elderly developed pneumonia. Dr. Waters felt more fatigue and despair. To cope, he started drinking alcohol and smoking more than usual. This began affecting his practice, because he would wake up with a debilitating hangover, report late to work, and keep his team waiting. Although he was supposed to visit the clinics in the field, he would not leave the compound anymore, delegating his fieldwork while making excuses that he had enough to do in the office. He became suspicious of his coworkers, believing that the other expatriates were planning his undoing. This affected his sleep. He began taking medication, and his alcohol intake increased. It was then that his two senior colleagues decided to intervene. They talked to him in confidence, indicating their concern for his emotional and physical well-being. They suggested that he take a break to seek help. However, he insinuated that they were envious and blamed them for all the things that were going wrong around him. That night, in a rage, he wrote his letter of resignation, faxed it to his unit head in another country, and flew home the following morning.*

Persistent Psychological Distress.   Although intrusive and avoidant responses may impair psychological well-being and functional performance in the theater of operation, such reactions are especially deleterious when they persist after repatriation. Perhaps the best current data on this question comes from follow-up studies of Norwegian UNIFIL soldiers (deployed to southern Lebanon) who were repatriated before the completion of their tour of duty (Weisæth et al., 1996). Repatriation was due to illness, injury, disciplinary reasons, and social or family problems. First, it is important to emphasize that 97% of the 15,931 Norwegian troops completed their UNIFIL assignment as planned, and regarded it as an extremely valuable and enlightening experience that had enhanced both their self-reliance and their capacity to cope with stress.

Among the 530 repatriated soldiers, however, comparative outcomes were decidedly negative, with higher rates of depression, alcoholism, suicides, death by accident, and psychosocial problems (Egge et al., 1996; Weisæth et al., 1996). Similar problems were observed in a follow-up study of Dutch UNIFIL veterans, 5% of whom reported excessive psychosocial problems, years after their return from south Lebanon (Knoester, 1989). Finally, a longitudinal study of 514 Swedish peacekeepers who served in Bosnia found 10% who reported psychological problems one year after deployment (Michel, Lundin, & Larsson, submitted for publication).

Unfortunately, there are very few long-range studies of UN peacekeepers following deployment. We, therefore, rely on long-term follow-up studies on military veterans from World War II, the Korean War, and the Vietnam War to provide estimates of psychological problems. These studies have shown that psychological and psychiatric symptoms are not only persistent but are usually associated with alcoholism, functional impairment, and poor psychosocial adjustment (Kulka et al., 1990).

Posttraumatic stress disorder [PTSD] was first described in the DSM-III in 1980 as a constellation of symptoms that develop when individuals are exposed to an extreme (emotional) stressor (APA, 1980). In its original formulation, exposure to the personal vulnerability, deprivation, human suffering, and witnessing of ongoing trauma associated with many peacekeeping or humanitarian deployments, would have easily qualified as a "traumatic" experience. As reformulated in the DSM-IV in 1994 (APA, 1994), such events must produce an intense emotional response such as "fear, hopelessness, and horror" to meet the criterion for a traumatic experience. The DSM-IV's greater emphasis on an individual's subjective emotional response to a stressful event is especially pertinent to UN and NGO personnel, since under the old definition, almost all peacekeepers and humanitarian staff would have been "traumatized" simply by virtue of their assignment to a war zone or disaster site. Under the DSM-IV definition, however, only those personnel who have had an intense emotional reaction to their stressful surroundings would be considered "traumatized."

The best research on PTSD among UN or NGO personnel concerns men and women who participated in peacekeeping operations. Estimates of PTSD vary greatly for UN peacekeepers. Some of this variation is undoubtedly due to differences in the traumatic severity of the UN missions in question, while other variation may be due to methodological differences in the way in which PTSD was diagnosed. Here are some representative findings. Among both Norwegian and Dutch soldiers participating in the prolonged UNIFIL Lebanon operation, 5% had posttraumatic symptoms (Egge et al., 1996). Swedish soldiers deployed to Cyprus exhibited very little (0.5%) trauma-related psychiatric distress in contrast to 20% Canadian (Passey & Crocket, 1995) and 30% Danish (Madsen, 1995) personnel sent to Bosnia who exhibited PTSD symptoms. Among American men and women deployed to Somalia, 8% met criteria for PTSD (Litz, King, King, Orsillo, & Friedman, 1997; Litz et al., 1997).

In the only study on PTSD among NGO humanitarian personnel, 10% of returning staff met full diagnostic criteria for PTSD and about half (51.3%) reported moderate problems in at least one PTSD symptom cluster. Furthermore, higher levels of PTSD were generally associated with higher report of life-threat exposure (Eriksson et al., 2001). In addition, other anecdotal reports on traumatic stress and emotional distress among humanitarian personnel leave little doubt that such assignments carry a clear risk of long-term psychological problems, although it is impossible to speculate, in general, on the expected frequency of such adverse psychological outcomes (Smith et al., 1996). As with peacekeepers, the risk of acute or persistent psychological problems will depend, in part, on the severity, duration, and unique aspects of each distinct UN or NGO mission.

The risk of acute or persistent problems will also depend on the preventive and intervention strategies that are implemented in the field or immediately after repatriation, as will be discussed below.

Persistent Functional Impairment. Finally, the ultimate cost of such delcterious psychological consequences can be enormous. There are significant differences in long-term function and achievement between mentally healthy and well-adjusted individuals and those with PTSD, depression, alcoholism, and other psychological problems. Such deficits include lower levels of performance in educational attainment, marital stability, family function, vocational achievement, and societal engagement.

It appears that attention to prevention of and early intervention to reduce UN or NGO mission-related intense emotional responses can be expected to have a long-term payoff with regard to the mental health, quality of life, and personal achievements of former peacekeepers and civilian field personnel.

Consequences to UN or NGO Mission. The success of UN or NGO missions is clearly affected by the performance of its personnel.

Stress-related deficits in cognition, judgment, motivation, functional capacity, and morale can reduce the productivity and efficiency of UN or NGO personnel in the field. When psychologically affected individuals can no longer perform at an acceptable level or tolerate the emotional demands of their assignment, they must be removed from the theater of operation so that their personal deficits do not endanger or interfere with the performance of colleagues. UN or NGO personnel who must be reassigned or repatriated for such reasons reduce the effective workforce and must be replaced. It also appears that a significant number of UN or NGO personnel who must be removed for psychological reasons may never resume such duties in the future. Thus from an institutional perspective, the attrition of previously effective personnel is a lost investment, since such highly-trained individuals might have been expected to provide much more service to UN or NGO missions. Indeed, such mission-based psychological problems increase the costs of UN and NGO operations because of performance deficits in the field of operations as well as the attrition of trained personnel. As these consequences mount, it becomes increasingly difficult to achieve the goals and objectives of UN and NGO missions. In a worst-case scenario, reduced performance and effectiveness by military and civilian field personnel affect the credibility of the UN and NGO, respectively.

The Importance of Culture

As reiterated throughout this book, there is a wide range of ethno-cultural expectations, explanations, and expressions of posttraumatic distress. Factors that must be considered include the cultural identity of the individual, culture-specific explanations for trauma-related emotional reactions, cultural factors related to the psychosocial environment in which peacekeeping or civilian missions must be carried out, cultural factors affecting the expectations and performance of professional responsibilities associated with the UN/NGO assignment, cultural factors that affect the recognition and acknowledgment of adverse psychological reactions, cultural factors affecting the willingness of distressed individuals to seek assistance, and cultural factors affecting the acceptability of different interventions for ameliorating such distress (Stamm & Friedman, 2000).

Given the cultural diversity among UN/NGO personnel, it is obvious that various conceptual models and intervention strategies will be better suited for some than for others. One useful way to characterize one dimension of cultural differences is the individualism-collectivism dichotomy (Keats, Munro, & Mann, 1989). People from more traditional cultures are often collectivists who perceive the self as part of a larger social unit, whereas individualists focus more on their own personal reactions

(Triandis, 1995). Therefore, the same event may be experienced and understood quite differently, since the collectivist may be most affected by its impact on the family, community, or tribe, whereas the individualist may be more distressed by his or her own personal symptoms and distress.

Such a cross-cultural perspective is not only crucial for understanding the psychological impact of posttraumatic stressors among different UN/NGO personnel, it is also essential for selecting the best and most culturally sensitive intervention strategy. Individualists are more likely to accept and respond to Western psychological approaches that focus on an individual's subjective symptoms. Collectivists may be more responsive to family interventions or ceremonies and rituals that involve the tribe or community at large. In this regard, it may be useful to think of UN/NGO military or civilian units as communities/tribes in which distressed personnel may benefit more from collective than from individual interventions. We will continue this discussion of culturally-sensitive approaches subsequently.

PREVENTION AND INTERVENTION

As illustrated in both vignettes, exposure to life-threatening danger and witnessing atrocities are inherent risks in many peacekeeping and civilian field humanitarian or social missions. Although it may be impossible to prevent such episodes, it is possible to minimize the short- and long-term emotional consequences of such experiences. Table 14.3 lists a number of

Table 14.3. Prevention and Intervention for UN Mission-Related Emotional Distress

Recruitment, Screening and Selection
Pre-deployment Training
  • Education About Stress
  • Preparation for Mission-Specific Stress Management
  • Preparation for General Stress Management
  • Preparation of Leaders
Self-help Interventions
  • Defusing
Formal/Professional Interventions
  • Debriefing/Other Acute Approaches
  • Frontline Treatment
  • Ceremonies and Rituals
Post-deployment Stabilization and Treatment
Organizational Response Plan

preventive strategies that have been utilized, mostly by military personnel and civilian disaster responders. Although systematic scientific evaluation of these approaches is at a relatively early stage, there is a growing experiential core of information to guide planning and to promote changes in current institutional policy and practice.

Recruitment, Screening, and Selection

In some future society, it may be possible to cite the known risk factors for maladaptive responding to extreme stress. Screening tools will have been devised to accurately identify those individuals most susceptible to stress at the point of entry into UN peacekeeping or civilian humanitarian or social institutions. In some cases, such individuals will not be permitted to participate because of irreversible vulnerabilities identified through this screening process. In other cases, individuals with reversible vulnerabilities will receive pre-deployment training that will fortify their capacity to cope with stress and make them suitable candidates for UN or NGO service.

At the present time, there is no information that might be used for such purposes. Although there are known vulnerabilities and risk factors for stress tolerance associated with a candidate's prior experiences and family history (Fairbank, Schlenger, Saigh, & Davidson, 1995; King, King, Foy, Keane, & Fairbank, 1999), such evidence has little practical utility because it cannot help predict which individuals will succumb to short-term or chronic stress under which conditions. This is due to the fact that the same event can have a different emotional impact upon different individuals. For this reason, in part, intervention targeted at the entire group seems most useful.

Predeployment Training

Predeployment training is the major opportunity for reducing mission-related stress reactions. Our discussion will focus on education about stress, preparation for mission-specific stress management, preparation for general stress management, and preparation of leaders.

Education about Stressors. The goal of this activity is to make sure that individuals learn about reactions to extreme stressors so that they will be prepared to recognize such responses in themselves if and when they occur. Such a proactive educational approach should help personnel understand that they are not losing their minds, that their constellation of symptoms has a specific name, that many people experience and

Table 14.4. Common Stress Reactions

Emotional	Biological
Shock	Fatigue
Anger	Insomnia
Disbelief	Hyperarousal
Terror	Somatic complaints
Guilt	Impaired immune response
Grief	Headaches
Irritability	Gastrointestinal problems
Helplessness	Decreased appetite
Despair	Decreased libido
Dissociation	Startle response
Loss of pleasure from regular activities	
Cognitive	Psychosocial
Impaired concentration	Alienation
Confusion	Social withdrawal
Distortion	Increased stress with relationships
Intrusive thoughts	Substance abuse
Decreased self-esteem	Vocational impairment
Decreased self-efficacy	
Self-blame	

Source: Young et al., 1998, p. 110

rapidly recover from such intense immediate emotional reactions, and that no stigma or shame should be associated with this kind of all-too-human response to an overwhelming experience. They need to understand that stress reactions typically include the emotional, biological, cognitive, and psychosocial symptoms shown in Table 14.4. Finally, they need to learn about potential sources of emotional and social support and where and when to seek counseling or other professional assistance.

Mission-Specific Stress Management. There should be a focus on stressors specifically related to the nature of the operation, such as combat exposure and the threat of death or capture, dealing with bodies and with wounded, exposure to mass human misery, prolonged separation from family and friends, sexual harassment or assault, issues related to collaborating with military or civilian field personnel from other nations and cultures, cultural isolation, or isolation from others due to working conditions and living arrangements.

General Stress Management. This component of stress management training focuses on stressors that are less directly related to the specific deployment under consideration. These include unit cohesion, morale, confidence in leadership, training and equipment, and social support during and after the deployment.

Realistic training and rehearsals should be used to develop both skills and confidence to reduce operational stress. Simulation of dangers involved will enable personnel to become familiar with anticipated stressors, and to develop appropriate coping skills. The more thorough the training, particularly the more rehearsed the drills to be implemented during critical events, the more automatic appropriate reactions will become in real circumstances.

Military research has consistently demonstrated that levels of cohesion, leadership, and morale are significant predictors of combat stress casualties and that units high in these characteristics function more effectively (Belenky, Noy, & Solomon, 1987). These factors may provide a social support system that allows personnel to express themselves after intensely stressful experiences, possibly providing a cathartic mechanism in coping with stress. However, *cohesion should be built prior to deployment for it to be effective during and after stressful events.*

Preparation of Leaders. It is especially important that leaders be able to recognize traumatic stress symptoms in themselves and others, since they not only have responsibility for the welfare of others but must also make the critical decisions that determine mission success and the safety of those they lead. Because of this, leaders are more susceptible to stress and are more affected by additional stressors than are subordinates. Following a group crisis, the leader is the person who must deal with the emotional needs of subordinates and restore group function. This is why pre-deployment training must place so much emphasis on the preparation of leaders.

The UN Office of Human Resources Management has published a booklet entitled *Mission Readiness and Stress Management* that includes specific sections on mission readiness, stress management, critical incident stress, and the post-deployment homecoming (United Nations Office of Human Resources Management, 1995). It is a clear, concise, and very accessible example of the kind of written educational material recommended for both pre-deployment training and post-deployment readjustment.

Frontline Treatment

Frontline treatment was developed in a military context and is extensively utilized by many UN member nations during peacekeeping deployments. There is no reason why this approach couldn't also be utilized by civilian field personnel.

As developed originally in 1919 by the military psychiatrist T.W. Salmon (1919), frontline treatment has always emphasized the importance of administering psychological interventions as close to the front as possible. This process has been modified over time (Artiss, 1963; Neria & Solomon, 1999) but has retained the three major principles of Proximity, Immediacy, and Expectancy (PIE). *Proximity* involves providing the intervention as close to the active (combat) zone as possible. *Immediacy* refers to providing the intervention as soon as possible after an acute stress reaction. *Expectancy* involves providing education that the acute stress reaction is a normal response to an overwhelming event, and emphasizes that rapid recovery and resumption of normal duties is expected. The other expectation is that there will be no long-term adverse consequences from this transient emotional reaction.

In military psychology, the most widely used interventions in the field of operations are defusing and debriefing (see below). Evidence favoring the effectiveness of frontline treatment is stronger than that favoring either defusing or psychological debriefing (Neria & Solomon, 1999; Solomon & Benbenishty, 1986). The difference may be due to more individualized, flexible, and intensive attention to emotional reactions provided by frontline treatment in comparison with these other approaches. Further research is needed on all of these interventions to determine their applicability and efficacy under a variety of circumstances.

Defusing. Defusing is a process developed for disaster workers (Young, Ford, Ruzek, Friedman, & Gusman, 1998) that is applicable for stress management of UN personnel. It is designed as a brief (10- to 30-minute) conversational intervention that can take place informally during a meal or while standing in line for services, etc. "Defusings are designed to give survivors an opportunity to receive support, reassurance and information. In addition, defusing provides...an opportunity to assess and refer individuals who may benefit from more in depth (support)" (Young et al., 1998, p. 40). When an individual appears preoccupied with thoughts about a stressful event and indicates a willingness to discuss such thoughts, a typical defusing intervention progresses through four stages: a) *Fact finding* ("Tell me what happened"); b) *Inquiring about thoughts* ("What thoughts have you had about this event?" "What was the worst part?" "What are your thoughts now?"); c) *Inquiry about feelings* ("How did you feel during the event?" "How do you feel now?"); and d) *Support and reassurance*: assisting colleagues to cope with current distress by reminding them of normal reactions to stress (e.g., Table 4) to help mitigate self-criticism and worry about stress-related emotional reactions.

The main goals of defusing are to reduce the intensity of acute stress reactions and to fortify coping mechanisms that have worked before. When provided by trained personnel, defusing can be a rapid and effective intervention. It is also a useful screening mechanism, since individuals who cannot benefit from a defusing or who become even more upset (as they attempt to recount the facts, thoughts, and feelings related to a stressful episode) may require a more intense intervention. As noted by Ørner (1995), the one-to-one counseling inherent in defusing "aims to ease the expression of feelings, promote understanding of (personal) reactions to critical incidents... (and) raise awareness of useful coping strategies" (p. 510).

There is evidence to suggest that early interventions provided by trained professional colleagues from the same unit, rather than by outside (mental health) professionals, are more effective and better accepted (Ørner et al., 2000). This would suggest that defusing may be a particularly useful intervention for peacekeepers or civilian field personnel. A recent report on 510 Swedish peacekeepers deployed to Bosnia shows the positive effect of defusing. One-third of these soldiers had experienced traumatic situations during service such as seeing wounded, maimed, or dead people, had witnessed violence between indigenous combatants, had been involved in a serious accident, or had been under attack. It was found that peer support followed by a defusing session led by the platoon commander (or similar leader) had a positive effect on the post-service mental health of the participants. Indeed, this approach had better results than peer support and defusing followed by a debriefing session led by a trained mental health professional who was not a member of the military unit (Larsson, Michel, & Lundin, 2000).

Debriefing.   *Psychological debriefing* began in military psychiatry and was later applied to support civilian disaster workers (Mitchell, 1983; Raphael, 1986). It is widely used, but evidence is mixed concerning its effectiveness (Bisson, McFarlane, & Rose, 2000; Neria & Solomon, 1999). Debriefing is a group-oriented intervention provided at the site of and shortly after the traumatic event to facilitate emotional recovery from acute distress. Although there are a number of variations on this approach, there are nine general components in a typical debriefing usually conducted in groups of 10–20 (Dyregov, 1989; Bisson, McFarlane, & Rose, 2000; Neria & Solomon, 1999).

Introduction: Leaders introduce themselves, describe the process, and emphasize confidentiality.

Facts: Participants are each encouraged to report what they witnessed and what happened to them, when, who else was involved, and their relationship to anyone else experiencing the event at the same time.

Thoughts: Participants recount their thoughts during the event and at present.

General Reactions: Participants recount impressions perceived through the five senses: sight, hearing, touch, smell, and taste. This is because re-experiencing the traumatic events is often triggered by sense reactions.

Emotional Reactions: Participants are encouraged to share painful and previously unexpressed emotional reactions to the stressful event, such as fear, helplessness, horror, grief, rage, or guilt.

Support Systems and Coping During the Event: Participants are encouraged to share positive factors, if any, that enhanced coping and/or survival. This helps to underscore and crystallize an appreciation for one's own coping skills and other support systems during stressful incidents.

Normalization: While sharing such intense emotions and ventilating powerful feelings, group members learn that others have had similar emotions to their own.

Future Planning/Coping: The debriefer informs the group that it is quite natural to have certain reactions to such an overwhelming event: for instance, insomnia, nightmares, jumpiness, etc. Group members are encouraged to discuss their symptoms as well as continue to examine internal coping mechanisms and external social support for quick recovery and future resiliency.

Disengagement: The debriefer reviews (and may hand out written material on) the normal human response to overwhelming stress. The expectation is strongly reinforced that the current intense distress is a transient emotional reaction that will subside within weeks. Group members are cautioned to consider professional assistance if current symptoms are intolerable or if such symptoms persist beyond a month. They are also offered a list of available mental health professionals if they wish to seek further assistance.

There is little empirical evidence supporting the efficacy of psychological debriefing or showing that it prevents PTSD. Indeed, some research suggests that debriefing may even exacerbate posttraumatic distress under certain conditions (Bisson, McFarlane, & Rose, 2000; Neria & Solomon, 1999). On the other hand, these same studies suggest that 50–90% of debriefing recipients report their belief that this intervention facilitated their recovery from the acute emotional distress caused by the stressful event. In addition, Deahl and associates (2000) have reported reduced alcohol misuse among debriefed British peacekeepers deployed to Bosnia in comparison to nondebriefed soldiers; they suggest that future trials of debriefing should monitor a wider range of outcome measures than PTSD symptoms. Despite unanswered questions about the usefulness of debriefing and mounting evidence that it may be deleterious under certain conditions, it has become a routine procedure in many settings for both disaster workers and military personnel. Further research is definitely needed to determine whether debriefing is effective and, if so, under what circumstances. We will return to these issues later.

Post-Exposure Interventions Reconsidered

Ørner and associates (Ørner, 1995; Ørner, King, Avery, Bretherton, Stolz, & Ormerod, 2000) have thoughtfully considered post-stress interventions for crisis workers from several original and heuristically rich perspectives. They have argued strongly against the routine and prescriptive use of debriefing following stressful episodes, emphasizing that most staff can be expected to cope successfully with mission-related stress and will probably require little or no special assistance to facilitate the transition to life at home. In addition, they suggest that early intervention should be provided by trained professional colleagues (as in defusing and front-line treatment) rather than by outside (mental health) professionals (who are often brought in to provide debriefing). Their results suggest that crisis workers prefer a flexible format for discussions about stressful events rather than the strict protocol utilized in debriefing. Furthermore, a majority of crisis workers report that nonverbal coping strategies, such as rest and relaxation, exercise, working hard, or using humor are more beneficial than talking about the traumatic event. In view of these observations, it is possible that the flexibility, individualization, non-verbal components, and administration by professional (military) colleagues may be important components that have contributed to the demonstrated effectiveness of frontline treatment.

Finally, Ørner (1995) states, "Ceremonies and rituals are integral to the culture of emergency services. They help define the relationship of each emergency service to its host community . . . to facilitate full reintegration of personal into their peer group" (p. 515). He cites as examples the healing and purification rituals of American Indian warriors seeking re-entry into their host tribes following warfare, and community (rather than Western individual) interventions "that take full account of the power and healing properties of group cohesion and belonging" (p. 516).

All of these factors are relevant to UN and NGO personnel. Indeed, there may be a number of approaches to post-stress interventions, from Western-style interventions involving group discussions to traditional non-verbal ceremonies and rituals. As we strive to develop a suitable repertoire of culturally sensitive interventions, we need to examine how best to harness the power of groups, family, and community to promote coping and recovery from the psychological impact of UN mission-related stress reactions.

In response "to the sharp increase in traumatic and prolonged periods of stress suffered by World Food Programme [WFP] staff and their families over the past few years," WFP initiated a program to "help reduce the harmful effects of stress and trauma experienced by WFP staff members" (Dufresne-Klaus, 2000). The objectives of this program are: a) to react quickly and effectively at the onset of emergencies; b) to prepare WFP staff members and managers prior to emergency startup and staff redeployment; and c) to prepare and strengthen WFP's future response to emergencies by training a cohort of pre-screened and pre-trained staff who are prepared for deployment to an emergency site within 24 or 48 hours' notice.

This program was launched January 10, 2000. Its goal is to train 80 Peer Support Volunteers within the first two years, and 18 staff had completed the two-week training workshop by April, 2000. Topics covered in the workshop included: communication skills, effective helping styles, being a Peer Support Volunteer in a multicultural environment, stress management techniques for self and others, the impact of trauma and posttraumatic stress, coping with loss and death, crisis management (how to handle emergencies), a (post-trauma) defusing model, intervention and referral, requirements and support for Peer Support Volunteers, advocacy issues, and "taking care of yourself" (Dufresne-Klaus, 2000).

We have detailed the WFP Peer Support Program to illustrate how one UN organization has acted proactively and decisively to systematically address mission-related stress that was clearly having a deleterious impact on the mental health of its staff and an adverse effect on its capacity to achieve its goals. Early feedback suggests to WFP that this program is working quite successfully (Dufresne-Klaus, personal communication, July 20, 2000).

As noted by Diana Russler (see UN Voice), "UNSECOORD has been given the mandate to develop a comprehensive United Nations policy" regarding stress management for UN personnel, especially those exposed to traumatic situations such as hostage-taking, evacuation, or the violent death of a staff member. UNSECOORD has designed a program by which "stress counseling and stress management training has been integrated ... (into its) ... security management training program and offered to all staff working within the UN system." Such a program exemplifies the critical ingredients of adequate pre-deployment education and preparation along with the capacity to provide timely interventions for traumatized field personnel requiring appropriate counseling or other kinds of support. OCHA is also increasingly attending to the needs of their staff. They now offer training in recognizing and coping with traumatic stress, as well as post-deployment interventions (see Mark Bowden's UN Voice).

As UN humanitarian, social, and military missions become more numerous and more complex, we anticipate that stress management programs such as those currently implemented by WFP and UNSECOORD will continue to be established and to expand.

Post-Repatriation Stabilization and Treatment

Periodic post-repatriation follow-up should be a routine procedure to monitor the physical and psychological well-being of individuals who have participated in UN missions. In the vignette on the Kibeho massacre, it should be noted that every member of the Australian medical contingent received a follow-up letter 6 and 12 months after their return home.

Professional mental health resources should be available to the minority of UN and NGO personnel who, following deployment, remain troubled or continue to exhibit the types of stress-related problems listed in Table 14.2. Individuals who did not benefit from defusing, frontline treatment, or other acute interventions may benefit from counseling, psychotherapy, or medication. It is already noted that UN peacekeepers who must be repatriated before completion of their tour of duty are a very high-risk group for long-term psychiatric disorders, alcoholism, and suicide (Egge et al., 1996; Weisæth et al., 1996). They should receive a thorough psychiatric evaluation and follow-up after repatriation. There are many effective treatments for stress-related symptoms. It is beyond the scope of this chapter to review such approaches; more information can be found in Chapter 4 and elsewhere (Foa, Keane, & Friedman, 2000).

Because lasting psychosocial dysfunction can arise from stress-related psychopathology, considerable effort should be focused on helping returning individuals assume a useful social and occupational role. Involvement in regular social activities and the development of an interpersonal network with appropriate supports is important to reduce the risk of relapse. Special rehabilitation programs may therefore need to be provided.

Organizational Response Plan. In their manual on mental health services for civilian disaster workers, Young and colleagues (1996) have proposed a six-point organizational response plan to support personnel who will be exposed to stressful events in the line of duty:

Provide pre-deployment training, as described previously.

Provide outreach to staff since people who usually accept such hazardous duties are not likely to seek psychological support on their own.

Expect and prepare to address an increase in personnel problems such as alcoholism, substance abuse, marital conflict, family dysfunction, and financial concerns.

Train leaders and administrators to recognize the impact of stress-related problems on job performance with regard to on-the-job accidents, changes in productivity, and increased tension among personnel.

Provide formal recognition for contributions to the UN mission.

Offer a wide range of services, including written materials (e.g., newsletters, brochures, bulletin boards), educational presentations (on the impact of stress), information on available stress-management resources (e.g., self-help groups, counseling, mental health professionals), and training and opportunities for defusing, debriefing, and front-line treatment.

In April 1995, 300 members of an Australian medical contingent deployed to Rwanda to provide health care to the peacekeeping force (UNAMIR) were confronted by a massacre. The victorious Rwandan Patriotic Army (RPA) was convinced that many of the perpetrators of the previous year's genocide had taken refuge in the camp for internally displaced persons (IDPs) at Kibeho. For five consecutive days, thousands of Rwandan IDPs, packed into the small area of the camp, were surrounded by two RPA battalions. A sense of panic and desperation grew among the IDPs because RPA soldiers occasionally fired into the crowd, killing or wounding dozens by direct gunfire and dozens more from trampling as the terror-stricken crowd of IDPs stampeded towards safety. In addition, the RPA siege had prevented IDPs from receiving food at any time during these five days. On April 22, frantic and starving IDPs ran to find shelter from an approaching thunderstorm. RPA troops misinterpreted this sudden mass movement as an attack and began to fire into the crowd for an hour, killing 130 people. The Australian medical team worked furiously, treating those whom they thought had a chance for survival, until later that afternoon when an RPA platoon again opened fire into the crowd with heavy machine guns and rocket-propelled grenades. At this point, all medical work had to be suspended as UN staff sought protective cover in the bunkers. The massacre continued throughout the night. At first light the next day, Australian medical personnel counted 4,000 dead IDPs and an additional 650 who had been wounded.

Because his troops were so angry, frustrated, and horrified by what they had witnessed at Kibeho, the Australian Force Medical Officer (FMO) put in place a comprehensive stress management program that included debriefing by commanders, doctors, psychologists, and the chaplain. In addition, just before the return to Australia, army psychologists conducted group and individual debriefings, and everyone was followed by letter at the 6- and 12- month markers back home.

The FMO had been concerned about both acute and post-deployment emotional responses. Acutely, he feared that failure of UN personnel to control their intense anger and hatred against the RPA would provoke furious retaliation and more bloodshed. With regard to long-term consequences, a dozen Australian troops were quickly identified through these proactive measures who were having difficulty resolving the experiences to which they had been subjected. At least one of these individuals was referred for psychiatric support on immediate return to Australia.

In summary, more than half the Australian contingent served during that savage month at Kibeho. The contingent's planning, presence, military discipline, and compassion saved many hundreds of lives and almost certainly prevented a catastrophe during both the massacre and the final sad days of the siege. Prompt attention to the psychological distress of UN personnel with professional and timely stress debriefing facilitated acute and long-term recovery from the emotional impact of that episode (Warfe, 1998).

RESEARCH NEEDED

· Promote research to understand *which factors protect* against the emotional impact of stress on peacekeepers and civilian field personnel and *which factors make individuals more vulnerable.*

Emphasize research that focuses on *coping and adaptive strategies* that minimize the impact of stressful situations on these groups.

Conduct research on the effectiveness of *preventive strategies (including education)* that could be applied in pre-deployment training.

Prioritize research on the *applicability and efficacy of specific acute on-site interventions* such as defusing, debriefing, ceremonies, rituals, or other procedures that may be applied to individuals or groups.

Emphasize research on the efficacy of follow-up interventions such as education, stabilization, ceremonies, rituals, counseling, alcohol/drug abuse rehabilitation, psychotherapy (especially cognitive-behavioral therapy), pharmacotherapy, marital/family therapy, and psychosocial rehabilitation. Such interventions should be tested in psychosocial (e.g., community, tribal, professional) units as well as in family/kinship and individual contexts.

RECOMMENDATIONS

- Carry out pre- and post-deployment monitoring and assessment in order to have an ongoing record of the psychological status and functional capacity of personnel who participate in UN peacekeeping or civilian humanitarian/social missions.
- Modify institutional structures and procedures in keeping with the Organization Response Plan outlined above in order to provide better pre-deployment preparation and post-deployment support for UN and NGO personnel.
- Ensure that needed education and training are included in all pre-deployment preparation.
- Provide psychological support during deployments in order to promote better coping and function.
- Promote post-repatriation stabilization and intervention (when necessary) for at-risk or prematurely repatriated personnel through psychosocial rehabilitation and/or mental health treatment.
- Follow-up returned personnel to monitor psychosocial well-being. Such an approach will make it possible to detect individuals with poor post-deployment psychological function in order to refer them for appropriate mental health services.

REFERENCES

American Psychiatric Association (1980). *Diagnostic and statistical manual of mental disorders* (3rd ed.). Washington, DC: Author.

American Psychiatric Association (1994). *Diagnostic and statistical manual of mental disorders* (4th ed.). Washington, DC: Author.

Artiss, K.L. (1963). Human behavior under stress: From combat to social psychiatry. *Military Medicine, 128,* 1011–1015.

Belenky, G.L., Noy, S., & Solomon, Z. (1987). Battle stress, morale, "cohesion," combat effectiveness, heroism and psychiatric casualties: The Israeli experience. In G. Lucas (Ed.), *Contemporary studies in combat psychiatry* (pp. 11–20). Westport, CT: Greenwood Press.

Bisson, J.I., McFarlane, A.C., & Rose, S. (2000). Psychological debriefing. In E.B. Foa, T.M. Keane, & M.J. Friedman (Eds.), *Effective treatments for PTSD: Practice guidelines from the International Society for Traumatic Stress Studies* (pp. 39–59). New York: Guilford.

Danieli, Y. (1984). Psychotherapists' participation in the conspiracy of silence about the Holocaust. *Psychoanalytic Psychology, 1,* 23–42.

Deahl, M.P., Srinivasan, M., Jones, N., Neblett, C., & Jolly, A. (2000). Preventing psychological trauma in soldiers: The role of operational stress training and psychological debriefing. *British Journal of Medical Psychology, 73,* 77–85.

Dufresne-Klaus, D. (2000). *Staff and peer support program.* Memorandum: May 29, 2000; World Food Programme.

Dyregov, A. (1989). Caring for helpers in disaster situations: Psychological debriefing. *Disaster Management, 2,* 25–30.

Egge, B., Mortensen, M.S., & Weisæth, L. (1996). Soldiers for peace: Ordeals and stress. In Y. Danieli, N. Rodley, & L. Weisæth (Eds.), *International responses to traumatic stress* (pp. 257–282). Amityville, NY: Baywood.

Eriksson, C.B., Van De Kemp, H., Gorsuch, R., Hoke, S., & Foy, D.W. (2001). Trauma exposure and PTSD symptoms in international relief and development personnel. *Journal of Traumatic Stress, 14,* 205–212.

Fairbank, J.A., Schlenger, W.E., Saigh, P.A., & Davidson, J.R.T. (1995). An epidemiologic profile of post-traumatic stress disorder: Prevalence, comorbidity, and risk factors. In M.J. Friedman, D.S. Charney, & A.Y. Deutch (Eds.), *Neurobiological and clinical consequences of stress: From normal adaptation to PTSD* (pp. 415–427). Philadelphia, PA: Lippincott-Raven.

Figley, C.R. (Ed.). (1995). *Compassion fatigue: Secondary traumatic stress disorders from treating the traumatized.* New York: Brunner/Mazel.

Foa, E.M., Keane, T.M., & Friedman, M.F. (Eds.). (2000). *Effective treatments for PTSD: Practice guidelines from the International Society for Traumatic Stress Studies.* New York: Guilford.

Keats, D.M., Munro, D., & Mann, L. (Eds.). (1989). *Heterogeneity in cross-cultural psychology: Selected papers from the Ninth International Conference of the International Association for Cross Cultural Psychology.* Newcastle, Australia. Amsterdam: Swets & Zeitlinger.

King, D.W., King, L.A., Foy, D.W., Keane, T.M., & Fairbank, J.A. (1999). Posttraumatic stress disorder in a national sample of female and male Vietnam veterans: Risk factors, warzone stressors, and resilience-recovery variables. *Journal of Abnormal Psychology, 108,* 164–170.

Knoester, J.P. (1989). Traumatische ervaringen en ex-Unifil militarien. Een literatuur—en dossieronderzoek, Doc nr GW 89-12 Doctoraalscriptie, Vrije Universiteit, Amsterdam.

Kulka, R.A., Schlenger, W.E., Fairbank, J.A., Hough, R.L., Jordan, B.K., Marmar, C.R., & Weiss, D.S. (Eds.). (1990). *Trauma and the Vietnam War generation: Report on the findings from the National Vietnam Veterans Readjustment Study.* New York: Brunner/Mazel.

Larsson, G., Michel, P.O., & Lundin, T. (2000). Systematic assessment of mental health following various types of posttrauma support. *Military Psychology, 12,* 121–135.

Litz, B.T. (1996). The psychological demands of peacekeeping for military personnel. *National Center for Post-Traumatic Stress Disorder Clinical Quarterly, 6,* 1–8.

Litz, B.T., King, L.A., King, D.W., Orsillo, S.M., & Friedman, M.J. (1997). Warriors as peacekeepers: Features of the Somalia experience and PTSD. *Journal of Consulting and Clinical Psychology, 65,* 1001–1010.

Litz, B.T., Orsillo, S.M., Friedman, M., Ehlich, P., & Batres, A. (1997). Posttraumatic stress disorder associated with peacekeeping duty in Somalia for US military personnel. *American Journal of Psychiatry, 154,* 178–184.

Lundin, T., & Otto, U. (1992). Swedish UN soldiers in Cyprus, UNFICYP: Their psychological and social situation. *Psychotherapy and Psychosomatics, 57,* 187–193.

Madsen, J.P. (1995). Stresspavirking under FN-tjeneste. *Militaert Tidsskrift, 1,* 4–10.

McCann, L.L., & Pearlman, L.A. (1990). Vicarious traumatization: A framework for understanding the psychological effects of working with victims. *Journal of Traumatic Stress, 3,* 131–150.

Michel, P.O., Lundin, T., & Larsson, G. (2000). Stress reactions among Swedish peacekeeping soldiers serving in Bosnia: A longitudinal study. Manuscript submitted for publication.

Mitchell, J.T. (1983). When disaster strikes. *Journal of Emergency Medical Services, 8,* 36–39.

Neria, Y., & Solomon, Z. (1999). Prevention of posttraumatic reactions: Debriefing and frontline treatment. In P.A. Saigh & J.D. Bremner (Eds.), *Posttraumatic stress disorder: A comprehensive text* (pp. 309–326). Boston: Allyn & Bacon.

Ørner, R.J. (1995). Intervention strategies for emergency response groups: A new conceptual framework. In S.E. Hobfoll & M.W. De Vries (Eds.), *Extreme stress and communities: Impact and intervention* (pp. 499–521). The Netherlands: Kluwer Academic Publishers.

Ørner, R.J., King, S., Avery, A., Bretherton, R., Stolz, P., & Ormerod, J. (2000, March). The search for a new evidence base for early intervention after trauma: Learning from high risk occupational groups. Presented at Third World Conference for the International Society for Traumatic Stress Studies, Melbourne, Australia.

Orsillo, S.M., Roemer, L., Litz, B.T., Ehlich, P., & Friedman, M.J. (1998). Psychiatric symptomatology associated with contemporary peacekeeping: An examination of post-mission functioning among peacekeepers in Somalia. *Journal of Traumatic Stress, 11,* 611–625.

Passey, G., & Crocket, D. (1995, November). Psychological consequences of Canadian UN peacekeeping in Croatia and Bosnia. Paper presented at the Annual Meeting of the International Society of Traumatic Stress Studies, Boston, MA.

Raphael, B. (1986). *When disaster strikes: A handbook for caring professions.* London: Hutchinson.

Salmon, T.W. (1919). War neuroses and their lesson. *New York Medical Journal, 109,* 993–994.

Smith, B., Agger, I., Danieli, Y., & Weisæth, L. (1996). Emotional responses of international humanitarian aid workers. In Y. Danieli, N. Rodley, & L. Weisæth (Eds.), *International responses to traumatic stress* (pp. 397–423). Amityville, NY: Baywood.

Solomon, Z., & Benbenishty, R. (1986). The role of proximity, immediacy and expectancy in frontline treatment of combat stress reaction among Israelis in the Lebanon War. *American Journal of Psychiatry, 143,* 613–617.

Stamm, B.H. (1997). Work-related secondary traumatic stress. *PTSD Research Quarterly, 8,* 1–6.

Stamm, B.H., & Friedman, M.J. (2000). Cultural diversity in the appraisal and expression of trauma. In A.Y. Shalev, R. Yehuda, & A.C. McFarlane (Eds.), *International handbook of human response to trauma* (pp. 69–85). New York: Kluwer/Plenum.

Triandis, H.C. (1995). *Individualism and collectivism.* Boulder, CO: Westview Press.

United Nations Office of Human Resources Management (1995). *Mission readiness and stress management*. New York: United Nations.

Warfe, P.G. (1998). Stress and peacekeeping: Experiences in Rwanda. *Australian Military Medicine, 7*, 11–14.

Weisæth, L., Mehlum, L., & Mortensen, M.S. (1996). Peacekeeper stress: New and different? *National Center for Post-Traumatic Stress Disorder Clinical Quarterly, 6*, 1–8.

Young, B.H., Ford, J.D., Ruzek, J.I., Friedman, M.J., & Gusman, F.D. (1998). *Disaster mental health services: A guidebook for clinicians and administrators*. Palo Alto, CA/White River Junction, VT: National Center for PTSD.

Part **V**

Summary and Conclusion

WORLD BANK: AN OVERVIEW AND SOME NEXT STEPS

The World Bank is committed to a world free from poverty. It is clear, now more than ever before, that efforts to achieve this must address the effects of traumatic events. On one level, poverty exacerbates traumatic events; poor families selling their girls off into prostitution is just one example. On another level, wars, conflicts, and natural disasters hinder development.

This book provides a timely and excellent discourse on the subject of trauma in war and peace. It provides a comprehensive overview of the concept, discussing stressors, communities at risk, and emotional reactions. It examines intervention options, addresses the needs of special populations including women, children, the elderly, refugees, and survivors of mass violence and torture, and discusses child abuse in peacetime. Gender is mainstreamed effectively throughout, and there is an emphasis on culturally appropriate interventions. The case vignettes in each of the chapters lighten the reading while effectively illustrating different issues and diverse cultural settings. The problem of poverty is a constant thread running throughout, as it heightens the risks for experiencing trauma and also affects the ability to marshal an effective response—a phenomenon of particular concern to the World Bank as it envisions a world free of poverty.

Attention to the needs of staff assisting traumatized populations in post-conflict or disaster situations is especially welcome. The individual and institutional cost of inadequate support to staff is noted as "decreased productivity, low morale, attrition of trained personnel, and higher monetary expenses, all of which jeopardize the successful completion of the mission as well as the reputation of the organization." The recommendations made are within the reach of development and emergency agencies and include screening and selection at recruitment, pre-deployment training, mission-specific stress management including outreach to staff, defusion and debriefing, post-stress interventions, and post-deployment stabilization and treatment.

Although each chapter provides an excellent reference list, the need for more research is stressed. More evidence-based research is especially needed on the economic burden of traumatic stress. We need to know more clearly how traumatic experiences affect the functioning, productivity, and overall development of affected populations. We need to know whether poverty can be truly eliminated without due attention to psychological distress. These lacunae are not due to any shortcoming on the part of the authors so much as to a paucity of data —underscoring the need for further research that would establish an empirical foundation for wisely-targeted mental health and psychosocial interventions among populations affected by traumatic events.

The book *Trauma Interventions in War and Peace: Prevention, Practice, and Policy* is a ground-breaking piece of work that is long overdue. It will not only inform the practice of agencies working in this field, but will also influence the direction of future research.

FLORENCE BAINGANA
Mental Health Specialist
HDNHE, World Bank
Washington DC

Chapter 15

A Call to Action
Responding to Social and Humanitarian Crises

Terence M. Keane

Creating order out of chaos is the first component of a systematic and successful response to a traumatic event. Safety, food, shelter, and clothing are the fundamentals needed by all survivors of communitywide disastrous events. Yet this may not be a sufficiently comprehensive strategy for integrating individuals back into the community, or for integrating the community into the larger Society. Increasingly, it is recognized that the psychosocial needs of the individual and the community are key to future adaptation across all dimensions: individual, family, community, nation, and the international society (at large). The need for planned, culturally appropriate psychosocial interventions is particularly salient when the ordinary and usual sources of support have been torn asunder.

The need for appropriate intervention is no less critical in situations of violence and abuse that occur to individuals one by one—sometimes in their own homes, perpetrated by family members, and sometimes perpetuated by the State, as in social injustice or torture. Interpersonal violence, physical abuse, rape, and trafficking take a huge toll as well. These types of events need to be addressed by Society at all levels, from prevention to responding to victims and affected communities.

In addition to these public or private traumatic events and situations, large portions of the world population are routinely subjected to ongoing sources of stress such as poverty, social oppression, and discrimination due to gender, ethnicity, racial grouping, or religious beliefs. While different from direct or specific traumatic stressors in many ways, these experiences nonetheless can result in adverse health and mental health outcomes. This is particularly true when traumatic stressors such as torture, war, and sexual assault are superimposed upon subgroups living in chronically stressful conditions, and when these groups lack access to resources that can help them. Data substantiating the rates of distress in low economy countries following traumatic events are only now appearing in the scientific literature (e.g., De Jong et al., 2001). These studies affirm the need for psychosocial interventions for these populations to ensure the viability of their economies, cultures, health, and mental health.

The purpose of this book is to summarize the extant literature across each of 10 areas of traumatic stress exposure selected for their potential relevance to the mission of the United Nations and its partners—NGOs, national governments, and peacekeeping contingents-that respond to the problems endemic in the world today. International experts drawn from developed and developing countries contributed to the synopses of the literature and developed recommendations that cross legal, policy, community empowerment, health care delivery, and treatment domains. They have proposed recommendations that call for policy changes, cooperation, collaboration, increased emphasis on planning, the involvement of the communities affected, and an emphasis on ethnocultural considerations while avoiding cultural centrism. They also call for the use of culturally sensitive methods of delivery of psychosocial services and emphasize the need for technology to deliver training and education to community leaders.

Each of the chapters estimate the numbers of people affected by these adverse events. The numbers are, indeed, staggering. How can psychosocial interventions be most effectively delivered to these masses of humanity? There are principles that can be derived from the empirical literature and from the experience of groups dispatched to deliver psychosocial interventions and services to communities that are traumatized. These principles appear to be robust across countries, including those that have little mental health infrastructure, are low in economic development and low in literacy, and have little exposure to Western methods of healing. In all cases, cost-effective interventions receive the highest priority.

Within a spectrum of culturally diverse ways of managing traumatic stress, some core principles are emerging. It is widely acknowledged, for example, that: (a) the psychosocial problems of communities transcend time and even generations, requiring intervention so that violence is not recapitulated; (b) the problems of those exposed to traumatic stress bear some consistency across cultures, perhaps owing to the severity of the threat and the attendant biological and cognitive dimensions of the responses; (c) interventions based on skill development are nearly universally acceptable as methods for improving stressful conditions; (d) early intervention can reduce the severity of the reactions, lend hope for recovery, and prevent a deterioration of the psychological status of the individual; (e) the use of community leaders and health care providers is optimal for delivery of services; (f) "train the trainer" models provide a useful method for defining the roles of external support and the indigenous deliverers of services; (g) to the extent possible, the identification of culturally specific expressions of distress and culturally acceptable methods of intervention will assist planners in providing optimal approaches; and (h) collaboration with the affected communities is critical to the long-term effectiveness of the approach, particularly when external support and resources begin to be withdrawn.

PUBLIC HEALTH MODELS OF INTERVENTION

Delivering effective services to the greatest number of people affected is the premise of this volume. Since nearly all people suffer following a crisis or traumatic event, the most rational allocation from an economic and societal perspective is to allocate scarce resources to those programs that will do the most good for the largest number of people. The model of intervention proposed by Fairbank et al. in Chapter 4 presents a system of mental health service delivery that specifies that resources directed at the largest number should be the first deployed. Resources expended for smaller, more affected segments of the population are only distributed as they become available. The *inverted pyramid* model preserves resources, with the primary objective of delivering interventions that have the maximal impact at the least cost.

One might speculate that public policy, even in the light of a social or humanitarian crisis, would have as its highest priority the delivery of effective educational and psychosocial interventions to as many people as possible. Thus, this level of intervention can be perceived as being at the top of the inverted pyramid. Individual psychotherapy or medication delivered by a professionally trained psychologist or psychiatrist would affect the fewest number of people and thereby reside at the lowest level of the inverted pyramid. It would be, then, the lowest priority for use when countries and governments face large-scale collective disasters and war, or high rates of more individualized and interpersonal traumatic experiences, even though clearly indicated for some individuals.

This model also places a premium on prevention. Unquestionably, preventing traumatic events is the most desirable goal for a government or agency, yet this is not always possible. Other models that share a public health and mental health perspective describe interventions that minimize the adverse impact of traumatic events and social deprivation by implementing initiatives that afford protection through education, preparation, and other large-scale social programs. Examples of this type of preventative approach abound in the various chapters.

For the United Nations, national governments, and organizations dedicated to promoting policies that enhance the well-being of the populace (e.g., NGOs), the adoption of a prevention model for managing the occurrence of traumatic life events seems the most compelling course of action. Each of the chapters in this volume includes recommendations to assist in this effort. Defining prevention broadly permits those involved in an active response to view their actions from both short- and long-term perspectives. Thus, the simple action of providing food after a collective event, like a disaster, has the potential for the dual impact of preventing hunger in the short term, yet unfavorably affecting the usual functioning of a community. The question of how food is distributed thus becomes an important component of the preventive model. For example, relying upon the leaders of communities to participate in the planning and distribution of food results in re-establishing community infrastructure, empowering leadership, and building future capacity. Considering how assistance is provided may be just as important to the future development of a ravaged community as the material assistance itself.

COORDINATION OF RESPONSES TO TRAUMATIC EVENTS

Traumatic events elicit a multi-sectorial response. This may include health, education, humanitarian, social, criminal justice, and human rights personnel. The recommendations in this volume require considerable coordination to be successfully implemented. The United Nations and associated NGOs, like individual governments, consist of many components. To effectively provide a response to traumatic events and circumstances, it is paramount for all the components to operate in a coordinated manner. For this reason, the UN created the Office for Coordination of Humanitarian Affairs (OCHA). Those involved in responding to traumatic events and deprivation have different charters, different lines of authority, different funding mechanisms, and different objectives. This is the case even within the broad range of agencies directly or loosely tied to the United Nations. For example, the UN's Children's Fund (UNICEF) might well be considered a semi-autonomous component despite its inclusion within the overall efforts of the UN.

Despite the important step of creating OCHA, full cooperation, collaboration, and integration are ideals that are not yet realized. Ongoing monitoring and feedback to all components involved are needed; concomitantly, an openness to implementing new methods and processes to improve future responses is crucial to the success of efforts at coordination. To fully mobilize the multiple agencies and component programs of the UN and associated NGOs would require collaboration among many individuals and teams. Moreover, these agencies and components are located across the globe in places such as New York, Geneva, Vienna, and Washington. Coordination is therefore a major challenge. Continuing efforts are needed to arrive at a blueprint for managing the response to traumatic events; this best-practice strategy will ensure that resources are optimally allocated and employed for the maximal benefit of the affected populations.

INTEGRATING A TRAUMA PERSPECTIVE

Addressing the psychosocial effects of traumatic life events will improve outcomes at every level. The rage and the sense of injustice that so often accompany traumatic events lead to retaliation and to the promulgation of violence. We have sadly witnessed this in the Great Lakes region in Africa, the Balkans, the Middle and Far East, and recently in the United States, as well as many other places in the world in the past decade. Sensitive interventions can assist in overcoming these obstacles to recovery and minimize the intergenerational transmission of racial, religious, and ethnic hatreds. These are fundamental goals of the interventions we are proposing.

Traumatic stress and PTSD are known to be debilitating from a psychosocial and medical point of view. A broad array of dysfunction is associated with traumatic reactions, including individual, marital, family, health, and community consequences that are empirically documented (see Chapter 2). Less well known is that these reactions have economic effects as well. Recent studies indicate that of all the anxiety disorders, PTSD is the most costly in terms of its overall economic impact on the individual and the community at large. People with PTSD earn significantly less and are more disabled and less productive than their non-PTSD counterparts. Simple extrapolation would indicate that communities that are traumatized would be less economically viable, and that nations wracked by traumatic events would similarly be less able to function in the highly competitive global marketplace.

In a report commissioned by the World Bank, Murray and Lopes (1996) found that four of the top fifteen causes of disability worldwide were psychological in nature, with depression ranking as the second most important. Similarly, in the United States a recent *Surgeon General's Report* (2000) focused upon the mental health needs of the American population, focusing on the impact of violence and victimization, depression, suicide, and behavioral contributors to disease states. It provides a clarion call to the world's remaining superpower to address in systematic ways the mental health needs of those exposed to the adversities of life. The present volume extends the focus of the report of the Surgeon General to the broader population of the world. With the strikingly high rates of traumatic events in the lives of individuals in high-, middle-, and low-income countries alike, it is imperative for resources to be directed at the prevention and amelioration of the psychological distress that is attendant to adverse life experiences. Psychosocial interventions are available, effective, and viable. In each of our chapters, we urge that such interventions be used to alleviate suffering across international boundaries and borders. In that regard, we believe that this book represents the latest addition to a series of reports from experts advocating for a more comprehensive and thoughtful response to traumatic life events and circumstances (e.g., Danieli, 2001; Danieli, Rodley, & Weisaeth, 1996; De Jong, 2002; Desjarlais, Eisenberg, Good, & Kleinman, 1995).

Increasingly, the empirical evidence suggests the important role that mental health plays in the overall productivity of an individual, a family, a community, and the Society at large. When exposed to conditions of social deprivation and traumatic events, all involved suffer emotionally. It is key to the proposed interventions that once exposed, efforts to facilitate recovery and a rapid return to the normal societal roles of parent, caretaker, worker, and wage earner should be a priority. The evidence is striking, and it is incumbent upon those of us responsible for the mobilization of resources to advocate for the inclusion of psychosocial interventions among the health services available in the wake of traumatic events.

For all these reasons, it is critical that mental health needs be given priority. The costs of not providing psychosocial interventions far outweigh the price of the interventions proposed. Clearly, there is a need to promote change. Psychosocial services should be incorporated into the international protocols for responding to traumatic events. Coordination of these services with other health care services (e.g., primary care) and with all levels of assistance is imperative.

CONCEPTUALIZING TRAUMATIC STRESS

While it is apparent from the research data that the development of PTSD is one important outcome of exposure to traumatic events, there are in fact many other directions that an individual's life can take. PTSD is relatively rare, ranging from 25–60% (e.g., DeGirolamo & McFarlane, 1996; Green, 1994; Kessler, Sonnega, Bromet, Hughes, & Nelson, 1995) among those exposed to a particular traumatic event (with combat and rape among the highest). Yet most people can and do recover from exposure to even the greatest adversities.

One of the major conceptual limitations in the field of psychological trauma, however, is the over-reliance upon a diagnostic label such as PTSD. Debates abound regarding the relative merits of the psychiatric nomenclature. Among the most prominent concerns is that conceptualizing the mental health effects of traumatic events as a psychiatric condition promotes medicalization of what is fundamentally a human rights issue. Some argue that PTSD is exclusively a Western concept minimizing the importance of symptoms other than those included in the PTSD criteria. While the scientific evidence is clear that PTSD occurs in African and Asian societies and among populations of developing countries as well, it is also clear that there are other conditions and expressions of distress that follow exposure to deprivation and stressful situations. Truly, the impact of traumatic events touches all dimensions of the human condition, transcending boundaries of institutions and systems. More work is needed to ensure that all individuals with psychosocial distress (PTSD and other Western diagnostic conditions notwithstanding) receive the necessary services to promote recovery and minimize prolonged distress.

A second PTSD-related issue is the extent to which the PTSD diagnostic criteria capture the range of reactions to traumatic life events. Epidemiological and clinical studies suggest that the diagnostic criteria may be limited in their usefulness and may minimize our understanding of the broad-based impact of traumatic stressors. In a presentation to the World Congress of the International Society for Traumatic Stress Studies (ISTSS), Friedman (2000) reiterated the importance and value of expanding our notions of the traumatic response. In this way we will develop a more thorough and comprehensive view of the adversity associated with exposure to traumatic events. More importantly, we will expand our view of the services that are warranted and needed to support communities so affected.

Still others view traumatic stress issues purely from a criminal justice perspective, preferring the use of courts to extract truth and deliver punishment. The development of truth and reconciliation commissions to manage the aftermath of interpersonal violence, war, and oppression is another mechanism for societies that experience devastation. These efforts are fundamental for addressing some portion of the psychosocial needs of the Society as a whole. They may not be sufficient for the individuals most directly affected by the reign of violence, abuse, disaster, and destruction. Truly, the impact of traumatic events touches all dimensions of the human condition and transcends the boundaries of institutions and systems. All approaches have something to contribute; all have inherent limitations. The answer to the problem really lies in coordination and collaboration among a range of options.

CULTURAL CONSIDERATIONS IN MOBILIZING RESOURCES

While virtually every chapter in this volume has addressed cultural considerations in the development of interventions following traumatic events, this issue is so fundamentally important that it bears mentioning in this epilogue. Psychosocial responses to traumatic events need to be viewed from a culturally respectful lens. Similarly, psychosocial programs need to be drawn from the culture and be culturally sensitive to the community's mores.

This can best be achieved by knowing the culture and by supporting the resources within the culture to address the needs of the individual, the family, the community and the Society as a whole. Relying upon the leadership of communities to develop interventions is perhaps the most telling lesson learned from the efforts of twentieth-century scholars and clinicians to address the sequelae of traumatic life events. Collaborating with the communities seems to be the way to ensure the most appropriate and acceptable interventions.

Finally, the capacity to recognize culturally-based manifestations of distress and knowledge of the customary routes for addressing psychological malaise will permit more people to access any services that are provided in a nation. Facilitating the work of indigenous healthcare providers and educators is one way to promote utilization of available services, services that are known to be helpful to people recovering from exposure to traumatic events. Destigmatizing or normalizing the use of these resources should be a priority among those responsible for establishing the programs.

LIMITS OF THE REPORT

Inherent in any report of this type are limitations, whether they be limitations on the topics addressed, the depth in which they are explored, or the empirical evidence available to support conclusions and recommendations. We have chosen a broad canvas. In so doing, we have not focused upon one source of traumatic stress, one survivor group, or a single geographic area, but instead have attempted an examination across many sources, groups, and geographic areas. We have examined specific traumatic stressors and their genesis in chronic stressful living conditions. Our intention is to stimulate a broad debate and discussion, one that would be reflected ultimately in the development of effective policies for intervention and prevention worldwide.

We have also chosen to focus this volume on what can be done in both high- and low-income countries. Systems of response to traumatic events are quite well developed in many if not most of the high-economic countries, yet not all citizens of these countries have equal access to these services. We project that this report will also be useful for countries where health care and mental health care, in particular, are rudimentary in nature. Thus, our recommendations are relevant for developing countries and the parallel subpopulations of disenfranchised and minority subgroups in the most developed and wealthy countries. In these countries, minority populations often have limited access to services and interventions when traumatic stressors strike and are thus less likely to derive benefit from the interventions and services that are in place. These subpopulations in high-economy countries also live with high rates of community and domestic violence, compared to the population at large. They, therefore, share many characteristics of the larger populations in low economy countries.

A limitation of this book is the specific set of topics included. Our holistic approach and the topics selected have been guided by focus groups conducted with stakeholders from the Division of Social Development and the Office for Coordination of Humanitarian Affairs during meetings at the United Nations in New York. We have attempted to mainstream gender and human rights perspectives throughout the text, in keeping with United Nations practices. We were unable to delve more into certain topics, particularly the traumatic impact of racism, xenophobia, youth violence and gang wars, the AIDS pandemic, and industrial and occupational disasters and injuries, and we hope that future work will also focus on these major areas of concern. A second limitation of the present volume is the lack of focus on substance abuse and the addictions. While some see the addictions as one consequence of exposure to traumatic events, there is also evidence that living the lifestyle associated with alcohol and drug addiction can lead to exposure to myriad traumatic events as well. This has certainly been the case in South and Central America as well as in Asia, North America, and Europe. Problems of violence associated with the production and marketing of drugs are epidemic in several countries in these regions of the world. Moreover, the addiction to alcohol and drugs can complicate recovery and lead to additional violence in the home and in the community. Managing and controlling alcohol use and drug abuse is fundamental to treating the aftereffects of traumatic exposure. While the impact of traumatic events is often seen as disproportionately affecting women and children, this observed difference might be, in part, a function of the tendency of men to abuse substances in the aftermath of traumatic events. Successful programs will focus on this means of expressing distress so that the problems associated with addictions do not cascade through the family and the community, adversely affecting the recovery of all.

Finally, no book could possibly address all the possible events that might occur. There will inevitably be new types of traumatic events and different circumstances that agencies must address. By selecting exemplars, the editors and authors intended to derive fundamental principles that could be extrapolated to new and different experiences. No two disasters, no two adverse, violent, or abusive circumstances are alike. Nor are the affected populations. Professionals responsible for mobilizing resources to assist exposed communities and individuals would do well to adopt these principles in order to marshal effective responses. Remaining flexible and examining response options when entering a new situation is the key to successful implementation of a psychosocial intervention or program.

CONCLUSION

Dissemination of the information contained within this volume is one remaining priority. How can the information contained herein on responses to social deprivation and traumatic events be most effectively and efficiently distributed to stakeholders responsible for planning interventions? Clearly, having many agencies and components of the UN involved in developing these recommendations and guidelines was a strategy that we recognized from the outset. We also solicited input from a wide range of agencies and personnel on all written documents. With this diversity of perspectives, our recommendations and guidelines are more likely to be accessed and utilized.

Yet, much more work needs to be done to increase the use of the current recommendations, and of future recommendations, from international experts. We view this volume as an additional step that will lead to future iterations and updates as the science and practice of responding to traumatic events grow. With opportunities for input from the field and from new evaluation efforts, the goal of up-to-date knowledge can be realized.

In summary, the work of the International Work Group on Traumatic Stress has as its primary objective the recognition and treatment of the global consequences of traumatic events. The impact of these experiences is often grave and long-lasting. Psychological, societal, and economic effects are observed following these life stressors. The level of disability and dysfunction can be profound. But there is hope. Countries that adopt public policies addressing the psychosocial needs of survivors will reap economic and social benefits, given empirical evidence that psychosocial and educational interventions can ease the psychological burden on the individual, the family, and the community. As a caring and concerned Society, it is imperative that we address these needs in systematic ways to concomitantly promote adjustment while we minimize the psychological damage secondary to violence, deprivation, and trauma. Provision of these services is one important form of justice for those who are affected, and without justice, future peace and prosperity are potentially compromised, if not jeopardized.

REFERENCES

Danieli, Y. (Ed.). (2001). *Sharing the front line and the back hills: International protectors and providers: Peacekeepers, humanitarian aid workers and the media in the midst of crisis.* Amityville, NY: Baywood.

Danieli, Y., Rodley, N.S., & Weisaeth, L. (Eds.). (1996). *International responses to traumatic stress: Humanitarian, human rights, justice, peace and development contributions, collaborative actions and future initiatives.* Amityville, New York: Baywood.

De Girolamo, G., & McFarlane, A. (1996). The epidemiology of PTSD: A comprehensive review of the international literature. In A.J. Marsella, M.J. Friedman, E.T. Gerrity, & R.M. Scurfield (Eds.), *Ethnocultural aspects of posttraumatic stress disorder: Issues, research, and clinical applications* (pp. 33–85). Washington, D.C.: American Psychological Association.

De Jong, J.T.V.M. (Ed.) (2002). *Trauma, war, and violence: Public mental health in socio-cultural context.* New York: Kluwer/Plenum.

De Jong, J.T.V.M., Komproe, I.H., Van Ommeren, M., El Masri, M., Mesfin, A., Khaled, N., Somasundaram, D., & Van de Put, W.A.M. (2001). Lifetime events and post-traumatic stress disorder in four post-conflict settings. *Journal of the American Medical Association, 286,* 555–62.

Desjarlais, R., Eisenberg, L., Good, B., & Kleinman, A. (Eds.). (1995). *World mental health: Problems and minorities in low income countries.* New York: Oxford University Press, p. 247.

Friedman, M. (2000). *Post-traumatic syndromes in the 21st century: Does PTSD have a future?* Presented at the 3rd World Congress of the International Society for Traumatic Stress Studies, Melbourne, Australia, March 16–19.

Green, B.L. (1994). Psychosocial research in traumatic stress: An update. *Journal of Traumatic Stress, 7,* 341–362.

Kessler, B.C., Sonnega, A., Bromet, E., Hughes, M., & Nelson, C.B. (1995). Posttraumatic stress disorder in the National Comorbidity Survey. *Archives of General Psychiatry, 52,* 1048–1060.

Murray, C.J.L., & Lopes, A.D. (Eds.) 1996. *The global burden of disease: A comprehensive assessment of mortality and disability from diseases, injuries, and risk factors in 1990 and projected to 2020.* Harvard School of Public Health on behalf of WHO and the World Bank (distributed by Harvard University Press).

Surgeon General's Report (2000). www.surgeongeneral.gov/library/mentalhealth/

Index

Aboriginal women, 174–175
Abortion, unsafe, 5, 26, 46
Absolute poverty, 39, 44, 45, 48
Abused Deaf Women's Advocacy Services (ADWAS), 147
Accountability, 117, 121
Acquired immune deficiency syndrome (AIDS): *see* AIDS/HIV
Action on Elder Abuse (UK), 107
Acupuncture, 66
Acute respiratory infections, 46
Acute stress disorder (ASD), 276
Adolescents, in armed conflict, 220, 223, 224, 225
Adoption, international, 221, 236, 240
Adrenergic activity inhibitors, 68
Adult protective services, 117–118, 123
Advocacy
    for abused women, 171–172
    for elderly, 118, 121, 125
ADWAS: *see* Abused Deaf Women's Advocacy Services
Afghanistan, 3
    children in armed conflict in, 226, 227, 234
    refugees from, 226, 227, 244, 248
Africa, 53, 355; *see also* Sub-Saharan Africa; *specific countries*
    AIDS/HIV in, 115–116
    child mortality rates in, 46
    children in armed conflict in, 224
    child sexual abuse in, 81
    cultural presentation of problems in, 250
    disabled persons in, 132, 136
    disasters in, 292
    elder abuse in, 107, 112–113, 114

Africa (*cont.*)
    female genital mutilation in, 80
    life expectancy in, 45
    poverty in, 39
    psychiatric villages in, 13
    PTSD in, 357
    refugees and IDP in, 244, 246, 253, 283
    religion in, 27
    restorative justice in, 172
African Americans
    disasters and, 300
    unemployment in, 48–49
Age, disaster response and, 300–301; *see also* Children; Elderly
Ageism, 112, 125
Agriculture, 51
AIDS/HIV, 26, 52, 115–116, 359
    child prostitution and, 87
    poverty and, 41, 46–47
    public education on, 63–64
    in rape victims, 200
    in refugees and IDP, 249
    social deprivation and, 36, 37
Alaskan Native women, 157
Albania
    cultural issues and, 27
    refugees and IDP from, 195, 246, 255
Alcohol abuse, 8, 26, 299, 360; *see also* Substance abuse
    in abused women, 164
    elder abuse and, 111
    in former combatants, 276, 283
    public education on, 62
    in refugees and IDP, 263–264
    in UN personnel, 329, 340, 343